AESTHETIC SURGERY OF THE FOREHEAD AND UPPER THIRD OF THE FACE

Thomas Procedures in Facial Plastic Surgery

Anthony P. Sclafani, MD, FACS
Director of Facial Plastic Surgery
The New York Eye and Ear Infirmary
New York City, New York, USA

Professor
New York Medical College
Valhalla, New York, USA

2011
PEOPLE'S MEDICAL PUBLISHING HOUSE—USA
SHELTON, CONNECTICUT

People's Medical Publishing House-USA

2 Enterprise Drive, Suite 509
Shelton, CT 06484
Tel: 203-402-0646
Fax: 203-402-0854
E-mail: info@pmph-usa.com

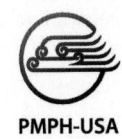

PMPH-USA

11 12 13 14/PMPH/9 8 7 6 5 4 3 2 1

ISBN-13: 978-1-60795-153-7
ISBN-10: 1-60795-153-3

Printed in China by People's Medical Publishing House
Copyeditor/Typesetter: Spearhead Global, Inc.
Cover designer: Mary McKeon

Library of Congress Cataloging-in-Publication Data
Sclafani, Anthony P.
    Aesthetic surgery of the forehead and upper third of the face : Thomas procedures in facial plastic surgery/
Anthony P. Sclafani.
        p. ; cm.

    Includes bibliographical references and index.
    ISBN-13: 978-1-60795-153-7
    ISBN-10: 1-60795-153-3
    I. Title.
    [DNLM: 1. Forehead—surgery.   2. Cosmetic Techniques.   3. Reconstructive Surgical Procedures—methods. WE
705]
    LC classification not assigned
    617.9'52—dc23

                                                                                                    2011031619

Sales and Distribution

Canada
McGraw-Hill Ryerson Education
Customer Care
300 Water St
Whitby, Ontario L1N 9B6
Canada
Tel: 1-800-565-5758
Fax: 1-800-463-5885
www.mcgrawhill.ca

Foreign Rights
John Scott & Company
International Publisher's Agency
P.O. Box 878
Kimberton, PA 19442
USA
Tel: 610-827-1640
Fax: 610-827-1671

Japan
United Publishers Services Limited
1-32-5 Higashi-Shinagawa
Shinagawa-ku, Tokyo 140-0002
Japan
Tel: 03-5479-7251
Fax: 03-5479-7307
Email: hayashi@ups.co.jp

United Kingdom, Europe, Middle East, Africa
McGraw Hill Education
Shoppenhangers Road
Maidenhead
Berkshire, SL6 2QL
England
Tel: 44-0-1628-502500
Fax: 44-0-1628-635895
www.mcgraw-hill.co.uk

Singapore, Thailand, Philippines, Indonesia
Vietnam, Pacific Rim, Korea
McGraw-Hill Education
60 Tuas Basin Link
Singapore 638775
Tel: 65-6863-1580
Fax: 65-6862-3354
www.mcgraw-hill.com.sg

*Australia, New Zealand, Papua New Guinea, Fiji, Tonga,
Solomon Islands, Cook Islands*
Woodslane Pty Limited
Unit 7/5 Vuko Place
Warriewood NSW 2102
Australia
Tel: 61-2-9970-5111
Fax: 61-2-9970-5002
www.woodslane.com.au

Brazil
SuperPedido Tecmedd
Beatriz Alves, Foreign Trade
Department
R. Sansao Alves dos Santos, 102 | 7th floor
Brooklin Novo
Sao Paolo 04571-090
Brazil
Tel: 55-16-3512-5539
www.superpedidotecmedd.com.br

India, Bangladesh, Pakistan, Sri Lanka, Malaysia
CBS Publishers
4819/X1 Prahlad Street 24
Ansari Road, Darya Ganj,
New Delhi-110002
India
Tel: 91-11-23266861/67
Fax: 91-11-23266818 Email:cbspubs@vsnl.com

People's Republic of China
People's Medical Publishing House
International Trade Department
No. 19, Pan Jia Yuan Nan Li
Chaoyang District
Beijing 100021
P.R. China
Tel: 8610-67653342
Fax: 8610-67691034
www.pmph.com/en/

ACKNOWLEDGMENTS

The author would like to thank Peter A. Adamson, MD, and Calvin M. Johnson, Jr., MD, for providing suggestions and photographs for Chapters 6 and 7. Special thanks is offered to J. Regan Thomas, MD, for the opportunity to contribute to this work, but especially for the mentoring and friendship he has generously offered to me over the past 16 years.

Most especially, I would like to thank Anthony, James, and Matthew, and most of all, my dearest Peggy, for tolerating not only the months of papers strewn about the house but also the time this work took. Throughout the process of writing this volume, they consistently supported me in this endeavor. Without their encouragement and support, I would never have even dreamed I could complete this work. It was only with their support, advice, tolerance, encouragement, suggestions, ideas, and most of all, their love that I have been able to finish this work, and I don't think I can ever thank them enough for all their help. It is in their eyes and faces that I see the ideals and perfection of internal and external beauty that rests at the heart of, and is the true inspiration of, this text, and it is to them that I dedicate this work.

Anthony P. Sclafani, MD, FACS

PREFACE

The best way to become acquainted with a subject is to write a book about it.

Benjamin Disraeli (1804–1881)

From the moment I picked up your book until I laid it down, I was convulsed with laughter. Some day I intend reading it.

Groucho Marx (1890–1977)

The forehead and eyebrows, despite occupying approximately a third of the face, have been relatively neglected in the facial plastic surgery literature. Whereas the visual focus of the face is the eyes and periorbital region, we do have a number of emotional and moral value judgments related to the upper third of the face: high foreheads are colloquially considered a sign of intelligence, as is the pursuit of "highbrow" interests. Great achievements are won by the sweat of one's brow. Finally, the position of the eyebrows and the contour of the forehead can convey anger, sadness, surprise, glee, inquisitiveness, and suspicion, among other emotions.

In contrast to the mid or lower face, relatively little has been written about the upper third of the face until recently. Patients were more apt to modify the appearance of the brow and forehead with cosmetics, hairstyling and eyebrow plucking, penciling or tattooing. These self-treatments stand as testament that patients are and have always been interested in improving the appearance of this area. Over the last 25 to 30 years, we have seen a progression and expansion in our understanding of brow aesthetics, anatomy, and physiology, and this has led to more thoughtful and logical procedures for forehead and brow rejuvenation. Recent workers have synthesized elements of older, less effective procedures and added newer approaches, techniques, and devices to produce better, longer-lasting, and more aesthetic results with fewer, smaller, and less noticeable incisions and more rapid recovery for the patient.

The task of tackling the subject of aesthetic surgery of the forehead, although daunting at first, becomes all the more so as one looks further into the topic. Many procedures have been described over the past 90 years of modern aesthetic surgery, and whereas modern surgeons may scoff at the simplicity (and, in some cases, "incorrectness" and naïveté), it became clear to me as I researched forehead and brow procedures that an understanding of each step along the path toward the forehead and brow surgery of the early 21st century allows the surgeon to better comprehend the specific anatomic, physiologic, and pathologic details of this area. With this knowledge, the surgeon can better evaluate current procedures and develop newer, better techniques. It has also become more plain to me that dogmatic adherence to a specific procedure for all patients is unacceptable and counterproductive. What some surgeons have dismissed as "outdated" or "ineffective" procedures may indeed have a place in the surgical armamentarium for specific circumstances; alternatively, "new" procedures may be knowingly or unknowingly based on procedures described decades ago. Only a familiarity with each of these can educate the surgeon sufficiently so that he or she can rationally choose the most appropriate procedure for the individual patient.

It is with this in mind that this volume has taken its current shape; emphasis has been placed on providing simple access to key preoperative issues of indications, risks, and alternatives, important elements of the procedures and postoperative care. Procedures have been illustrated by drawings, photographs, and surgical videos. I have attempted to couch the discussion of each surgical technique in terms of our knowledge of the patho- and chrono-physiology of the brow and expected wound healing. References provided at the end of each chapter are not intended to be comprehensive but broadly representative of each topic and would provide additional valuable information to the reader.

As a fellow consumer of medical literature, I understand the premium we as surgeons place on time devoted to additional learning, and I hope you find this text a useful guide to aesthetic evaluation and treatment of the upper third of the face, and I hope by the end you agree more with Disraeli than with Marx.

Table of Contents

Aesthetics of the Forehead and Brow

Anthony P. Sclafani, MD, FACS

Judgement of beauty can err, what with the wine and the dark.

Ovid (43 BC–AD17)

Introduction

Whereas a complete discussion of facial aesthetics is beyond the scope of this volume, a focused understanding of aesthetic issues related to the forehead and brow is essential when adjusting the appearance of the brow. Indeed, in this area of the face, minimal surgical changes in position and angulation of the brow can not only drastically change the appearance but also impart specific emotive expressions to the face. A thorough comprehension of general facial aesthetics, forehead- and brow-specific aesthetics, and how these two interact is an essential foundation upon which any forehead or brow procedure should be built.

General Facial Aesthetics

Although there is some ebb and flow to the concepts of facial beauty, certain aspects have been fairly constant over the three millennia of descriptions and depictions of facial attractiveness. A beautiful face is a balanced face. It should be well proportioned to other elements of the face as well as to the face as a whole. The natural smooth contours of adjacent areas should be smoothly contiguous or complementary to the sagittal and coronal convexity of the forehead and the arch of the brow. The dorsal nasal line should continue along the orbital rim as the contour of the brow.

Classic and neoclassic concepts of facial and brow aesthetics propose that the forehead represents approximately one third of the total facial height

(**Figure 1-1**). This "rule of thirds" states that the distance of the hairline to the glabella (most anterior projection of the forehead on lateral view) is equal to both the distance of the glabella to the subnasale (point where the columella meets the upper lip) and the distance of the subnasale to the menton (most inferior point of the chin on lateral view).

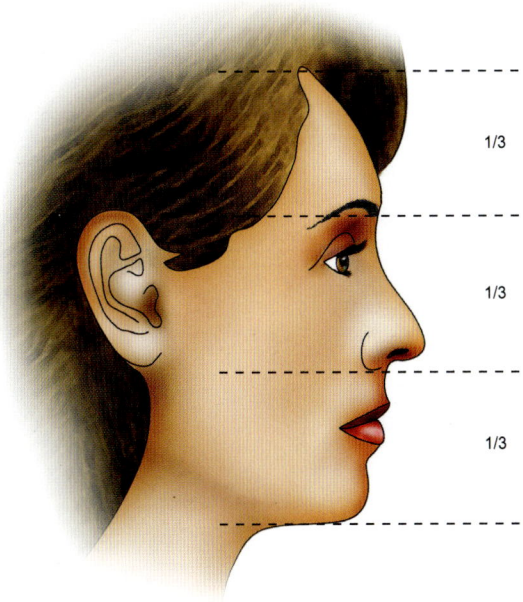

1/3

1/3

1/3

1/3

Figure 1-1. Ideally, the facial height is divided into three equal segments, from the hairline (trichion) to the junction of the columella and the upper lip (subnasale) and ending at the low point of the chin (menton).

Horizontally, the "rule of fifths" divides the width of the face into five equal segments, with the intercanthal distance equal to the palpebral distance and the distance between the pinna and the lateral canthus.

In addition, the bizygomatic facial width should be approximately 10% greater than the bitemporal width.[2] This highlighting of the cheek bones enhances the ovalness of the face (**Figure 1-2**).

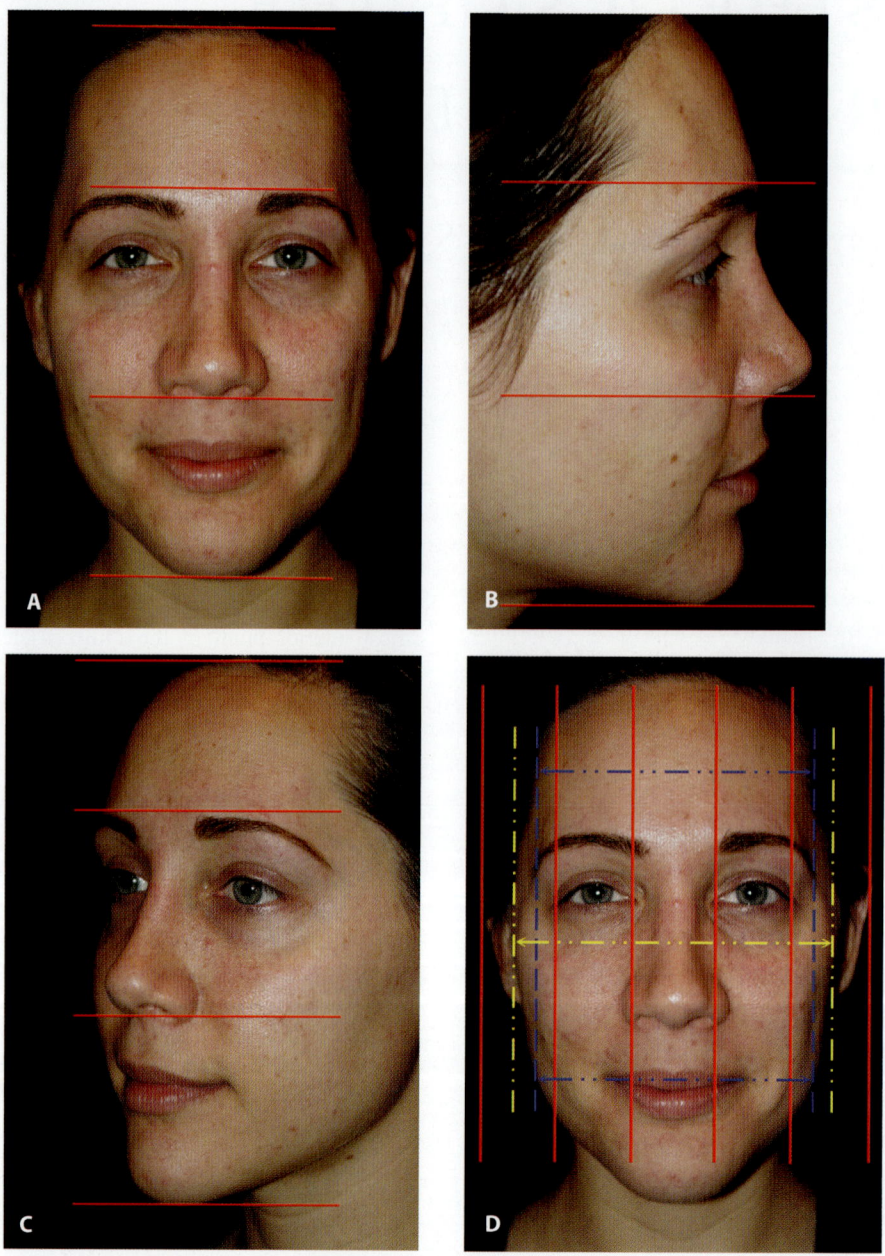

Figure 1-2. (A–C) The balanced face has a vertical height divided into *roughly* equal thirds, beginning at the trichion and ending at the menton. The boundary between the upper and the middle thirds is located at the most anterior projection of the forehead (glabella), and the junction of the middle and lower thirds is at the subnasale. (D) The face can be divided into approximately fifths *(solid red lines),* from the helical rim to the lateral canthus, the lateral to the medial canthus, and the medial canthus to the medial canthus. Ideally, the bizygomatic width *(interrupted yellow lines)* is approximately 10% greater than the bitemporal or bigonial *(interrupted blue lines)* facial width, giving prominence to the midface and making the face more "oval."

The interplay of facial height and width determines the overall shape of the face. Four basic shapes have been described: oval, round, square, and long. The oval face is commonly accepted as most cosmetically pleasing. Round faces typically show less malar definition and appear heavier and fuller, especially in the mid and lower face. The square face is a more masculine face, typically with greater prominence of the gonion and lower jawline. Finally, the long face changes the dimension of the face by drawing the eye more vertically. General imbalances between facial elements will affect the ways the brow and forehead are integrated into the facial appearance as a whole.

General inspection of the upper face shows that the degree of convexity of the forehead can significantly affect perceived forehead height (**Figure 1-3**). A patient with a flat or protruding forehead will appear to have a shorter forehead than one with a posteriorly sloping forehead, even with identical positions of the brow and the anterior hairline. Ideally, on a lateral view, the forehead should have a gently convex surface extending from the top of the head toward the brow. The most anterior point of the forehead (glabella) should lie just above the nasion. The angle formed by line from the glabella to the nasion and a line along the nasal dorsum (nasofrontal angle) should normally be between 115° and 135°.

Certain aspects of forehead attractiveness have changed over time—compare the high, sloped foreheads of the early Renaissance artists with today's standards. However, we can characterize current general aesthetics. Farkas and Kolar[3] studied the relationship between forehead height and attractiveness. These workers noted that when patients are stratified by facial attractiveness, attractive patients have shorter than average forehead heights, with *very attractive* patients having the shortest foreheads of all.

Brow Facial Aesthetics

Hair

The brow hairs are ideally situated to course as a gentle, arching continuation of the nasal dorsal aesthetic line near the supraorbital rim. The hairs are uniquely angled (**Figure 1-4**), changing orientation as the brow runs laterally. At the medial head of the brow, the hairs extend more vertically, turning and running more parallel to the course of the brow itself in the central and lateral brow.

Shape and Position

The classic description of brow shape was outlined by Westmore,[1] an aesthetician, in a presentation in 1975. He defined brow shape and position in relation to the orbital rim, nasal ala, and lateral canthus (**Figure 1-5A**). Medially, the brow begins along a vertical line running tangent to the nasal ala and medial canthus. If the eyes are more widely spaced than

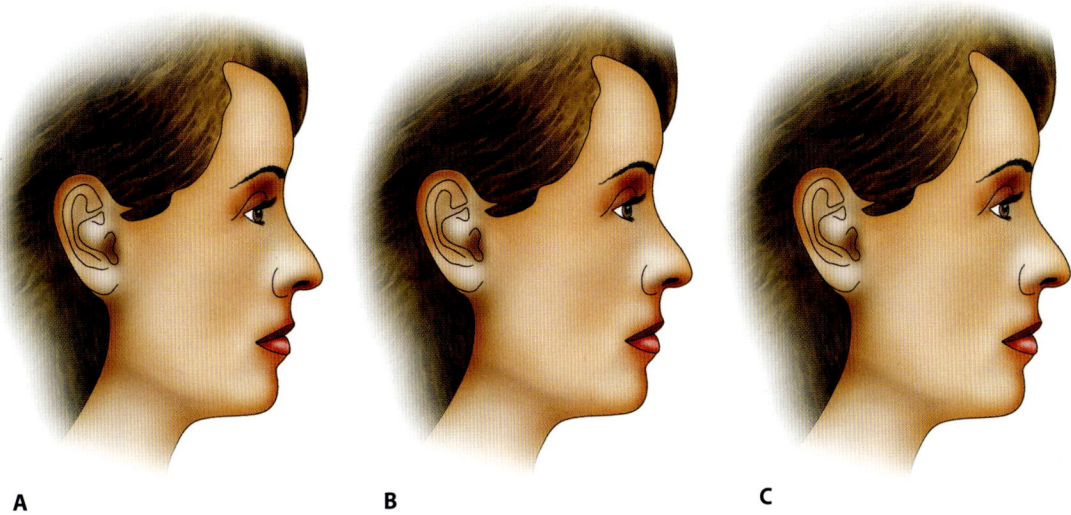

A **B** **C**

Figure 1-3. (A–C) The forehead slope can affect the apparent height of the hairline. As the forehead slopes more posteriorly (B and C), the hairline appears to recede and lends more prominence to the forehead.

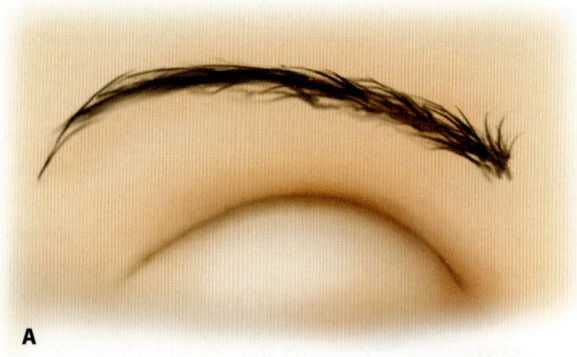
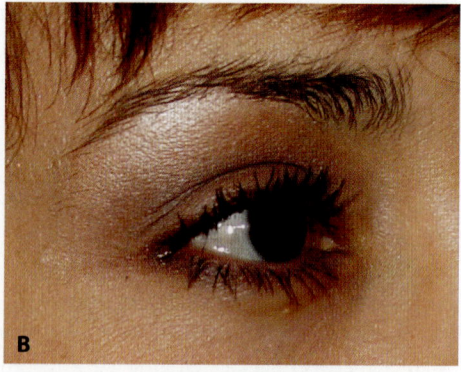

Figure 1-4. (A, B) The brow hairs are mediovertically oriented in the medial clubhead of the brow and run progressively more laterally (eventually inferolaterally) in the central and lateral brow.

normal, the medial end of the brow will continue more medially than the medial canthus. Laterally, the brow tapers to an end at a point on a line running from the alar crease and continuing through the lateral canthus. The medial and lateral ends of the brow rest at the same vertical height, and the brow peak is centered over a tangent passing along the lateral limbus. Subsequent workers have moved the brow peak as far laterally as the lateral canthus (**Figure 1-5B**), but Baker and coworkers[4] have argued that the ideal position of the brow peak is best "fiine-tuned" based upon the facial shape. These workers compared images of the same subject digitally altered to produce an oval, round, square, or long facial shape. For each of these, brows were then drawn either based on Westmore's standard[1] or by an aesthetician. Images in each pair were then rated by independent observers. There was no significant difference between attractiveness of the aesthetician's brow and Westmore's brow in the oval or round faces. However, the aesthetician's brow in the long face (straighter with a flatter arch) and in the square face (softer, more curved arch with a peak lateral to the lateral limbus) was rated as more attractive than the brow created by strictly applying the Westmore standard. This study highlights the importance of considering specific facial shape and features when determining the ideal brow for a given patient.

In general, the medial brow should be at or slightly above the orbital rim, arching upward as it travels laterally. The lower border of the brow should lie over or just superior to the supraorbital notch as it courses toward its peak and then gently descend laterally. It is acceptable for the male brow to be lower and flatter than the female brow, and it can be thicker and less tapered laterally (**Figure 1-5C**).

Brow height has been defined in a number of ways. The upper edge of the central brow should be about 25 mm from the midpupil, and the lower edge of the brow should be at least 15 mm from the supratarsal crease. Superiorly, the upper edge of the brow should be no more than 50 mm (in women) or 60 mm (in men) from the hairline. In the case of male pattern baldness, the brow height is measured from the highest transverse forehead rhytid (**Figure 1-6**). On average, there is typically 6 to 8 mm of brow movement from repose to maximal elevation in healthy adults. Sclafani and Jung[5] described the brow shape as having the lateral brow at the same height as the medial brow in women, but approximately 8 mm lower than the medial brow in men. These workers also found the ideal brow peak was located approximately 2/3 of the distance from the medial to lateral brow ends, or at 90% of the distance from medial to lateral canthi. Additionally, these workers examined the movement of the brows and found that the average maximum excursion of the brow (maximal elevation to maximal contraction) at the midpupillary line was only 15 mm, and the under the same conditions the medial brows moved horizontally only about 4 mm. These data reinforce that subtle changes are essential in forehead surgery to avoid unnatural results.

The upper brow border should be at least 25 mm above the midpupil; smaller distances are indications for a brow-lifting procedure. Alternatively, in cases in which the distance from hairline to upper brow edge is greater than 50 mm (women) or 60 mm (men), brow elevation is also indicated. If these distances are exceeded and the hairline is receded, procedures that can advance the hairline anteriorly should be chosen.

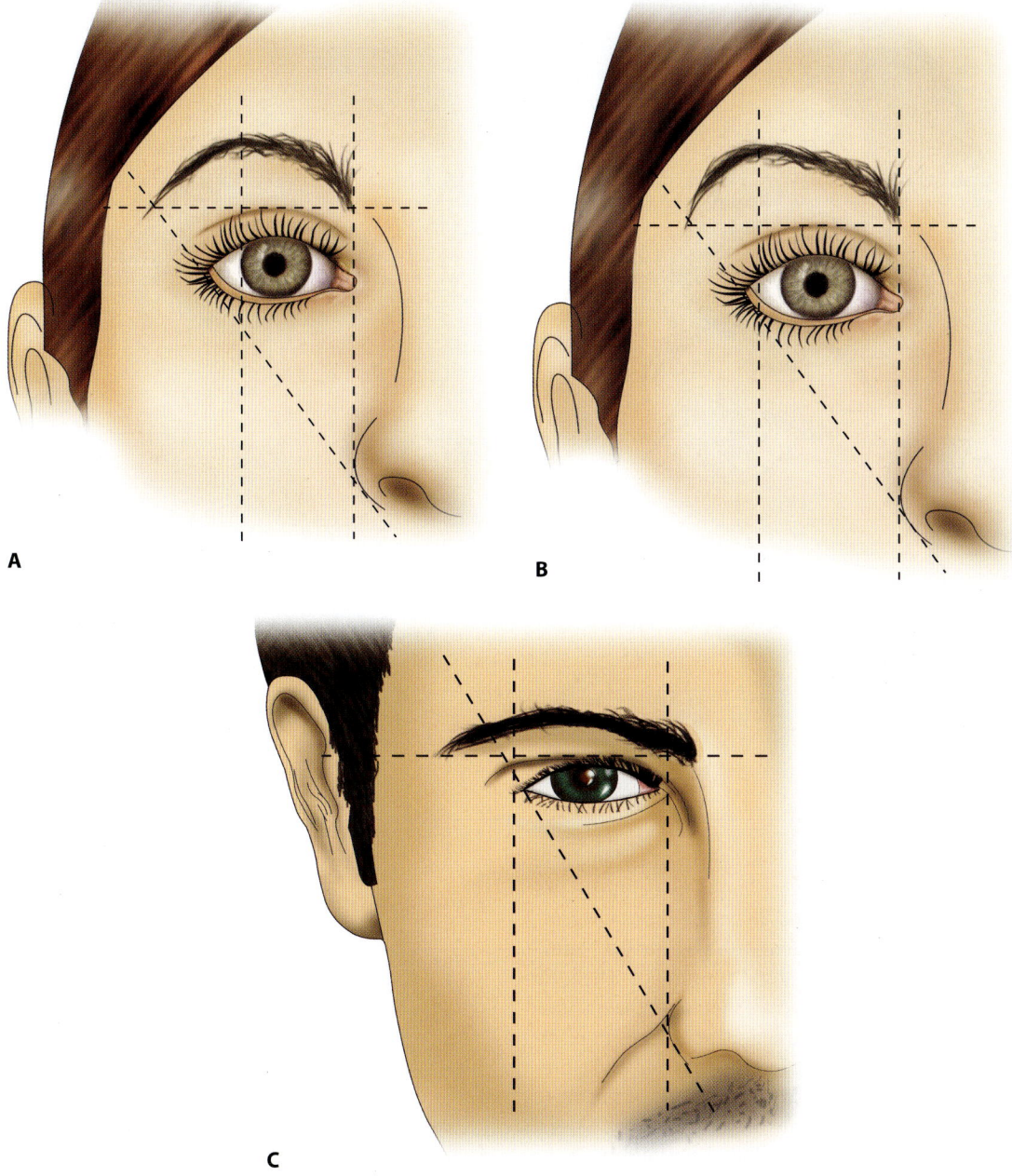

Figure 1-5. (A) The brow position and shape was classically described by Westmore in 1975.[1] The medial end of the brow lies on a tangent through the nasal ala and medial canthus; the brow tail ends along a tangent through the nasal ala and lateral canthus. The medial and lateral ends of the brow fall along the same horizontal line, and the brow peak lies on a vertical line through the lateral limbus. (B) In recent years, many have advocated a more lateral brow peak position over the lateral canthus. (C) The male brow is typically thicker, lower, and much less arched than the female brow and tapers less at its lateral end.

Conclusion

The position and shape of the brow can impart powerful emotive expression to the face. With aging, brow malposition can leave the patient with a "tired," "angry," or "sad" appearance. Brow and forehead

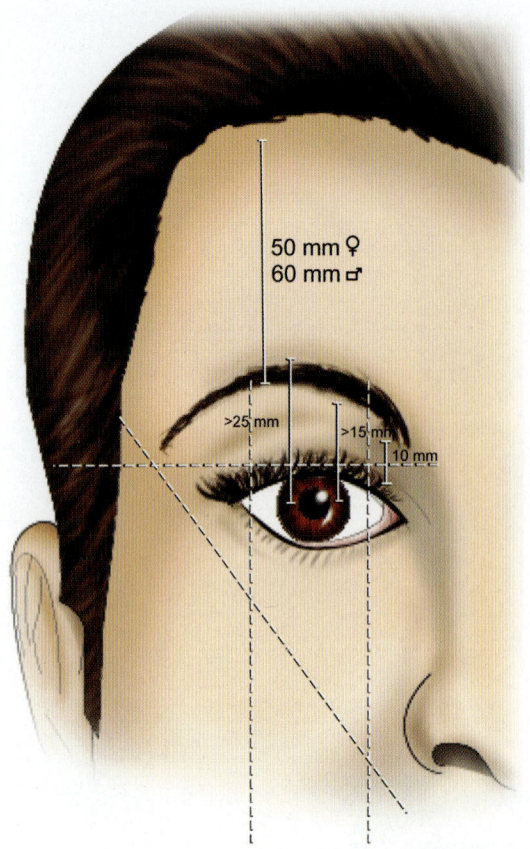

Figure 1-6. The brow should lie at or above the orbital rim. The lower border of the brow should be at least 15 mm from the midpupil. The distance from the top of the brow to the anterior hairline should be no more than 50 mm in women and 60 mm in men. If these distances are exceeded, a forehead-shortening brow procedure should be considered.

procedures can correct this malposition and improve facial aesthetics. However, "more" is definitely not necessarily "better," especially in the brow. Overcorrection can leave the patient with a "surprised," "quizzical," or otherwise unnatural appearance. The ideal brow and forehead procedure should produce a brow with an aesthetically pleasing shape and position, absence of active and static forehead rhytids, and elimination of frontalis hyperactivity, ptosis of the brow, glabellar furrows, and any brow asymmetry. Several guidelines for surgeons exist to help determine brow shaping and positioning. The final decision should be based on the surgeon's appreciation of each patient's specific facial features and shapes and ultimately depends upon the artistic vision of the surgeon.

Beauty is the purgation of superfluities.
　　　　　Michelangelo Buonarroti (1475–1564)

Suggested Readings

1. Westmore MG. Facial cosmetics in conjunction with surgery. Course presented at the Aesthetic Plastic Surgery Society Meeting, Vancouver, British Columbia, May 1975.
2. Powell N, Humphreys B. Proportions of the Aesthetic Face. New York, Thieme-Stratton, 1984.
3. Farkas LG, Kolar JC. Anthropometrics and art in the aesthetics of women's faces. Clin Plast Surg 1987;14:599–616.
4. Baker SB, Dayan JH, Crane A, Kim S. The influence of brow shape on the perception of facial form and brow aesthetics. Plast Reconstr Surg 2007;119: 2240–2247.
5. Sclafani, AP, Jung M. Desired position, shape and dynamic range of the normal adult eyebrow. Arch Facial Plast Surg 2010;12:123–127.

2

Surgical Anatomy and Physiology of the Forehead and Brow

Anthony P. Sclafani, MD, FACS

Anatomy is destiny.

Sigmund Freud (1856–1939)

Introduction

The brow and the forehead are seemingly simple areas in which basic anatomy can be mastered quickly and easily, usually given little more than a few passing comments in medical school (and, too often, facial plastic surgery) training. Whereas the basic anatomy is relatively simple, the surgical anatomy is more complex, intricate, and detailed. Furthermore, the brow is rarely thought of in a physiologic sense, and hence, the structures of the forehead and brow and the forces acting upon them have been fairly ignored except in the extreme case of facial paralysis. However, if the facial plastic surgeon is to venture to alter, adjust, or correct these structures, it is imperative to understand not only the basic layers of the forehead, brow, and temple but also how each layer differs at different positions and how each relates to the other. In an area in which changes of as little as 1 to 2 mm can make the difference between an excellent result and a disfiguring one, the successful surgeon will appreciate the anatomy of the forehead and brow and modify these areas in a way that harmonizes with the natural structure of the forehead and brow.

In understanding the anatomy of the forehead, temple, and brow, it is important to know not only the anatomic layers but also the way they interrelate. This discussion considers each of these areas separately, but the surgeon must recognize that, frequently, the way structures in these areas interact will determine brow position and forehead aesthetics.

Bones

For the purposes of this chapter, the forehead is considered to be that area from the crown of the head to the superior orbital rim, lying between vertical lines extending from the lateral canthi. The deep surface of this area is primarily composed of the frontal bone, although there is a small contribution of the parietal bones at the superolateral limits of this area (**Figure 2-1**). The frontal bone will contain a bilateral frontal sinus in 80% and a unilateral frontal sinus in an additional 10% of patients. The frontal bone thickness, especially important when cranial fixation is used, ranges from 4.9 mm at the inferior temporal line to approximately 7.5 mm near the midline. In the midline, the sagittal sinus runs just below the bone, and venous lakes (lacunae lateralis) can focally thin the inner cortex as well (**Figure 2-2**).

The frontal bone articulates with the frontal process of the zygoma at the superolateral orbital rim (frontozygomatic suture); slightly more posterior, the frontal bone articulates with the greater wing of the sphenoid bone, and the posterior border of the frontal bone joins with the parietal bones at

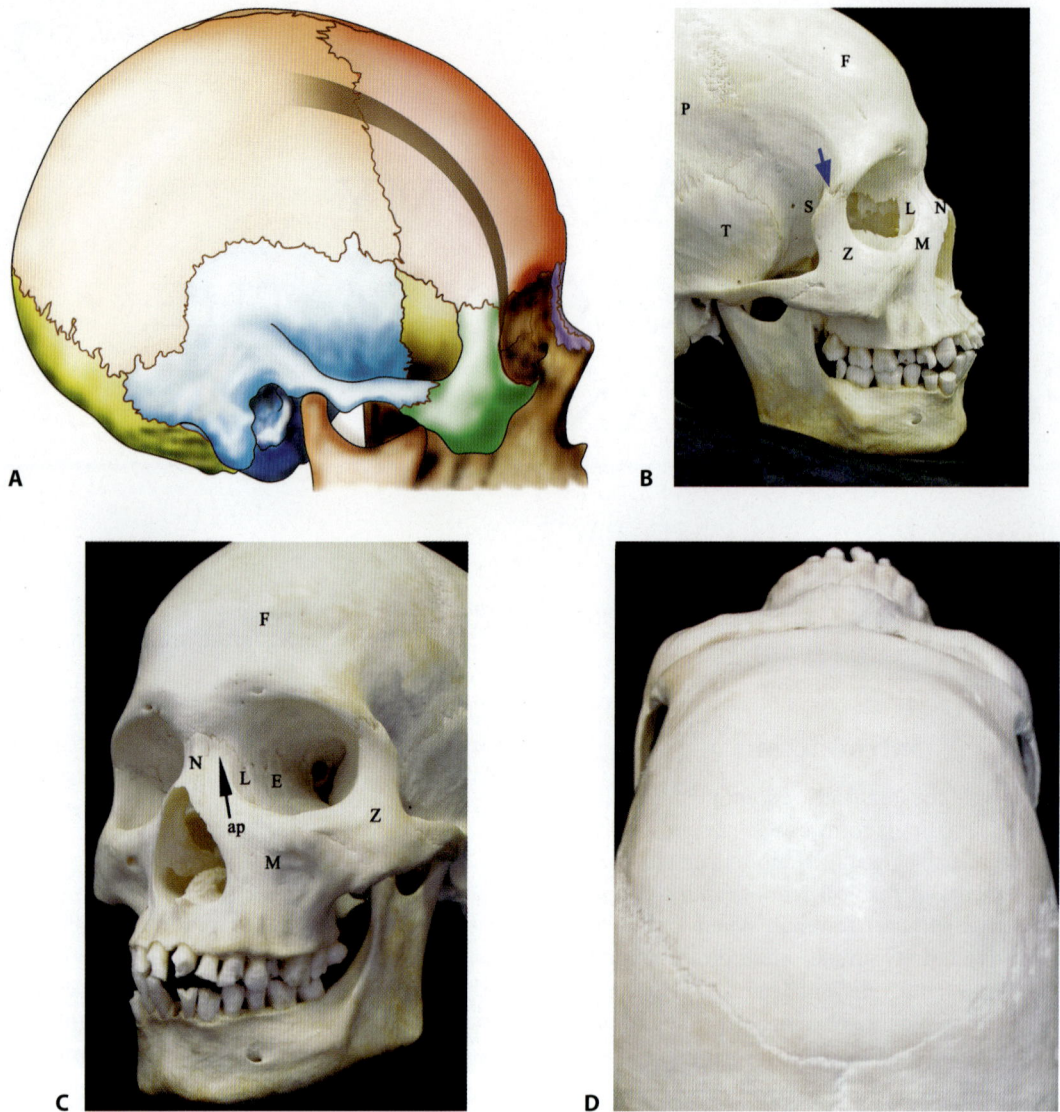

Figure 2-1. (A) The bones of the frontotemporal area include the parietal and frontal bones, zygoma, greater and lesser wings of the sphenoid bone, nasal bones, ascending process of the maxilla, squamous portion of the temporal bone, and ethmoid bone. Lateral (B), oblique (C), and bird's eye (D) views of the skull. ap = ascending process of the maxilla; E = wthmold bone; F = frontal bone; L = lacrimal bone; M = maxilla; N = nasal bone; P = parietal bone; S = greater wing of sphenold bone; T = squamosa of the temporal bone; Z = zygoma. *Arrow* points to the frontozygomatic suture. A zone of fixation of fascia exists just medial to the superior temporal line (shaded).

the coronal suture. More medial, the frontal bone abuts the nasal bones and frontal (ascending) process of the maxilla. The frontal bone additionally articulates with the lacrimal bone, the lesser wing of the sphenoid, and the ethmoid bone.

The frontal bone is smoothly contoured with a gentle convexity angling down toward the orbital rims. A few surface structures will affect surgical procedures and serve as important anatomic landmarks. The supraorbital ridges lie below the main convexity of the frontal bone and rise anteriorly to meet the orbital rims (**Figure 2-3**). These are generally more pronounced in men and, occasionally, may be distinct enough to require osteoplasty to reduce brow prominence.

Laterally, the superior orbital rim articulates with the frontal process of the zygoma. Just above this articulation, the temporal crest courses posteriorly, eventually splitting into the inferior and superior temporal lines above the temporal fossa

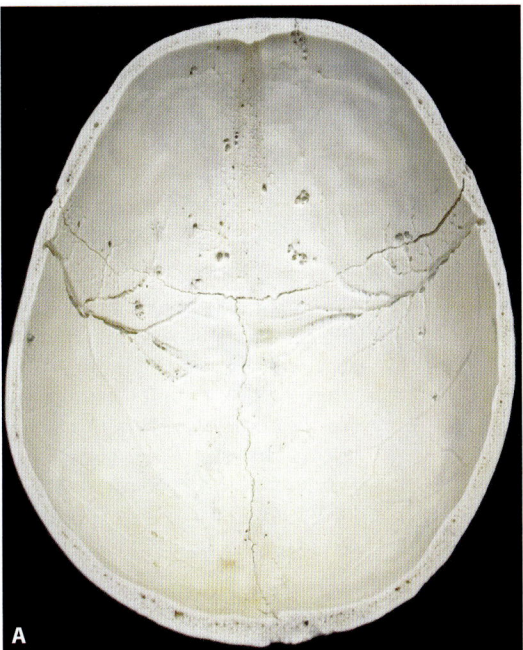

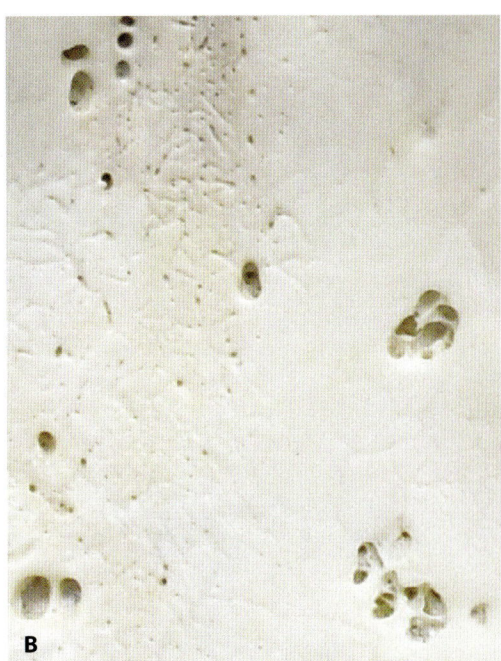

Figure 2-2. Views of the inner table of the calvarium. (A) Sagittal and coronal suture lines visible, along with impressions of middle meningeal arteries. Also seen are lacunae lateralis (venous lakes), which can focally cause significant thinning of the calvarium. (B) Close-up of the lacunae lateralis.

(**Figure 2-4**). Along the medial superior orbital rim, there may be a notch or groove for the exit of the supratrochlear nerve (**Figure 2-5A**). Slightly more laterally, the supraorbital nerve exits through either a distinct foramen or a notch (**see Figure 2-5B**). Bilateral supraorbital foramina are present in approximately one third of patients; bilateral notches occur in roughly half of all patients; and one notch and one foramen appear in the remaining patients. These neurovascular bundles, on average, exit the skull 14 to 17 mm (supratrochlear) and 24 to 27 mm (supraorbital) from the midline. Occasionally, multiple supraorbital foramina may be present and can be found up to 4 cm above the orbital rim (**Figure 2-6**).

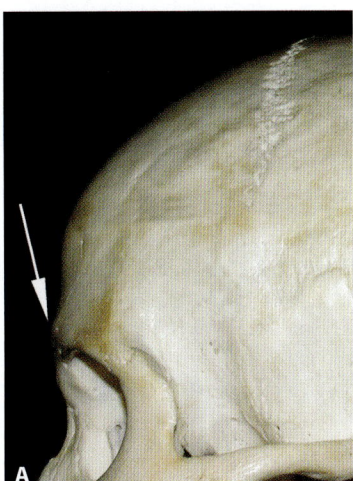

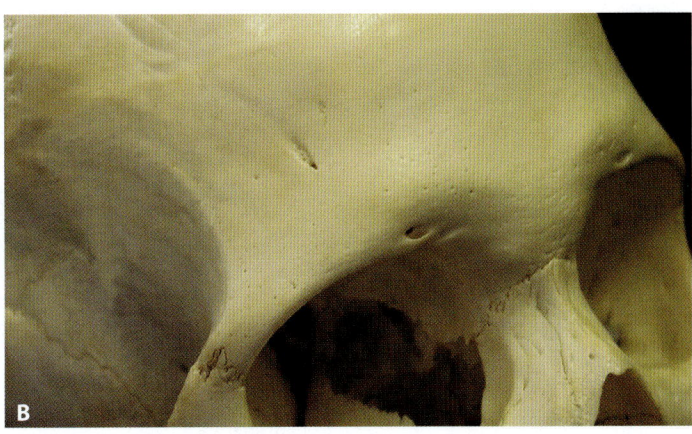

Figure 2-3. (A, B) The supraorbital ridge (arrow) rises away from the frontal bone and may be pneumatized by ethmoid or frontal sinus air cells. The convexity of the ridge allows the brows (especially medially) to appear more elevated, because the brow hairs are angled more anterosuperiorly.

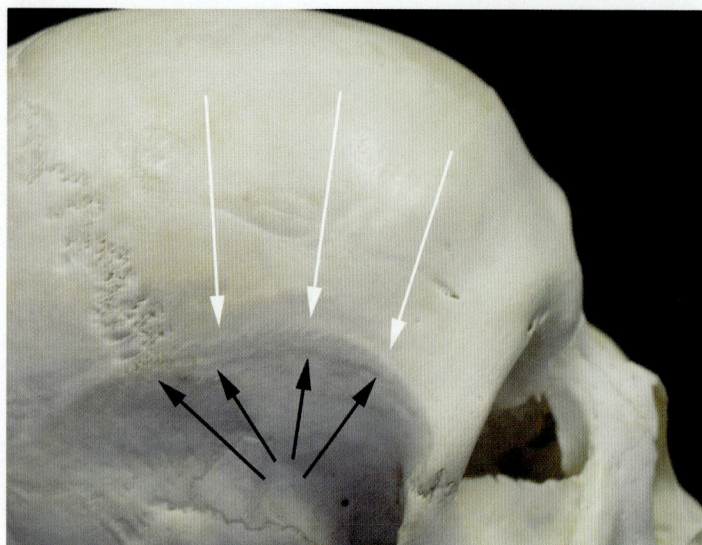

Figure 2-4. The temporalis muscle originates from the temporal bone, with the upper limits of its attachments at the inferior temporal line *(black arrows)*. The various layers of temporal fascia begin to fuse together to periosteum at the superior temporal line *(white arrows)*.

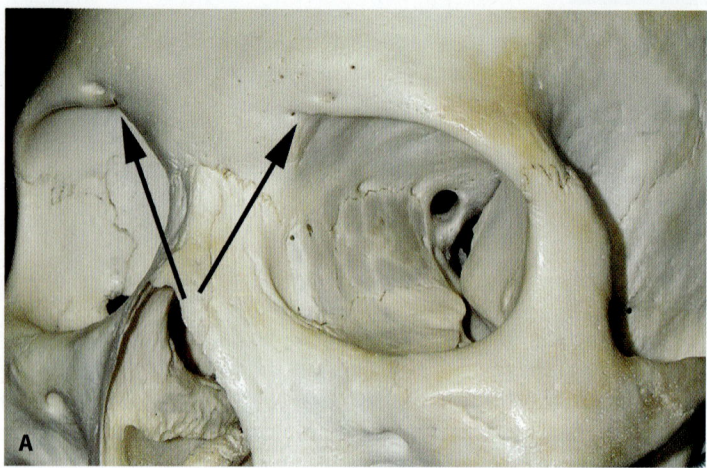

A

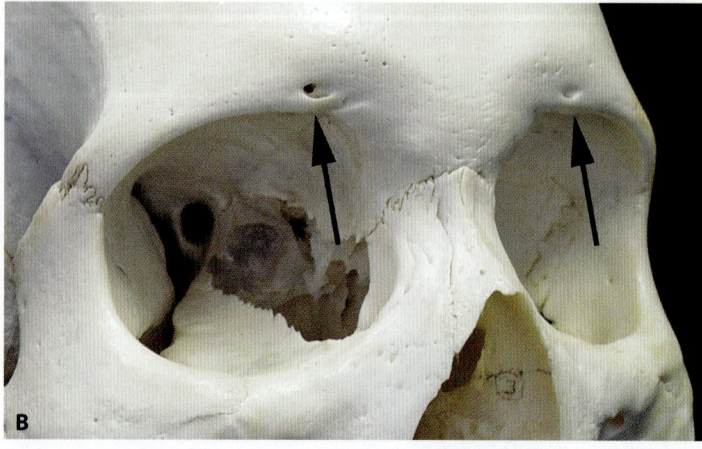

B

Figure 2-5. Close-up of the orbital rim. (A) *Arrows* indicate grooves in the medial orbital rim through which the supratrochlear neurovascular bundles exit. (B) *Arrows* indicate bilateral supraorbital foramina, through which the supraorbital neurovascular pedicles pass. Bilateral foramina are present in about one third of patients.

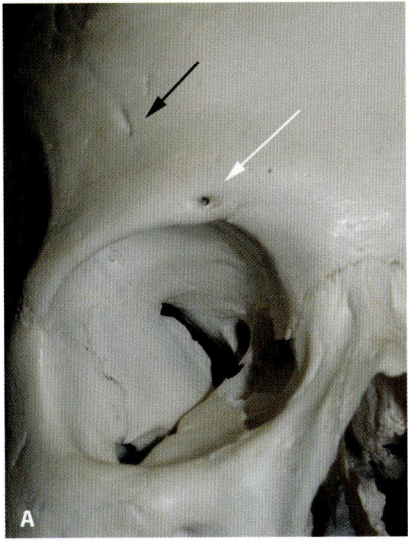 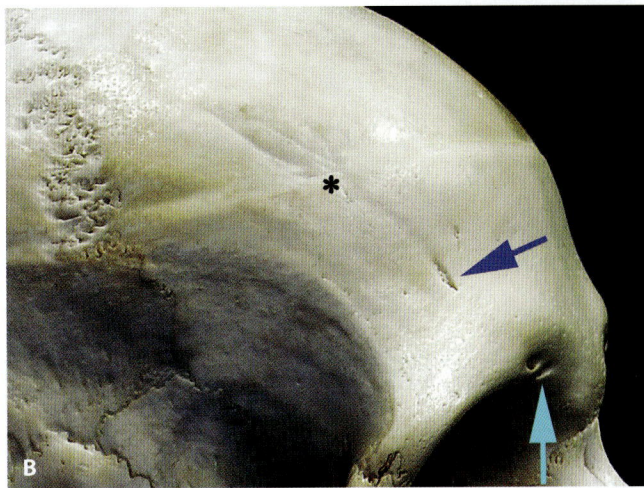

Figure 2-6. The supraorbital nerves may exit through multiple foramina. (A) Frontal view of the right orbital rim and forehead. The main trunk of the supraorbital nerve will exit a notch or foramen *(white arrow)* at the orbital rim, but additional foramina may be present up to 4 cm above the rim through which the deep branch of the supraorbital nerve *(black arrow)* can emerge. (B) Oblique view of the right supraorbital rim and forehead shows the supraorbital foramen *(dark blue arrow)* and supratrochlear notch *(light blue arrow)* along with an accessory supraorbital nerve foramen for the deep branch of the supraorbital nerve, which runs superolaterally just medial to the zone of fixation. More distally (*), impressions in the bone shows the main nerve branches as it runs superiorly to provide sensation to the posthairline forehead.

Muscles

The muscles of interest in the forehead are the paired orbicularis oculi, corrugator supercilii, and depressor supercilii muscles and the frontalis and procerus muscles, all in the central forehead, and the paired temporalis muscles laterally (**Figure 2-7**).

The frontalis muscle originates from the deep layer of the galea aponeurotica, which extends over the crown as a thick layer after enveloping the occipitalis muscle posteriorly. The frontalis muscle runs vertically (at a slight angle) as bilateral muscle bellies; superiorly, there is a fibrous midline, devoid of muscle, but the muscle bellies are in contact more inferiorly. The frontalis fibers interdigitate with the orbicularis oculi muscle inferiorly, and it is primarily by elevating the insertions of the orbicularis oculi fibers to the overlying dermis that the frontalis muscle elevates the brow. The frontalis is innervated by the temporal branch of the facial nerve, which enters the midportion of the muscle laterally.

The orbicularis oculi muscle is a horseshoe-shaped muscle originating from the medial orbit and medial canthal tendon. The pretarsal and preseptal portions of this muscle course over the tarsus and septum orbitale, respectively. The orbital portion of the orbicularis oculi extends approximately 1.5 cm beyond the orbital rim and covers the temporalis fascia laterally. The medial head of the orbicularis originates from the medial canthal tendon and covers the corrugator supercilii. Dermal insertions of the orbicularis allow contraction of this muscle to move the eyelid and eyebrow skin centripetally toward the pupil. This contraction contributes to an inferior vector of pull along the length of the eyebrow. The medial head of the orbital portion of the orbicularis attaches to the dermis under the medial head of the brow, but it is a lesser contributor to the formation of glabellar furrows than the depressor and corrugator supercilii muscles. Superiorly, the fibers of the orbital portion of the orbicularis muscle interdigitate and blend with the inferior frontalis muscle. The orbicularis oculi muscle is innervated by branches of both the temporal and the zygomatic branches of the facial nerve.

The corrugator supercilii muscle is a rectangular muscle that originates from the frontal bone at the superomedial orbital rim, anterior to and above the trochlea. The corrugator measures about 5 cm in length, and Park and coworkers[1] have described a set of "muscle sheets" running parallel to each other in a

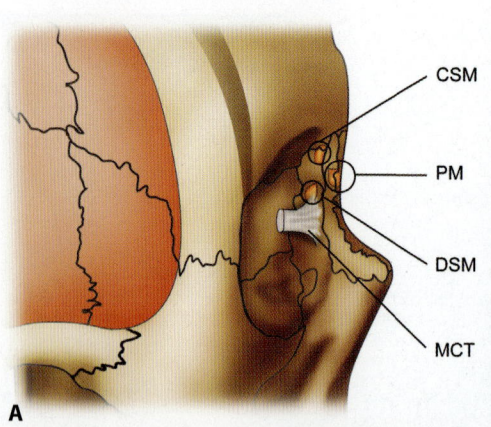

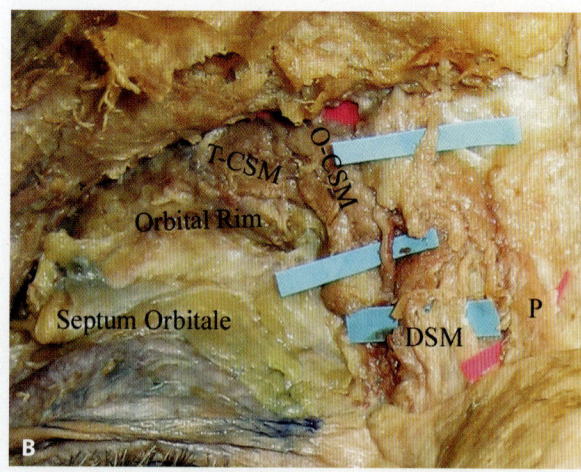

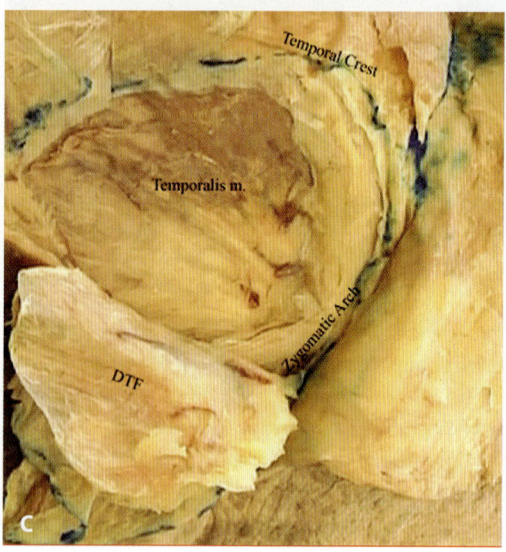

Figure 2-7 Muscles of the forehead, brow, and temple. (A) Pertinent muscle origins in the temple and brow. CSM = corrugator supercilii muscle; DSM = depressor supercilii muscle; MCT = medial canthal tendon; PM = procerus muscle; TM = temporalis muscle. (B) Cadaver dissection of the medial and superior orbital rim. O-CSM = oblique head of the corrugator supercilii muscle; T-CSM = transverse head of the corrugator supercilii muscle. The supratrochlear artery is seen emerging over a blue tag in between the O-CSM and the DSM, and branches of the supratrochlear nerve can be seen superficially lateral to the O-CSM *(blue tag)* as well as above the DSM and PM. (C) Right temple dissection, from above. The TM is seen originating from the temporal bone below the inferior temporal line and coursing below the zygomatic arch. DTF = deep temporal fascia; *superior blue ink* = temporal crest.

laminar fashion. As the muscle courses laterally, it becomes more superficial. Initially, the corrugator runs just above the periosteum and below the depressor supercilii, but it rises superficially as it travels laterally and blends with fibers of the orbicularis and frontalis muscles. It generally terminates above the midbrow (at least 1 cm lateral to the supraorbital notch).

The corrugator supercilii has two heads. The oblique head courses more vertically, inserting into the dermis of the medial brow and is a strong depressor of this portion of the brow.[2] The oblique head of the corrugator is innervated by fibers from the zygomatic branch of the facial nerve. The transverse head runs more transversely and inserts into the dermis immediately superior to the midbrow. In contrast to the oblique head, the transverse head of the corrugator

supercilii is innervated by branches of the temporal branch of the facial nerve, which enters this portion of the muscle at its superolateral extent.

The depressor supercilii muscle also originates from the superomedial orbital rim and runs parallel but superficial to the oblique head of the corrugator to insert into the dermis under the medial end of the brow; it is innervated by the zygomatic branch of the facial nerve. The depressor supercilii and the oblique head of the corrugator are the primary depressor muscles of the medial brow.

Most medially, the procerus muscle is a trapezoid-shaped muscle originating from the dorsal nasal bones. The procerus widens as it runs superiorly, lying over the medial extent of the frontalis muscle bellies as it inserts into glabellar dermis. The procerus is innervated superiorly by the temporal branch and inferiorly by the zygomatic branches of the facial nerve.

The temporalis muscle does not directly affect the position of the brow, but it is in the surgical field of many forehead and brow procedures. The temporalis muscle originates from the frontal and parietal bones inferior to the inferior temporal line and inserts onto the coronoid process and the anterior part of the mandibular ramus after crossing deep to the zygomatic arch.

Vascular Supply

The forehead and brows are well supplied by a network of vessels from the internal and external carotid artery systems (**Figure 2-8**), with multiple anastomoses within the galea and superficial temporalis fascia. Posteriorly, the occipital arteries anastomose freely with the superficial temporal artery and posterior auricular artery; more anteriorly, the supratrochlear, supraorbital, and superficial temporal arteries interconnect as well. This vascular network also sends branches to the subdermal plexus, and terminally, these vessels themselves become subdermal. This rich system of vascular interconnections allows a variety of substantial incisions and large flaps without compromising skin vascularity.[3]

The supratrochlear and supraorbital arteries are terminal branches of the ophthalmic artery, itself a terminal branch of the internal carotid artery. The supratrochlear artery exits the superomedial orbit adjacent to the supratrochlear nerve. These structures can be found exiting from the orbit 14 to 17 mm from the midline across the superomedial orbital rim. After emerging from the orbit, the supratrochlear artery wraps over the rim and then enters the corrugator muscle and emerges superiorly to run over the surface of the frontalis muscle. The supratrochlear artery anastomoses with branches of the supraorbital artery in the superficial galea and subdermal plexus.

The supraorbital artery emerges from the superior orbit 24 to 27 mm lateral to the midline, and typically, multiple branches penetrate the corrugator muscle. This artery, like the supratrochlear artery, then runs in the superficial layer of the galea and anastomoses with the supratrochlear artery medially, the superficial temporal artery laterally, and the occipital arteries posteriorly.

The superficial temporal artery is a terminal branch of the external carotid artery system, arising near the temporomandibular joint between the superficial and the deep lobes of the parotid gland. Near its origin, the superficial temporal artery gives off the middle temporal artery, which runs superficial to the zygomatic arch and then enters the deep temporal fascia and then the transverse facial artery, which runs anteriorly, inferior and parallel to the zygomatic arch.[4] The superficial temporal artery runs superiorly, entering the temporoparietal fascia as it crosses the zygomatic arch. Coursing superiorly, the superficial temporal artery bifurcates approximately 2 cm above the zygomatic arch into anterior and posterior divisions, both of which send branches along and superficial (never deep) to the temporoparietal fascia. The branches of the superficial temporal artery enter the subdermal plane about two thirds of the distance from the zygomatic arch to the vertex. The superficial temporal vein runs parallel, 2 to 3 cm posterior and slightly superficial to the artery,[5] joining with the maxillary vein below the zygomatic arch to form the retromandibular vein.

Nerves

A firm understanding and appreciation of both the pertinent motor and the pertinent sensory nerves is mandatory to minimize postoperative complications of forehead procedures. The motor nerves of concern in the temple and forehead are the temporal branch of the facial nerve and, to a lesser degree, the zygomatic branch. Arising from the zygomaticotemporal division of the facial nerve, the temporal branch runs superiorly in the temporoparietal fascia after crossing the zygomatic arch (**Figure 2-9**). The temporal branch typically crosses the arch as two to five rami[6,7] (**Figure 2-10**). These rami generally span a 2- to 3-cm width of the middle third of the zygomatic arch. Ozersky and colleagues[8] identified anterior and posterior rami crossing the zygomatic arch 3 cm and 4 cm posterior to the lateral orbital rim, respectively. Bernstein and Nelson[9] described three to five rami that cross a 2- to 4-cm section over the middle third of the arch.

More superiorly, Ellis and Bakala[10] described three rami: an inferior ramus with multiple branches that run laterally toward the lateral canthus to supply the upper orbicularis oculi muscle; a superior ramus that runs superiorly, at least 2 cm anterior to the superficial temporal artery, and then turns into and supplies the frontalis muscle; and a middle ramus that extends superomedially, turning more medially 1 to 2 cm superior to the lateral

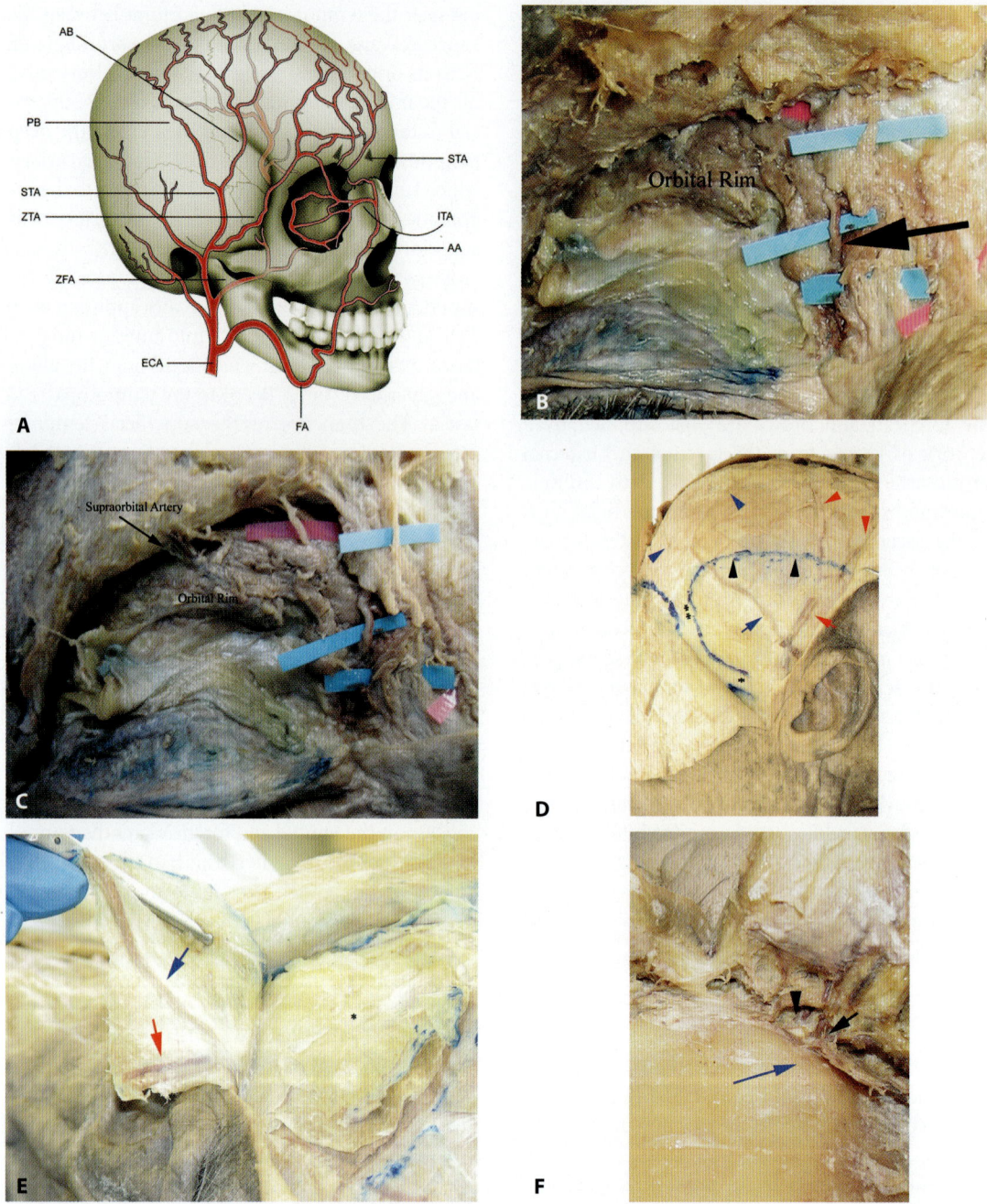

Figure 2-8. Vascular supply of the temple, brow, and forehead. (A) AA = angular artery; AB = anterior branch of the STA; ECA = external carotid artery; FA = facial artery; ITrA = infratrochlear artery; PB = posterior branch of the superficial temporal artery; SOA = supraorbital artery; STA = superficial temporal artery; STrA = supratrochlear artery; ZFA = zygomaticofacial artery; ZTA = zygomaticotemporal artery. (B) *Arrow* indicates the STrA emerging from the CSM near its origin. (C) Cadaveric dissection with the orbicularis oculi muscle (OOM) reflected, demonstrating the SOA coursing superiorly and superficially. (D) Lateral view of the temple. *Black arrowheads* mark the temporal crest, * = zygomatic arch; ** = lateral orbital rim; *blue arrow* = AB; *blue arrowheads* = branches of the AB; *red arrow* = PB; *red arrowheads* = branches of the PB. (E) Left temporoparietal fascia has been elevated, showing branches of the STA. *Blue arrow* = AB; *red arrow* = PB; * = superficial layer of the deep temporal fascia. (F) Right supraorbital subperiosteal dissection, seen from above. *Blue arrow* = supraorbital ridge; *black arrow* = supraorbital neurovascular pedicle; *black arrowhead* = supratrochlear vessels (after the CSM has been removed).

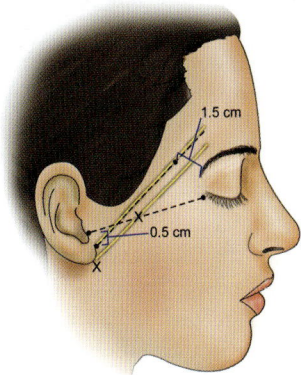

A

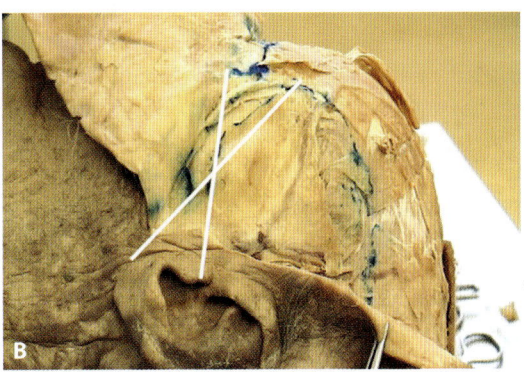

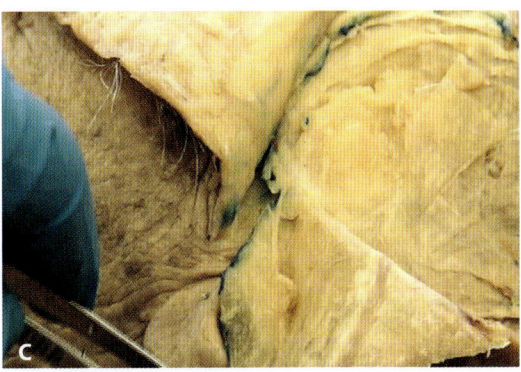

Figure 2-9. Path of the temporal branch of the facial nerve. (A) Two topographic methods of plotting course of the temporal branch of the facial nerve. Method 1: *Dotted lines* show Pitanguy's line: 5 mm below the tragus through a point 1.5 cm superolateral to the tail of the brow. Method 2: *Solid line* shows an alternate method: the line originating from the lowest point of the earlobe bisects a line from the tragus to the lateral canthus. (B) Cadaver dissection demonstrates method 2 plotted over the temporoparietal fascia (TPF). (C) TPF elevated. Close-up view shows the temporal branch on the undersurface of the elevated TPF close to the predicted location.

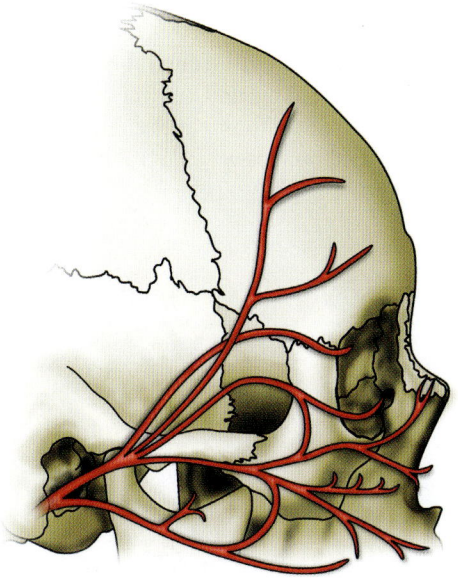

Figure 2-10. Temporal branch of the facial nerve crosses the middle third of the zygomatic arch with at least two rami. Branches then travel superiorly (to supply the transverse head of the corrugator supercilii muscle [T-CSM]) and laterally (to supply the orbicularis oculi muscle [OOM]). Zygomatic branches run below and parallel to the zygomatic arch to supply the medial OOM.

brow, and enters the lateral aspect of the transverse head of the corrugator supercilii muscle with multiple branches and also sends branches to innervate the superior procerus muscle. Inferiorly, the zygomatic branches run anteriorly below the zygomatic arch to curve superiorly and supply the inferior and medial orbicularis oculi, the depressor supercilii, and the inferior portion of the procerus muscles.

From a surgical perspective, accurately predicting the anticipated course of the branches of the facial nerve both enables maximal protection of the nerve and also allows raid dissection in safe zones. With respect to the facial nerve's temporal branch, Pitanguy and Ramos[11] used a line beginning 5 mm inferior to the tragus and ending 1.5 cm superolateral to the brow to predict the nerve's course. Sabini and associates[12] have further refined this method of topographic plotting of the nerve's course based on a series of cadaver dissections. They determined that the path of the temporal branch could be accurately predicted by first drawing a reference line from the tragus to the lateral canthus and then tracing the projected path of the nerve from the inferior earlobe through the halfway point of the tragus–lateral canthus line. These authors also pointed out that multiple branches of the temporal branch run in proximity (within 0–2 mm) to the medial zygomaticotemporal ("sentinel") vein, found routinely 1 cm lateral to the frontozygomatic suture.

The supratrochlear and supraorbital nerves are end branches of the ophthalmic division of the trigeminal nerve and wrap around the medial and central aspects of the supraorbital rims, respectively. As noted earlier (see "Bones"), the supratrochlear nerve exits the orbit along a groove or notch just medial to the origin of the corrugator supercilii muscle,[13] 14 to 17 mm from the midline.[14,15] The supratrochlear nerve divides into three or four main branches that run through the corrugator supercilii superiorly and subsequently penetrate and run atop the frontalis muscle to provide sensation to the midline and paramedian forehead. These fibers blend laterally with branches of the supraorbital nerve. The infratrochlear nerve, a branch of the nasociliary nerve, exits the orbit approximately 1 cm inferior to the supratrochlear nerve and innervates the glabella and the nasal root.

The supraorbital nerve exits the orbits between 24 and 27 mm from the midline[14,15] through either a notch or a foramen. Approximately half of patients will have bilateral supraorbital notches that can be easily palpated. The remaining patients will have at least one supraorbital foramen. Generally, the supraorbital nerve divides into multiple superficial branches and a deep division. The superficial branches penetrate the corrugator muscle and, like the supratrochlear nerve, run superiorly over the surface of the frontalis muscle to provide sensory in-nervation for the remaining forehead to the temporal crests below the vertex (**Figure 2-11**). The deep division of the supraorbital nerve generally exits the orbit together with the superficial division but, in approximately 10% of patients, will exit through a separate foramen located within 2 cm of the orbital rim. Rather than ascend into a superficial plane, the deep division of the supraorbital nerve runs obliquely under the transverse head of the corrugator supercilii muscle before turning superiorly and running just medial and parallel to the superior temporal line. In the lower half of the forehead, the deep division of the supraorbital nerve runs just above the periosteum, but more superiorly, it rises into the subcutaneous plane to provide sensation to the post-trichial frontoparietal scalp.

Laterally, two branches of the maxillary division of the trigeminal nerve, the zygomaticofacial and the zygomaticotemporal nerves, provide sensation to the lateral orbital rim and malar eminence. The zygomaticotemporal nerve courses around the lateral orbital rim near the frontozygomatic suture and provides sensation to a fan-shaped area behind the lateral orbital rim, whereas the zygomaticofacial nerve exits a bony foramen near the junction of the zygomatic arch and the malar eminence. More posteriorly, the auriculotemporal nerve, a branch of the mandibular division of the trigeminal nerve, crosses the zygomatic arch just behind the superficial temporal artery and vein and branches within the temporoparietal fascia to provide sensation to the skin over the temporal fossa.

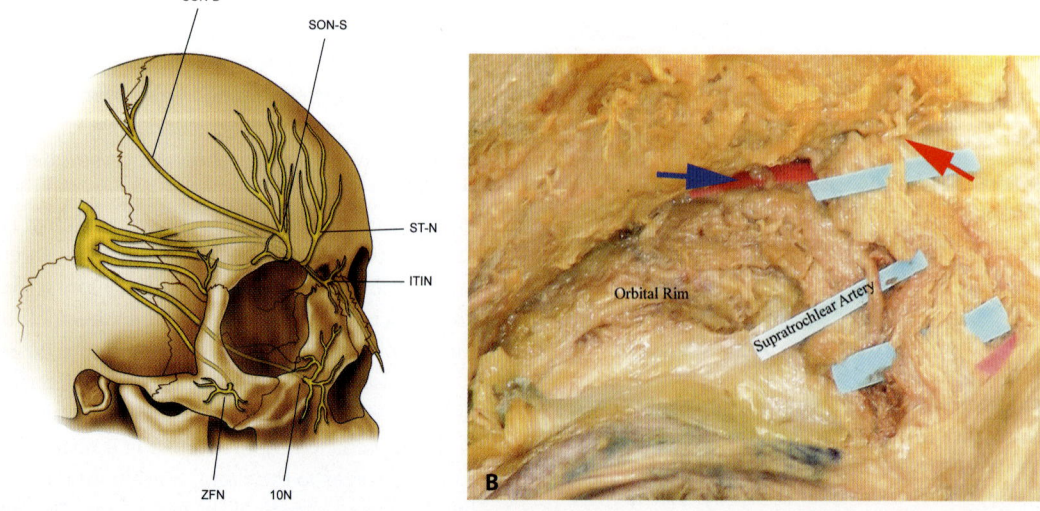

Figure 2-11. (A) Schematic of the sensory nerves of the forehead and brow. ION = infraorbital nerve; ITrN = infratrochlear nerve; SON-D = deep branch of supraorbital nerve; SON-S = superficial branch of supraorbital nerve; STrN = supratrochlear nerve; ZFN = zygomaticofacial nerve. (B) Cadaveric dissection demonstrates SON (*blue arrow*) and STrN (*red arrow*).

Fascial Layers

In the past, the fascial layers of the scalp had been oversimplified to "galea" and "loose connective tissues." However, several excellent works have more completely described the complex relationships between the fine but significant soft tissue components of the forehead and temple. In particular, the reader is referred to the works of Knize[16–19] for a more thorough description. This section is intended to provide the reader with a sufficient understanding of the soft tissues of the forehead that affect forehead function and relate to aesthetic forehead surgery (**Figure 2-12**).

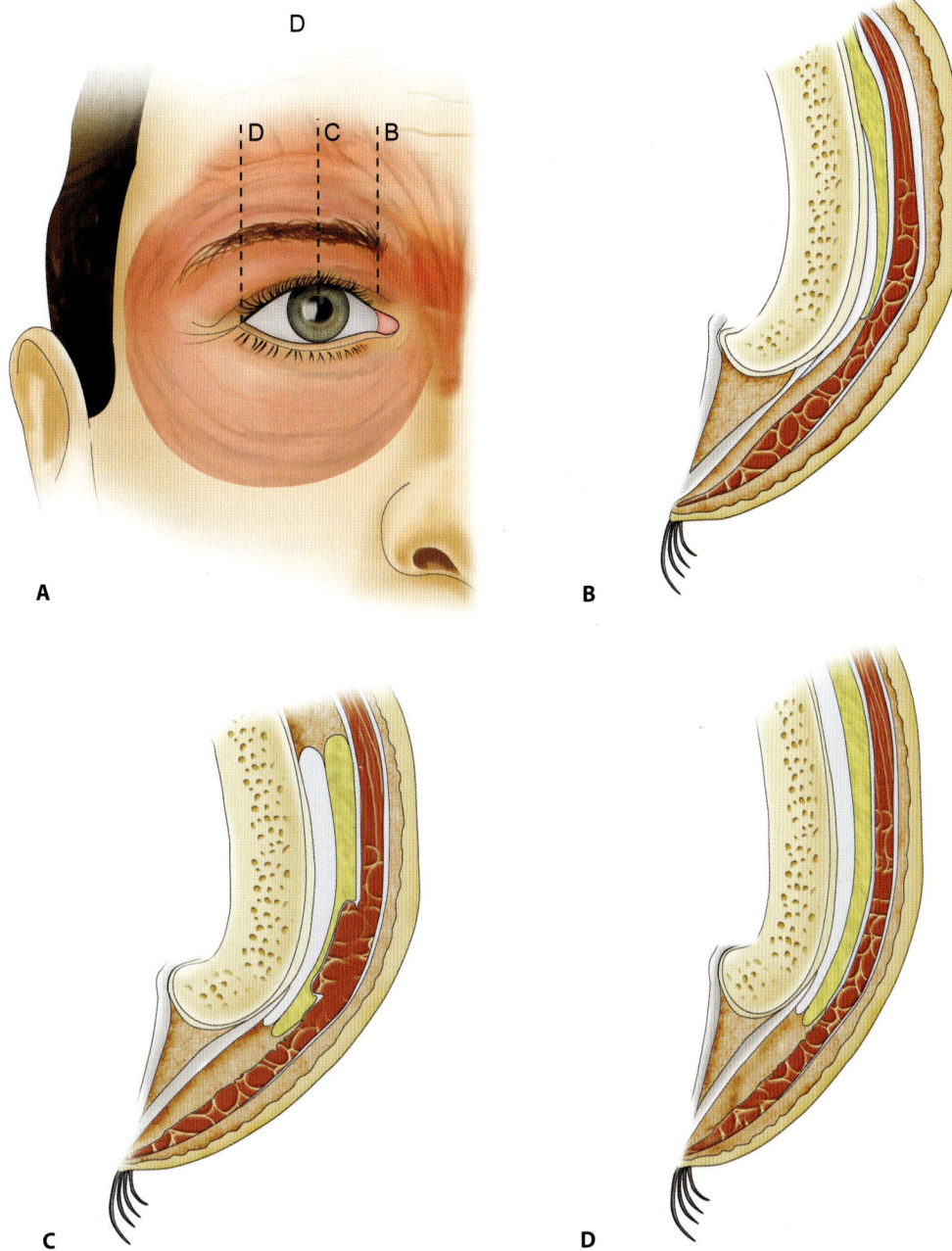

Figure 2-12. (A) Layers of the brow at the medial, central, and lateral brow. (B) Cross-section of the medial brow. The glide plane space allows movement of the lower forehead and brow. (C) Cross-section of the central brow. The corrugator muscle forms part of the roof of the galeal fat pad (GFP). (D) Cross-section of the lateral brow. The floor of the GFP can be less developed laterally, allowing inferior descent of the galeal fat.

Central Forehead

The galea aponeurotica surrounds the occipitalis muscle after it arises from the superior nuchal line and courses anteriorly over the vertex (**Figure 2-13**). At the superior edge of the frontalis muscle, the galea splits into a superficial and a deep layer to envelope the frontalis, with the muscle actually originating from the deep layer of the galea. Superior to the frontalis, the galea is a single, thicker layer with loose fibrous attachments to the underlying periosteum (**Figure 2-14**). The thin, superficial layer of galea continues inferiorly over the frontalis to also cover the orbicularis oculi muscle.

The deep galea subsequently splits a number of times to envelop significant structures and spaces in the lower half of the forehead (**Figure 2-15**). A portion of the deep galea continues inferiorly to form the suborbicularis fascia. Approximately 2.5 cm above the orbital rim, the deep galea splits to envelop the galeal fat pad, which extends the width of the superior orbital rims, extending more inferiorly at the lateral brow. The corrugator extends through and above the galeal fat pad as the muscle runs superolaterally to its insertion into the dermis above the central brow. Inferiorly, the galeal fat pad is separated from the preaponeurotic fat of the upper eyelid by only a thin layer of fascia that extends more inferiorly at the lateral brow; hence, the galeal fat pad may pseudoherniate and/or blend with preaponeurotic fat of the lateral upper eyelid.

The extension of deep galea deep to the galeal fat pad again splits into two layers to surround a space of loose connective fibers that extends the full width of the eyebrows. This glide plane space is narrow (~5 mm) in height medially but more significant laterally, extending 2 to 2.5 cm upward from the orbital rim. The inner aspect of this space is smoothly lined and allows "gliding" of the superficial tissues over the deep layer. Again, the transverse head of the corrugator muscle runs over this structure and contributes to part of the medial roof of the glide plane space. The deep layer of the glide plane space, beginning about 2 cm above the orbital rim, fuses tightly with the periosteum, and it is this adherence that makes true subgaleal dissection difficult inferior to this point. The deep division of the supraorbital nerve, which courses superolaterally after exiting the orbit, runs in this plane between periosteum and deep galea and is vulnerable to injury in this location. The deeper portions of the deep galea, together with the periosteum, contribute to the formation of the septum orbitale, whereas most of the more superficial leaves of the deep galea re-fuse at

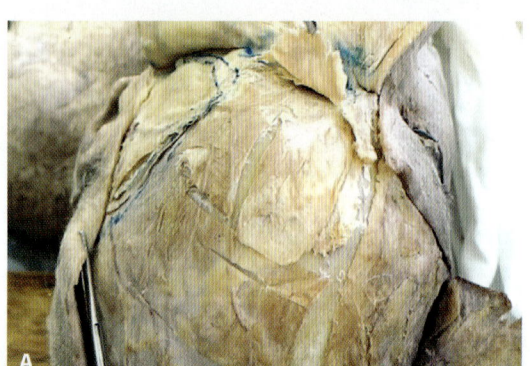

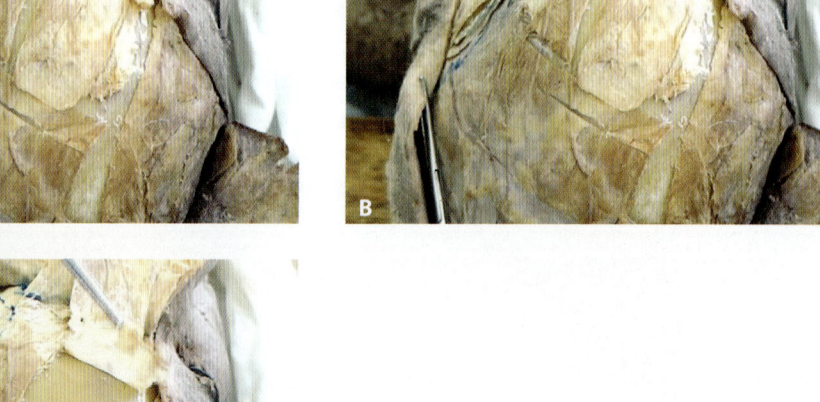

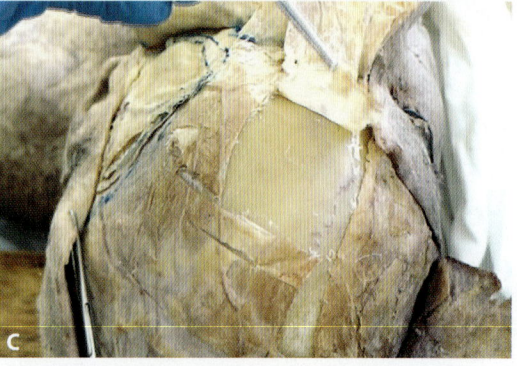

Figure 2-13. Cadaveric forehead dissection, seen from above. Frontalis muscle partially (A) and more fully (B) elevated. The galeal fat pad can be seen between the frontalis muscle and the periosteum. (C) Periosteum elevated.

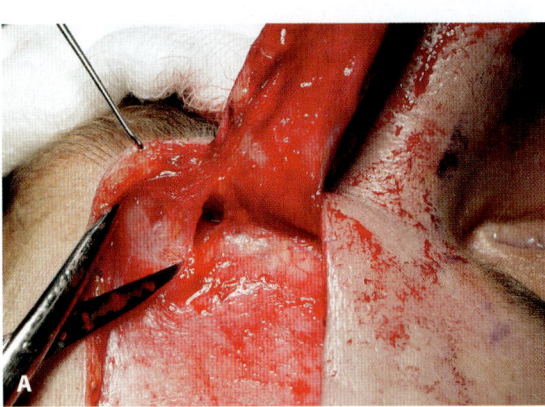 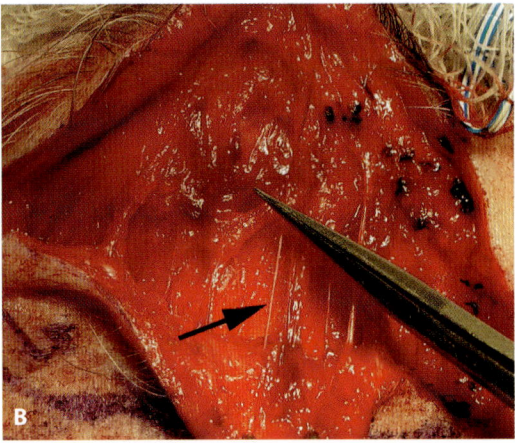

Figure 2-14. (A) Surgical dissection demonstrates the glide plane space between the periosteum and the subfrontalis muscle layer of the deep galea. (B) Dissection directly below the left brow shows multiple superficial branches of the supraorbital nerve (SON; *arrow*) and the corrugator supercilii muscle (CSM, pointer) obliquely covering a portion of the GFP.

the orbital rim. The exception is laterally, where the inferior boundary of the galea fat pad may be weak and the fat may prolapse inferiorly.

This unique multilaminar structure of the deep galea in the inferior forehead provides greater forehead mobility than exists in the upper forehead

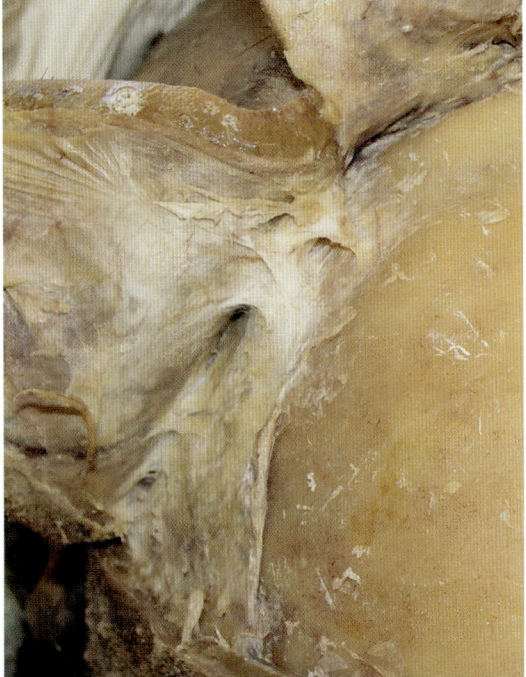

Figure 2-15. Cadaver dissection shows multiple fascial layers of the left temple fusing together and attaching densely at the zone of fixation.

(**Figure 2-16**). Mobility of the upper forehead skin is limited, generally no more than 5 to 10 mm. Conversely, lower forehead skin can slide up to 2 cm vertically. Whereas some of this lower forehead movement occurs at the galeal fat pad level, the glide plane space accounts for the majority of movement. The limited motion of the upper forehead occurs at the periosteum–deep galea level.

The fascia of the temple (**Figure 2-17**) is multilaminar and, although more straightforward than the galea, has significant relations with vital structures. Immediately below and densely adherent to the temporal subdermis, the temporoparietal fascia (superficial temporal fascia) is a temporal continuation of the galea. The temporoparietal fascia continues inferiorly over the zygomatic arch to blend with the superficial musculoaponeurotic system. Superiorly, the temporoparietal fascia fuses with the galea and layers of the deep temporal fascia at the zone of fixation, a strip approximately 5 to 6 mm in width, immediately medial to the superficial temporal line. The temporoparietal fascia is tightly adherent to the overlying skin superiorly, with multiple fibrous bands and vessels bridging between the skin and the temporoparietal fascia (**Figure 2-18A**). As mentioned earlier, the superficial temporal artery runs within the temporoparietal fascia (**see Figure 2-18B**) and gives off branches that also run within the fascia and into superficial tissues; there are no branches of the superficial temporal artery deeper than the temporoparietal fascia. The same holds true for the superficial temporal vein, which runs

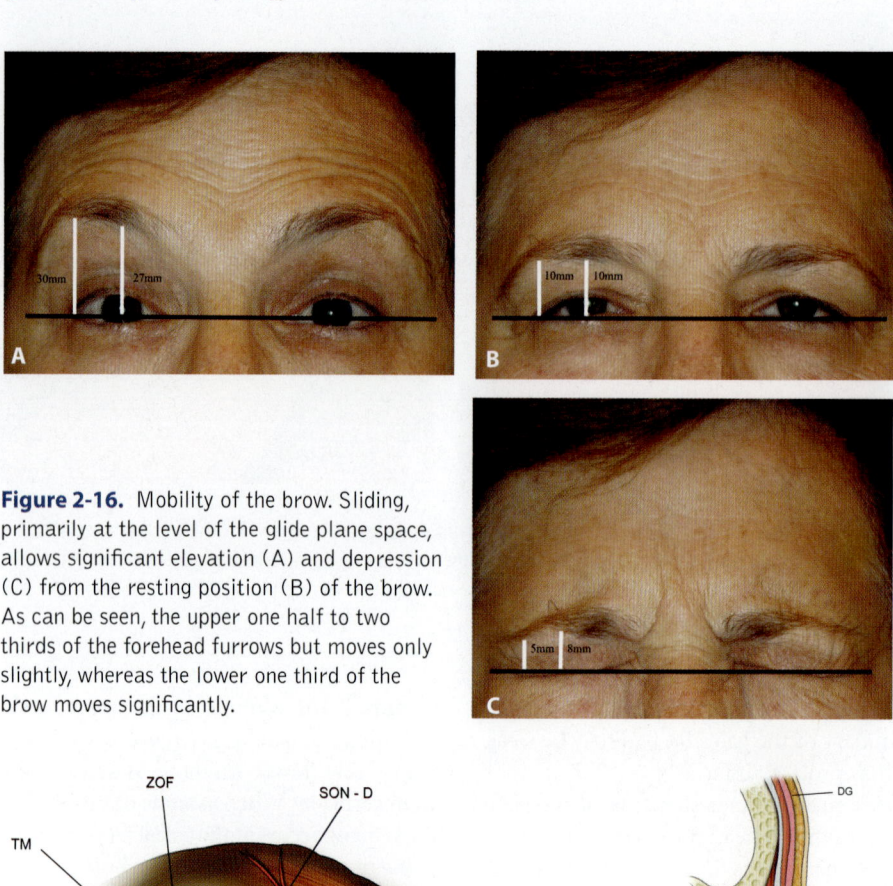

Figure 2-16. Mobility of the brow. Sliding, primarily at the level of the glide plane space, allows significant elevation (A) and depression (C) from the resting position (B) of the brow. As can be seen, the upper one half to two thirds of the forehead furrows but moves only slightly, whereas the lower one third of the brow moves significantly.

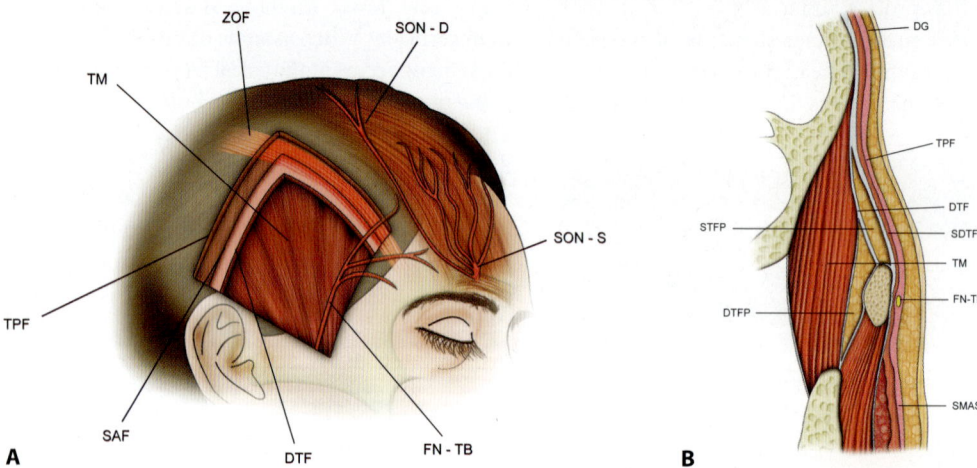

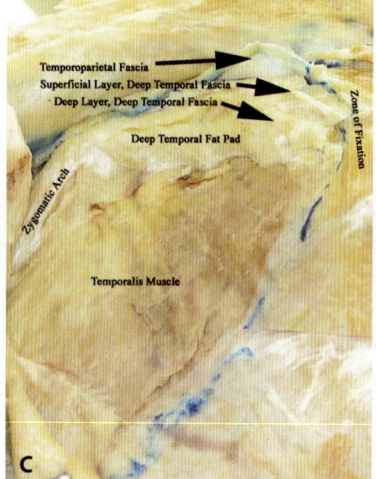

Figure 2-17. Fascial layers of the temple. (A) The multiple temporal fascial layers fuse at the zone of fixation (ZOF). The temporal branch of the facial nerve runs (FN-TB) runs on the undersurface of the temporoparietal fascia (TPF). DG = deep galea; DTF = deep layer of the deep temporal fascia; SON-D = deep division of the supraorbital nerve; SDTF = superficial layer of the deep temporal fascia; SON-S = superficial division of the supraorbital nerve; TM = temporalis muscle. (B) Cross-section through the temple shows layers of temporal fasciae and temporal fat pads. DTFP = deep temporal fat pad; SMAS = superficial musculoaponeurotic system; STFP = superficial temporal fat pad. (C) Layers of the left temporal fascia at the ZOF, as seen from above.

on top of, not within, the temporoparietal fascia. Immediately below the temporoparietal fascia exists a loose areolar plane; this loose layer and the lack of bridging vessels allow mobility of the superficial temporal tissues. Deep to the temporoparietal fascia lies the deep temporal fascia, which is an extension of the temporoparietal periosteum. This dense layer covers the temporalis muscle as a single layer superiorly but splits at the temporal fusion line (roughly at the level of the supraorbital ridge) into a superficial and a deep layer. The deep temporal fascia is densely attached to bone at the superior temporal line, along the lateral orbital rim and the upper border of the zygomatic arch, as well as along the posterior margin of the temporalis muscle.[20] The superficial layer of the deep temporal fascia typically inserts onto the lateral aspect of the arch (contiguous with the parotidomasseteric fascia), whereas the deep layer of the deep temporal fascia inserts onto the medial aspect of the arch. The superficial temporal fat pad can be found in between these layers of the deep temporal fascia, bounded superiorly by the temporal line of fusion and inferiorly by the zygomatic arch.

In a small but significant percentage of patients, the superficial and deep layers re-fuse up to 1 cm superior to the zygomatic arch before inserting on the superior border of the zygomatic arch. Deep to the deep layer of the deep temporal fascia, the deep temporal fat pad represents a superior extension of the buccal fat pad of Bichat (**see Figure 2-18C**) and lies directly on the temporalis muscle. Extensive dissection below either the superficial or the deep layers of the deep temporal fascia can cause postoperative fat necrosis of the superficial or deep temporal fat pads, respectively, presenting clinically as temporal wasting.

Three key areas require specific release to allow unfettered brow elevation. The zone of fixation has been extensively described by Knize.[16-19] It is a rectangular area just medial to the superior temporal line and extending inferiorly to the superolateral orbital rim. The zone of fixation is approximately 5 to 6 mm in width and is the area at which the layer of deep galea below the frontalis muscle becomes confluent with the temporoparietal fascia, the layer of deep galea below the galeal fat pad becomes confluent with the superficial

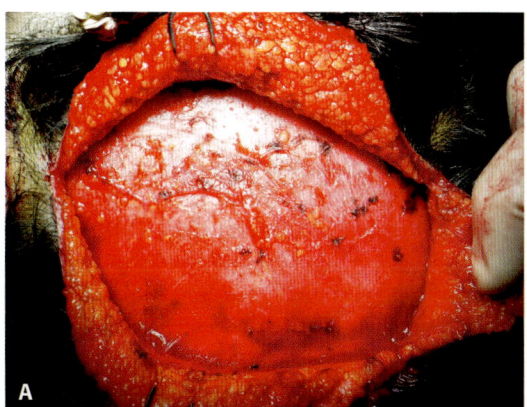

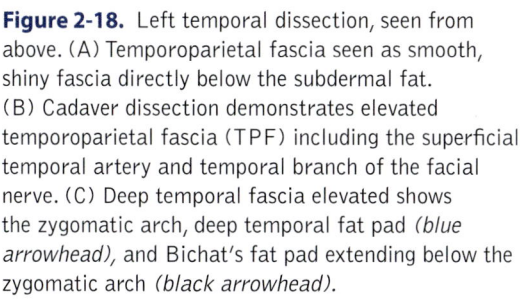

Figure 2-18. Left temporal dissection, seen from above. (A) Temporoparietal fascia seen as smooth, shiny fascia directly below the subdermal fat. (B) Cadaver dissection demonstrates elevated temporoparietal fascia (TPF) including the superficial temporal artery and temporal branch of the facial nerve. (C) Deep temporal fascia elevated shows the zygomatic arch, deep temporal fat pad (*blue arrowhead*), and Bichat's fat pad extending below the zygomatic arch (*black arrowhead*).

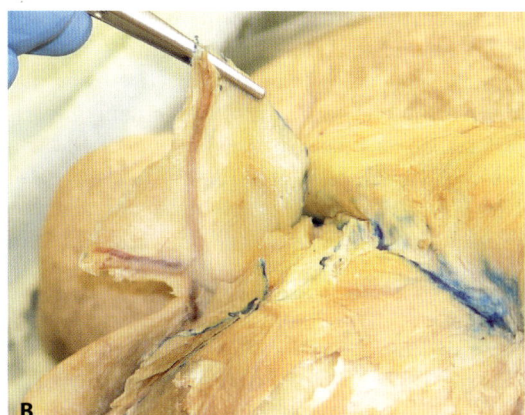

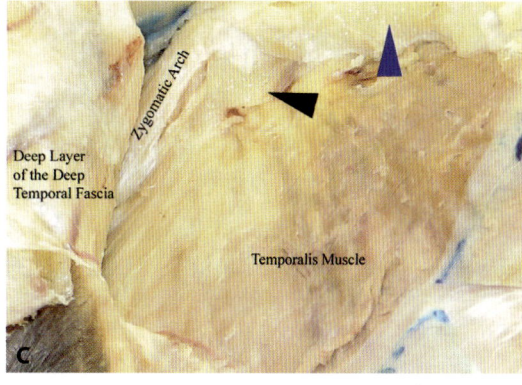

layer of the deep temporal fascia, and the periosteum becomes confluent with the deep layer of the deep temporal fascia. All three of these confluent tissue planes are themselves tightly bound to the calvarium at the zone of fixation. Effective mobilization of the scalp requires adequate elevation and release of these fascial layers at the zone of fixation, rendered somewhat more difficult by the proximity of the deep division of the supraorbital nerve as it runs superiorly toward the vertex.

The second area of specific release begins 2 to 2.5 cm above the supraorbital rim. As discussed earlier, the deepest layer of the deep galea is fused with the periosteum at this level and below, and this relationship explains the benefit of transitioning a subgaleal (actually, an intragaleal—see prior discussion of the layer of the deep galea) dissection to a subperiosteal plane at this point. Any "subgaleal" dissection inferior to this point is most likely in the glide plane space. The dense adherence of deep galea and periosteum to bone continues inferiorly to the orbital rim and the arcus marginalis, and this layer needs to be fully released at or slightly below the arcus to allow complete mobilization of the superficial brow tissues along both orbital rims and across the glabella.

Finally, the orbital ligament must be released at the superolateral orbital rim (**Figure 2-19**). The orbital ligament is a band of connective tissue that attaches the bony orbital rim to the temporoparietal fascia, essentially at the junction of the two previously mentioned areas. The orbital ligament restricts mobility of the lateral brow, and failure to release the orbital ligament will prevent full mobilization and repositioning of the tail of the brow.

Dynamic Theory of Brow Position and Form: The Four Dimensions

Brow position is classically thought of as static, dependent upon muscle attachments and skin elasticity only; with aging, loss of this elasticity allows gravity to inferiorly displace the brow. Photodamage and chronoaging of the skin lead to horizontal forehead and oblique glabellar rhytids.

However, improved understanding of the anatomy of the forehead, temple, and brow, coupled with the introduction of botulinum toxin A for chemodenervation, has led to a better understanding of how the brow works and how it ages. Specifically, the interaction of the forehead and

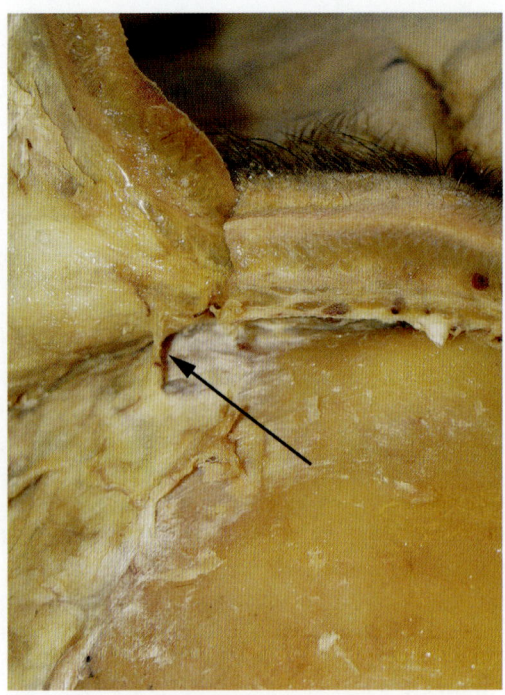

Figure 2-19. Orbital ligament (*arrow*) attaches the superficial and deep temporal fascia densely to the lateral orbital rim.

brow muscles determines to a great degree the appearance of the forehead and brow.

As with all muscles, those of the forehead and brow possess a certain tone[21] and maintain a degree of contraction at all times (**Figure 2-20A, B**). In response to external stimuli (e.g., bright light) or as a chronic habit (e.g., frowning), a muscle in this area may develop an elevated tone. This increased tone and contraction will pull the brow in the direction of that particular muscle's vector of force. If this force is great enough to affect the position of the brow, the other brow muscles will respond to maintain homeostasis of the position of the brow. The compensatory muscle reactions/contractions will cause several effects of their own and may ultimately involve all brow muscles. Brow ptosis will occur if the forces of depressor contraction outweigh those of the elevator (frontalis only) muscle (**see Figure 2-20C**). Even if there is no substantial inferior displacement of the brow, the frontalis muscle is still required to contract additionally to counterbalance the inferior pull of the depressor muscles. This will lead to contour irregularities and (eventually) rhytids across the central forehead (**see Figure 2-20D, E**). This can be demonstrated by asking a pa-

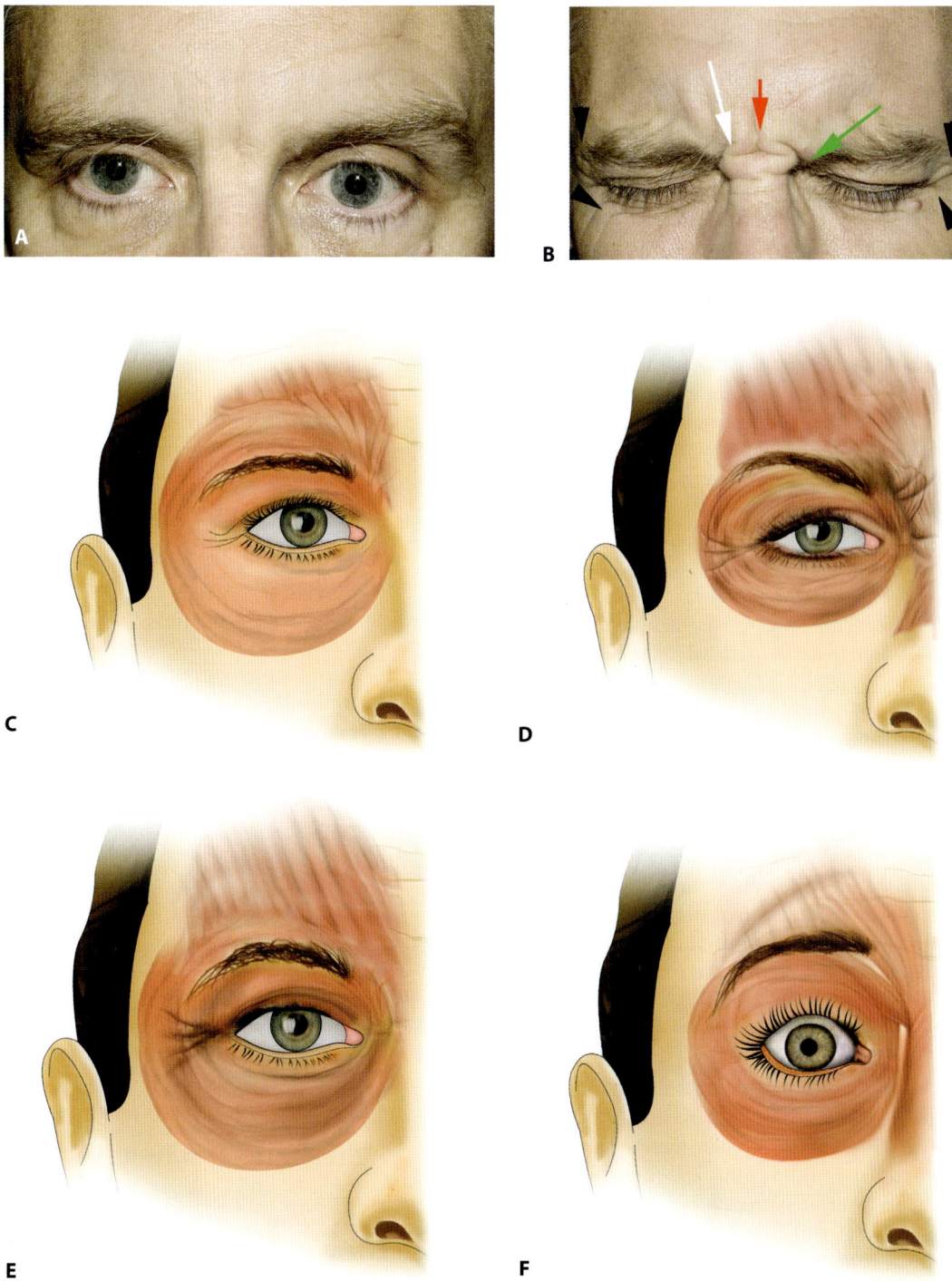

Figure 2-20. Muscular effects on the brow. (A) At rest. (B) Full contraction shows rhytids caused by the pull of the oblique head of the corrugator supercilii muscle (CSM; *white arrow*), transverse head of the CSM (*green arrow*), procerus muscle *(red arrow),* and orbicularis oculi muscle *(black arrows).* (C) Resting tone of the periorbital muscles contribute to the creation of periorbital rhytids and the position of the brow. (D) Elevated tone of corrugator and depressor supercilii, orbicularis oculi, and procerus muscles will increase brow ptosis. (E) Compensatory contraction of the frontalis muscle to elevate the brow enough to eliminate any visual field impairment will add forehead rhytids to those already present. (F) Overaggressive treatment of the brow depressor muscles may cause excessive brow elevation and undesired lateral drift of the medial brow.

tient with (an apparent) borderline brow ptosis to close her or his eyes. Once the subtle visual cues of brow ptosis (visual field shading by the descended brow) are removed, the frontalis muscle is allowed to more fully relax and the brows can be observed to gently descend. This is the *true, descended position of the brow,* and elevation should be planned from *this* point.

Following this point further, it stands to reason that changes in brow position after treatment can be anticipated based on this concept. As the sole brow elevator, disruption of the frontalis muscle would be expected to lead to *descent* of the brow; procedures in which there is extensive myoplasty or paralysis of the frontalis muscle must necessarily rely on some other, nonphysiologic, mechanism for brow elevation. Conversely, by restricting treatment of the frontalis muscle to its upper two thirds, the more mobile lower 2 cm remains intact and functional. Contraction of this segment is most effective in elevating the position of the brow; contraction of the more superior segment of the muscle produces transverse rhytids while stabilizing the forces more inferiorly.

The lateral orbicularis oculi muscle is a major source of depressor forces acting on the lateral brow; lessening this inferior pull (e.g., with botulinum toxin) will allow an intact frontalis pull to elevate this segment of the brow. Treating the corrugator/depressor supercilii muscle complex would reduce not only the brow depressor forces (generated by the oblique head of the corrugator supercilii and the depressor supercilii muscles) but also those forces directed inferomedially (by the transverse head of the corrugator muscle). Aggressive treatment in this area may overly lateralize the medial head of the brow (**see Figure 2-20F**).

In addition, with aging comes involutional skin changes and subcutaneous senescence. As skin elasticity decreases, the brow skin increasingly hangs down and herniates over the superior orbital rim. In patients with anatomically weak lateral floors of the galeal fat pad, this fat may herniated below the orbital rim and increase lateral hooding. Even patients who pluck the inferior hairs of the lateral brow still show obvious signs of aging in this area because the thicker brow and infrabrow skin now hangs down and rests over the upper eyelid. Other patients may experience atrophy of the brow soft tissues, including the galeal fat pad. Loss of this bulk will "flatten" the brow, angling the brow hairs

inferiorly and increasing the apparent ptosis of the brow. Restoration of this volume can seemingly rejuvenate the brow in excess of what would be expected based on brow height only.

In summary, brow position is highly dependent upon brow and forehead muscles, and the brow and forehead can be intelligently treated if sufficient forethought is given to the goals, risks, and techniques employed. Rhytids of the central forehead and/or the glabella or ptosis of the medial, central, and/or lateral segments of the brow can be corrected as long as the surgeon has a thorough understanding of not only the anatomy but also the physiology of the brow. Understanding these four mechanisms of brow aging (muscle contraction, dermal atrophy, fat atrophy, and gravity) is essential.

Summary

Although the anatomy of the forehead and temple is fairly simple, it is essential that the facial plastic surgeon has a firm understanding of these structures and layers and appreciates their interrelation. Only with this understanding can one fully evaluate, understand, and successfully execute forehead and brow rejuvenation procedures.

Whatever is in any way beautiful hath its source of beauty in itself, and is complete in itself; praise forms no part of it. So it is none the worse nor the better for being praised.

Marcus Aurelius Antoninus (AD 121–180)

Acknowledgments

The author would like to thank Matthew A. Pravetz, O.F.M., Ph.D., and Mr. Raymond Chang, Department of Cell Biology and Anatomy, for their assistance with cadaver dissections.

Suggested Readings

1. Park JI, Hoagland TM, Park MS. Anatomy of the corrugator supercilii muscle. Arch Facial Plast Surg 2003;5:412–415.
2. Walden JL, Brown CC, Klapper AJ, et al. An anatomic comparison of transpalpebral, endoscopic, and coronal approaches to demonstrate exposure and extent of brow depressor muscle resection. Plast Reconstr Surg 2005;116:1479–1487.
3. Tolhurst DE, Carstens MH, Greco RJ, Hurwitz DJ. The surgical anatomy of the scalp. Plast Reconstr Surg 1991;87:603–614.

4. Abul-Hassan HS, Ascher GvD, Acland RD. Surgical anatomy and blood supply of the fascial layers of the temporal region. Plast Reconstr Surg 1986;77:17–24.

5. Tremolada C, Candiani P, Signorini M, et al. The surgical anatomy of the subcutaneous fascial system of the scalp. Ann Plast Surg 1994;32:8–14.

6. Gosain AK, Sewall SR, Yousif NJ. The temporal branch of the facial nerve: how reliably can we predict its path? Plast Reconstr Surg 1997;99:1224–1233.

7. Utley DS, Goode RL. Radiofrequency ablation of the nerve to the corrugator muscle for elimination of glabellar furrowing. Arch Facial Plast Surg 1999;1:46–48.

8. Ozersky D, Baek SM, Biller HF. Percutaneous identification of the temporal branch of the facial nerve. Ann Plast Surg 1980;4:276–280.

9. Bernstein L, Nelson RH. Surgical anatomy of the extraparotid distribution of the facial nerve. Arch Otolaryngol 1984;110:177–183.

10. Ellis DAF, Bakala CD. Anatomy of the motor innervation of the corrugator supercilii muscle: clinical significance and development of a new surgical technique for frowning. J Otolaryngol 1998;27:222–227.

11. Pitanguy I, Ramos AS. The frontal branch of the facial nerve: the importance of its variations in face lifting. Plast Reconstr Surg 1966;38:352–356.

12. Sabini P, Wayne I, Quatela VC. Anatomical guides to precisely localize the frontal branch of the facial nerve. Arch Facial Plast Surg 2003;5:150–152.

13. Riefkohl R, Kosanin R, Georgiade GS. Complications of the forehead-brow lift. Aesthetic Plast Surg 1983;7:135–138.

14. Lorenc ZP, Ivy E, Aston SJ. Neurosensory preservation in endoscopic foreheadplasty. Aesthetic Plast Surg 1995;19:411–413.

15. Michelow BJ, Guyuron B. Rejuvenation of the upper face. A logical gamut of surgical options. Clin Plast Surg 1997;24:199–212.

16. Knize DM. An anatomically based study of the mechanism of eyebrow ptosis. Plast Reconstr Surg 1996; 97:1321–1333.

17. Knize DM. Anatomy of a frown: basis for a limited incision approach to trreatment of eyebrow ptosis and glabellar lines. Perspect Plast Surg 1996;10:1–37.

18. Knize DM. Transpalpebral approach to the corrugator supercilii and procerus muscles. Plast Reconstr Surg 1995;95:52–62.

19. Knize DM. Muscles that act on glabellar skin: a closer look. Plast Reconstr Surg 2000;105:350–361.

20. Dempsey PD, Oneal RM, Izenberg PH. Subperiosteal brow and midface lifts. Aesthetic Plast Surg 1995;19:59–68.

21. Pennock JD, Johnson PC, Mandeps EK, Van Sweanngen JM. Relationship between muscle actually of the frontalis and the associated brow displacement. PNS. 1999; 104:1789–1797.

3

Brief History of Aesthetic Forehead Surgery

We are like dwarfs on the shoulders of giants, so that we can see more than they, and things
at a great distance, not by virtue of any sight on our part, or any physical distinction,
but because we are carried high and raised up by their giant size.

Bernard of Chartres (12th Century AD)

The history of elective forehead and brow surgery is relatively short, beginning in the early 20th century. However, it is important to recognize that for medical and functional reasons, surgery of the scalp (and cranium) has been performed since the Neolithic age. In the *Iliad*, 6 of the 140 wounds described by Homer[1] involved the forehead and temple (interestingly, all victims were Trojan). In *The Histories*, Herodotus[2] described the Scythian method of scalping victims, essentially the same method attributed to Native Americans in the 18th century in New York by James Thatcher,[3] and in Tennessee by James Robertson.[4] These primitive procedures, although done in the context of "shock and awe" military campaigns, relied on an appreciation of the loose subgaleal plane (**Figure 3-1**) to tear the scalp off the calvarium after the skin and fascia had been circumferentially incised. Modern aesthetic forehead surgery, however, truly began after the advent of aseptic techniques and the era of antibiotics. A variety of approaches and techniques have been described,[5] with incisions situated for appropriate exposure and optimal safety and wound healing (**Figure 3-2**). It has evolved in four distinct but overlapping phases.

Tissue Suspension

Early techniques were based solely on skin excision and relied on mass tissue movement and a tension closure to reposition the brows. The primary concern

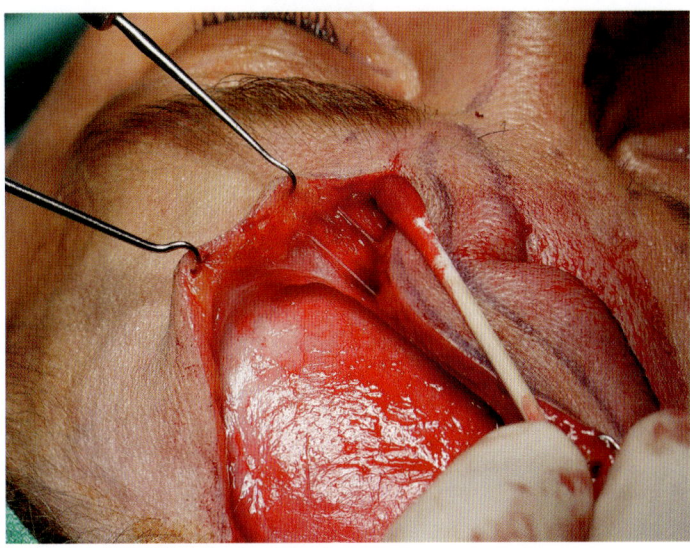

Figure 3-1. A loose plane between the deep galea and the periosteum can be established 2 cm above the orbital rim and higher and extends to the occiput.

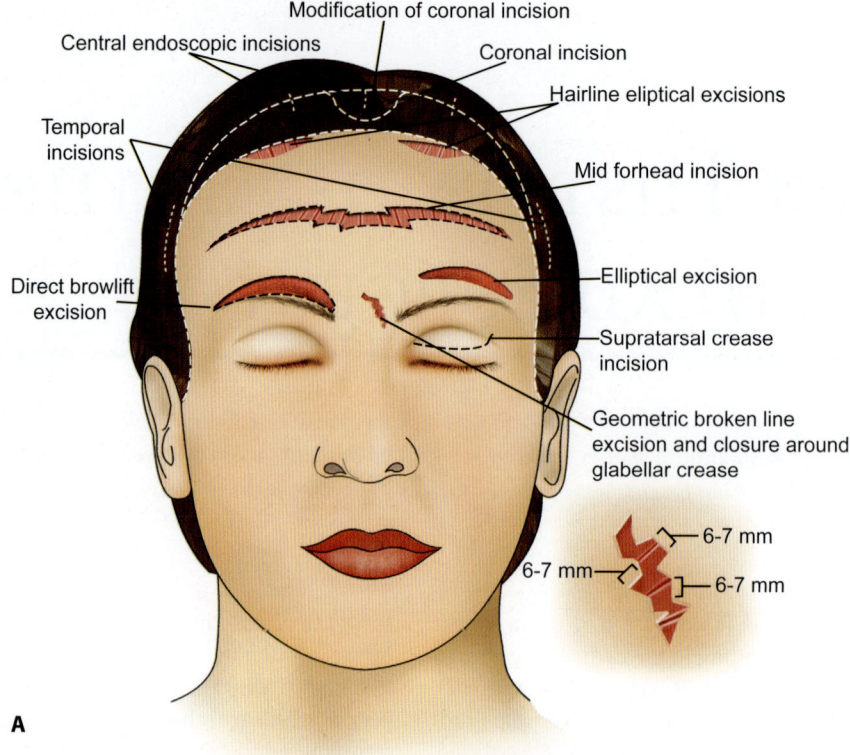

A

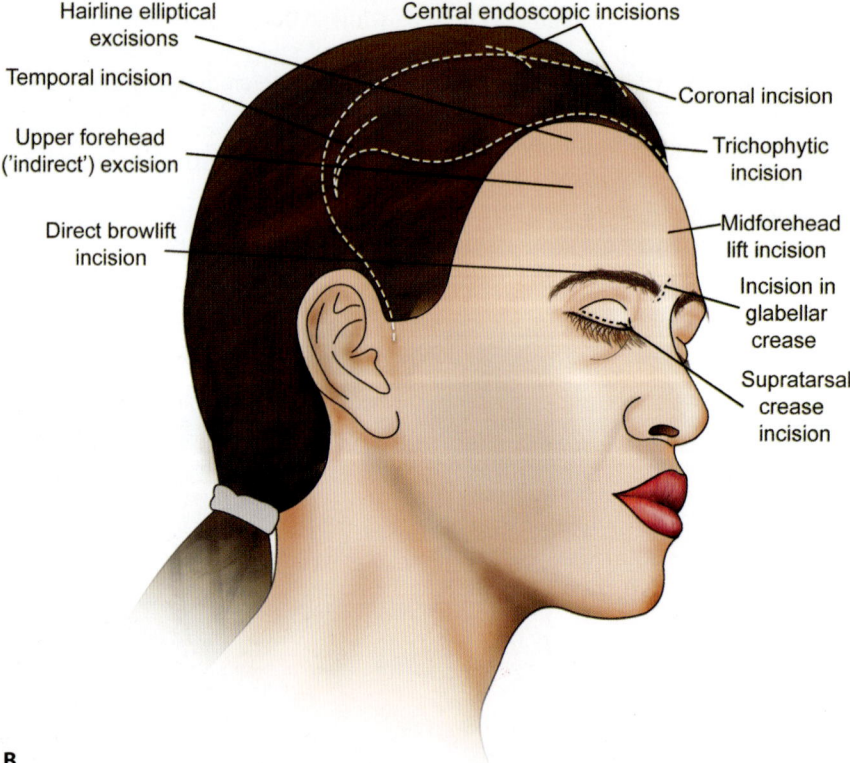

B

Figure 3-2. Frontal (A) and lateral (B) views of a variety of forehead, temple, and brow incisions.

of these procedures, beyond brow elevation, was the camouflage of the scar.

In 1919, Passot described a number of forehead skin elliptical excisions designed to elevate specific portions of the brow when the wound was closed. In 1924, Miller[6] further described a number of patterns of skin excisions, hidden behind the hairline. Like Passot, Miller also used the specific designs and locations of these excisions to affect different portions of the brow. Noel in 1926, and Lexer, Joseph, and Passot in 1931 all used more extensive hairline or post-trichial skin ellipses. Passot added temporal branch neurectomies to these procedures in 1933, an admission of the need for reduction in muscular activity to reduce rhytids. The midforehead lift is an extension of these early forehead procedures, with the incision hidden in a preexisting central forehead rhytid. It does, however, incorporate an incision through the frontalis muscle, elevation, and resuspension. Later on, glabellar myoplasties were added.[7] In this context, simpler forms of browlifting with less scarring and minimal recovery were constantly being attempted. In 1976, Parkes and coworkers[8] described suture suspension of the brow through small incisions as an in-office, static procedure to reset the brow nadir. This, as well as the more recent iterations with barbed suspension sutures, is a purely mechanical procedure that does not modify the vectors of pull on the brow, nor does it permanently reposition the brow.

Functional Browlifting

It was the introduction of the modern coronal forehead lift that significantly increased interest in forehead and brow surgery. In 1962, Gonzales-Ulloa[9] described a circumferential incision used to rejuvenate both the face and the forehead and brow. In 1969, Vinas presented his technique (subsequently published in 1976),[10] in which a (usually) post-trichial coronal incision is made and a subgaleal dissection is performed to the orbital rim. Glabellar rhytids were treated with corrugator excision, and a horizontal strip of frontalis muscle was excised from the upper frontalis muscle. This technique demonstrated an improved understanding of brow dynamics; depressor forces acting on the brow were eliminated (if only to treat glabellar wrinkles), but the brow elevator (frontalis muscle) was also weakened. As the procedure was refined in the 1970s and 1980s, an enhanced appreciation of forehead aesthetics provided better guidelines by which to

choose a post-trichial or trichophytic coronal incision. Aggressive frontalis myoplasty techniques (e.g., extensive resection, "checkerboard scoring") gave way to limited scoring of only the muscle directly underlying the deepest rhytid of the upper forehead. As Luckey[11] presciently wrote in 1981, "It seems that as we move towards the end of the 20th century, it is time to look beyond our simplistic effort at correction of the static changes of aging and attempt to modify the dynamic processes of the body to produce the effect desired by the physician and patient alike."[11]

Physiologic Browlifting

As the nuances of the coronal forehead lift were being elucidated, interest in endoscopic surgery had expanded from abdominal and pelvic surgery to head and neck and plastic surgery. This technique diverged from the mass tissue movement of the coronal lift and instead developed along the lines of a "physiologic" modification, relying mostly on muscle modifications for changing brow position. Aiache, Isse, Ramirez, and Vasconez all presented their techniques and results in 1992. In 1994, Chajchir[12] published a description of his technique of subperiosteal and temporal subfascial dissection followed by periosteal release at the orbital rim and myotomies. In 1994, Isse[13] dissected subperiosteally anteriorly but subgaleally posteriorly. Core and colleagues[14] and Isse[15] also published their works in 1995. Isse described several variations of the endoforehead lift, each with its own specific focus: elevation the lateral brow, with or without central forehead elevation. In that same year, Oslin and associates[16] and Ramirez[17] described techniques of endoforehead lifting that eliminated excessive hairline elevation. Over the subsequent 10 years, different authors debated the need for central fixation, its duration, and even the efficacy of the procedure itself. However, most surgeons have come to understand that with thorough elimination of brow depressor muscle tone, a reliable elevation of the brow can be achieved with the use of central forehead calvarial fixation and temporal fascial suspension sutures.

Focused Physiologic Browlifting

As our knowledge of brow and forehead anatomy has improved and our understanding of how the various structures of the brow interact, surgeons have sought to focally alter the brow dynamics through small incisions and with limited dissection.[18-26] Limited transtemporal procedures were developed to achieve brow changes with limited dissection and recovery. Several workers have described a transtemporal approach to release the brow and its retaining ligaments and resuspend the brow superolaterally. In addition, a transpalpebral approach can be added to access the medial brow depressors with relatively little additional morbidity or recovery time. A transpalpebral approach alone also can be used to modify the bulk of the brow or to reposition it. Through this approach, the medial brow depressors can be treated, the retaining ligaments of the brow released, and the brow fixed more superiorly.

Along the same lines, the shape and position of the brow can be modified by reducing or eliminating the vector(s) of pull of brow musculature. With the introduction of selective chemodenervation with botulinum toxin in 1994,[27] the reduction of crow's feet was soon followed by the "chemical brow lift,"[28-31] which could provide temporary elevation to specific areas of the brow. Current research on selective radiofrequency neurectomy may provide a more long-lasting, highly specific reduction in brow depressor activity, a far cry from the temporal branch neurectomy recommended by Passot in 1933 to reduce forehead wrinkles.

Conclusion

Aesthetic treatment of the brow has progressively evolved since the 1935s, beginning with the simple concept of simply pulling the brow superiorly, through various procedures to affect the overall forehead and brow muscle activity, and finally to surgical (open and closed) procedures and noninvasive treatments to selectively modify particular muscle vectors. In the future, procedures will become more specific, more accurate, and less invasive in improving the aesthetics of the brow and forehead.

The real voyage of discovery consists not in seeking new landscapes but in having new eyes.
                    Marcel Proust (1871–1922)

Suggested Readings

1. Homer. The Iliad. Samuel Butler (trans). St. Petersburg, FL, Red & Black Publishers, 2008.

2. Herodotus. The Histories. Aubrey De Selincourt (trans), London, Penguin Books, 2002.

3. Thatcher J. Excerpts from a military journal during the Revolutionary War. In Earle AS (ed). Surgery in America, 2nd ed. New York, Praeger, 1983, pp. 42–49.

4. Robertson J. Remarks in the management of the scalped-head. In Earle AS (ed). Surgery in America, 2nd ed. New York, Praeger, 1983, pp. 36–40.

5. Arneja JS, Larson DL, Gosain AK. Aesthetic and reconstructive brow lift: current techniques, indications, and applications. Ophthal Plast Surg 2005;21: 405–411.

6. Miller CC. Cosmetic Surgery. The correction of featural imperfections. Philadelphia, FA Davis, 1924, pp. 57–81.

7. Adamson PA. The forehead lift: refinements in technique. J Otolaryngol 1986;15:89– 93.

8. Parkes ML, Kamer FM, Bassilios M. Surgical treatment of the ptotic brow. Laryngoscope 1976;86:1435–1436.

9. Gonzalez-Ulloa M. Facial wrinkles. Integral elimination. Plast Reconstr Surg 1962;29:658–673.

10. Vinas JC, Caviglia C, Cortinas JL. Forehead rhytidoplasty and brow lifting. Plast Reconstr Surg 1976; 57:445–454.

11. Luckey RC. The forehead lift (letter). Plast Reconstr Surg 1981;68:645.

12. Chajchir A. Endoscopic subperiosteal forehead lift. Aesthetic Plast Surg 1994;18:269–274.

13. Isse NG. Endoscopic facial rejuvenation: endoforehead, the functional lift. Aesthetic Plast Surg 1994;18:21–29.

14. Core GB, Vasconez LO, Graham HD. Endoscopic browlift. Clin Plast Surg 1995;22:619–631.

15. Isse NG. Endoscopic forehead lift. Evolution and update. Clin Plast Surg 1995;22:661–673.

16. Oslin B, Core GB, Vasconez LO. The biplanar endoscopically assisted forehead lift. Clin Plast Surg 1995;22:633–638.

17. Ramirez OM. Endoscopically assisted biplanar forehead lift. Plast Reconstr Surg 1995;96:323–333.

18. Knize DM. Limited incision forehead lift for eyebrow elevation to enhance upper blepharoplasty. Plast Reconstr Surg 2001;108:564–567.

19. Knize DM. Transpalpebral approach to the corrugator supercilii and procerus muscles. Plast Reconstr Surg 1995;95:52–62.

20. Kikkawa DO, Miller SR, Batra MK, Lee AC. Small incision nonendoscopic browlift. Ophthal Plast Reconstr Surg 2000;1:28–33.

21. Paul MD. The surgical management of upper eyelid hooding. Aesthetic Plast Surg 1989;13: 183–187.

22. Paul MD. The evolution of the brow lift in aesthetic plastic surgery. Plast Reconstr Surg 2001;108:1409–1424.

23. McCord CD, Doxanas MT. Browplasty and browpexy: an adjunct to blepharoplasty. Plast Reconstr Surg 1990;86:248–254.

24. Sokol AB, Sokol TP. Transblepharoplasty brow suspension. Plast Reconstr Surg 1982;69:940–944.

25. Paul MD. Subperiosteal transblepharoplasty forehead lift. Aesthetic Plast Surg 1996;20:129–134.

26. Sclafani AP. Comprehensive periorbital rejuvenation with resorbable Endotine implants for trans-lid brow and midface elevation. Clin Facial Plast Surg 2007;15:255–264.

27. Keen M, Blitzer A, Aviv J, Binder W. Botulinum toxin A for hyperkinetic facial lines: results of a double-blind, placebo-controlled study. Plast Reconstr Surg 1994;94:94–99.

28. Frankel AS, Kamer FM. Chemical browlift. Arch Otolaryngol Head Neck Surg 1998;124:321–323.

29. Ahn MS, Catten M, Maas CS. Temporal brow lift using botulinum toxin A. Plast Reconstr Surg 2000;105:1129–1135.

30. Huang W, Rogachefsky AS, Foster JA. Browlift with botulinum toxin. Dermatol Surg 2000;26:55–60.

31. Tayani R, Rubin PA. Aesthetic periocular surgery including brow, midface, and upper face. Curr Opin Ophthalmol 1999;10:362–367.

4

Preoperative Evaluation and Perioperative Management of the Forehead Rejuvenation Patient

Beauty is the wonder of wonders. It is only the shallow people who do not judge by appearances.
Oscar Wilde (1854–1900), *The Picture of Dorian Gray*

Introduction

Patients considering cosmetic improvement of the upper face often are unclear as to their specific aesthetic needs. Because the eyes are the central visual focus of an individual's facial appearance, patients with periorbital aging will often present requesting upper blepharoplasty. However, in a substantial proportion of these patients, correction of brow ptosis is the principal surgical maneuver necessary for rejuvenation. The time leading up to surgery, from the moment the patient contacts the surgeon's office to the day of surgery, is the surgeon's opportunity to diagnose the patient's aesthetic needs and goals, assess the suitability of the patient for surgery, develop a surgical treatment plan and convey that plan to the patient, and physically, emotionally, and financially prepare the patient for surgery. Redundancy is deliberately built into the consultation visit: important concepts and policies introduced by the office staff to the patient are explained further by the physician and reiterated again by the patient care coordinator. These concepts are then supported in follow-up

documents mailed to the patient. By the time of surgery, the patient should feel completely comfortable with every aspect of the treatment process and should comprehend and accept the goals, expectations, and responsibilities of each member of the treatment team (surgeon, staff, and patient).

The Preconsultation

The patient's first interaction with the surgeon is through his or her telephone staff, and it is every patient's right to be greeted and treated courteously by the telephone receptionist. The receptionist should be familiar with the procedures performed by the staff and be available to answer basic questions about the physician (his or her training and credentials), procedures (in general), and approximate cost ranges for each. However, these conversations should be brief (≤10 min), and patients should be encouraged to bring a list of questions to the consultation. It is neither appropriate nor efficient to have reception staff answering questions in detail at this stage, and patients who expect this may be "doctor shopping." Staff is encouraged to note their general impressions of the patient at this and all points of interaction with the patient, especially if there is any question about the patient's suitability for treatment.

The Consultation

Consultation with the surgeon should be scheduled of sufficient length to ensure the surgeon can determine the patient's goals and aesthetic needs, formulate a surgical plan, and explain it to the patient along with pertinent risks. The physician's time with the patient can be maximally utilized by delegating some functions to the patient care coordinator. However, the surgeon should always keep in mind that she or he is ultimately responsible for every element of the patient's care and it is her or his reputation and good name at risk with each and every interaction the patient has with any part of her or his practice.

Initial Information

Patients are asked to come 15 minutes early to the office on the day of the consultation. Once the patient has completed a standard health history and financial and photography/videography release forms, the patient care coordinator introduces herself or himself to the patient and briefly describes the surgeon's training and qualifications, as well as principal focus of the practice, and then performs a directed interview of the patient to assess the patient's specific aesthetic goals. Because upper facial rejuvenation patients often assume their cosmetic issues are limited to the upper eyelids, they are counseled at this point that many patients may benefit from forehead surgery (with or without upper blepharoplasty) and that the surgeon will discuss this further with the patient if deemed appropriate. Introducing this concept at this time allows the patient to understand that this is not an uncommon scenario and avoids the surgeon appearing to advocate an additional but unnecessary procedure.

The patient is then specifically asked about any medical conditions or personal restrictions (particularly time available for recovery) that would contraindicate treatment or interfere with proper recovery. Specific to treatment of the upper facial third, it is essential to inquire directly about prior blepharoplasty or any other ophthalmologic conditions (especially symptomatic xerophthalmia). In this setting, patients are often more comfortable discussing with staff what they may perceive to be minor issues, such as a limited time available for recovery or an important social engagement by which they would like to be fully healed. Again, specific finances are not discussed, but the individual components of the patient's out-of-pocket expenses (e.g., surgeon's, anesthesiologist's and facility fees, medications) are explained to the patient and, based on this interview, more specific ranges of costs are provided to the patient.

Medical Consultation

It is useful if the surgeon first is briefed by the patient care coordinator on her or his conversation with the patient. Desired goals and any constraints are described, and the patient care coordinator should feel comfortable relating any concerns about the patient's motivation and appropriateness for surgery.

The essence of the patient's goals can usually be distilled in a few minutes by asking the patient focused questions and allowing him or her to answer in three or four sentences. The patient is asked to state his or her primary aesthetic concern, and the surgeon *must allow* the patient to answer without interruption. This simple step of listening helps put the patient at ease and signals to the patient that the surgeon is interested in a partnership to provide the best and most appropriate care for the patient. It also provides the surgeon with an opportunity to better understand the patient's goals, appreciate the degree of the patient's knowledge and misconceptions, and observe the patient's demeanor and affect. The surgeon can then evaluate the patient with a better comprehension of the specific changes the patient desires.

The surgeon should obtain a complete medical history from the patient including use of any prescription, over-the-counter, and/or homeopathic medications. A history of all prior surgery (aesthetic or noncosmetic), as well as nonsurgical facial plastic treatments (especially botulinum toxin), is also noted. Use of tobacco, alcohol, or any elicit drug is also recorded.

Even if the patient indicated an interest in only upper facial rejuvenation, a complete facial analysis and evaluation should be performed. The forehead and brow do not exist in isolation, and any surgery in these areas must be fundamentally considered as an integral part of the facial *whole*. Particular attention is given to facial symmetry and balance. The face is evaluated using the "rule of thirds" and the "rule of fifths," and significant deviations from the general norms of facial aesthetics should be brought to the patient's attention.

Brow Analysis

The analysis of the brow should always include a general impression of the brow, including its shape, bulk, and hair density, as well as height and positioning. Any asymmetry should be noted and pointed out to the patient. The brow is inspected more closely, noting areas of brow depilation by waxing or brow plucking (**Figure 4-1A**). The true shape and position of the brow should be considered to include these areas, because this skin (especially at the brow's lower border) is *brow* skin, distinctly thicker and more sebaceous than upper eyelid skin; failure to reposition this skin, even if hair can be removed, will leave brow skin unacceptably low and prolapsed over the thinner upper eyelid skin. As with the face as a whole, (a)symmetry of the brows should be noted, because 40% of patients will have a significant degree of asymmetry of the brows, with the right side lower 85% of the time (**see Figure 4-1B**). Up to half of patients who appear to have borderline to mild ptosis can be corrected by addressing the brow ptosis.

The brow is then considered more specifically, visually dividing the brow into three segments:

medial head (medial to the medial limbus), central (medial limbus to brow arch peak), and tail (lateral to the peak of the brow arch). Each segment should then be considered separately, in the context of facial shape and ideal brow shape and position. The segments of the brow typically need different degrees of elevation. Uniform elevation will generally lead to brow repositioning without a change in brow shape, and most patients need reshaping, not just repositioning, of the brow. Elevation of the central segment of the brow usually "opens" the palpebral height while also contributing somewhat to reshaping the peak of the brow arch, whereas treating the lateral segment addresses primarily the brow peak and temporal brow hooding. The medial head is chiefly affected by the glabellar muscles and must be considered to avoid leaving a postoperative "scowl" or "angry" appearance and glabellar rhytids.

It is imperative at this point to reiterate that many patients (up to 79% in one recent study) may be unaware of the need for brow and forehead treatment, instead mistakenly assuming treatment should be directed toward the upper eyelids. The appropriateness of brow and forehead treatment can be demonstrated to the patient using a fine ear curet bent with a gentle curve to roll the redundant skin herniated over the upper lid into the superior sulcus. By improving the upper lid contour and defining the supratarsal crease without correcting brow ptosis,

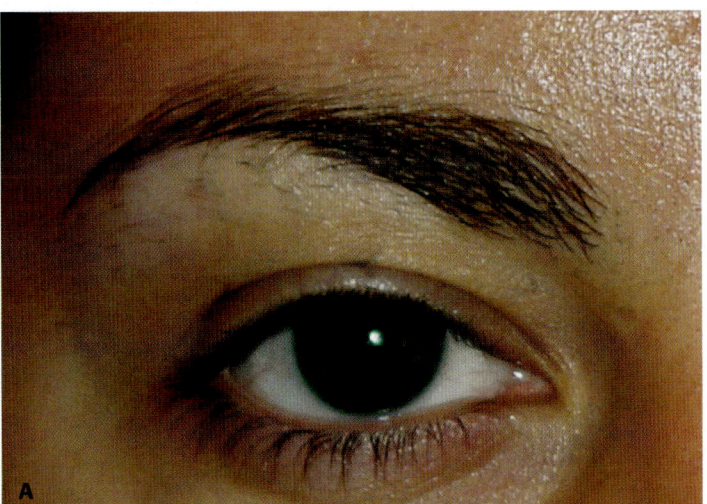 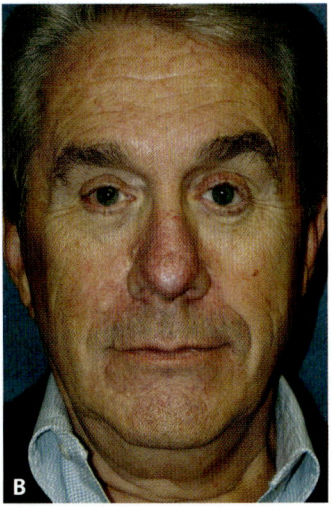

Figure 4-1. (A) Patients with brow ptosis may pluck the lower hairs of the eyebrow, making the brow seem higher. However, the thicker brow skin extending onto the upper lid still causes a "tired"-appearing eye and brow. A Patient who plucks the lower hairs of the lateral two thirds of the brow. Although the brow arch is enhanced, the thicker ptotic brow skin still lies over the upper lid even in this young patient. (B) Patients frequently are unaware of significant brow asymmetry. This should be discussed with the patient preoperatively.

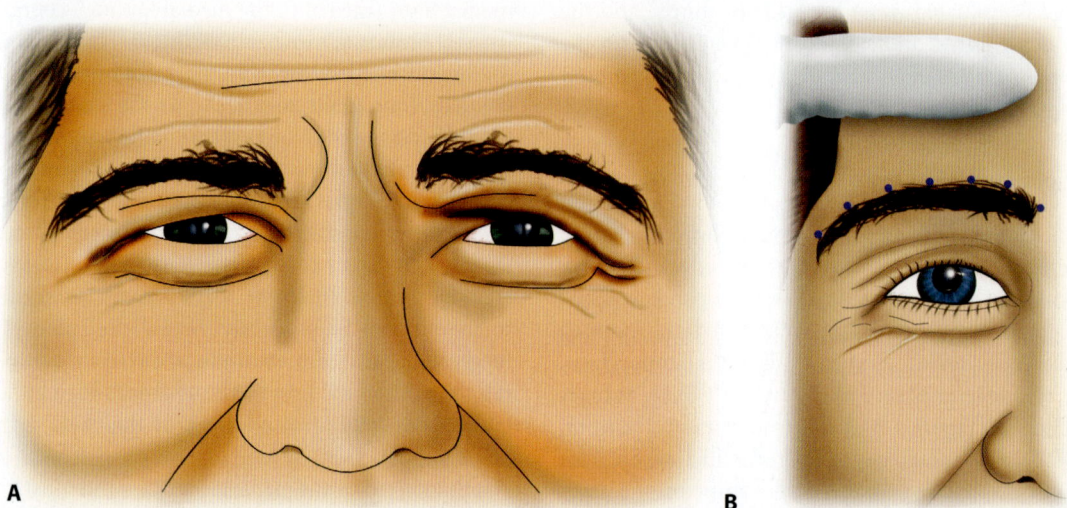

Figure 4-2. (A) Patients with significant brow ptosis will often present requesting upper blepharoplasty to eliminate excessive skin between the brow hairs and the eyelashes. (B) The surgeon demonstrates to the patient the need for brow elevation by manually lifting the brow, which improves the appearance of the eyes and brow. Only after the brow is positioned aesthetically should upper lid skin redundancy be evaluated.

the patient can visualize in a mirror the "frowned" appearance that even a properly performed upper blepharoplasty would create. By failing to establish an appropriate distance between the brows and the eyelashes, the brow appears to frown, often worsening the periorbital appearance. Having done this, the surgeon should then demonstrate the beneficial effect of brow repositioning (**Figure 4-2**). The surgeon stands behind the patient and uses the index, middle, and ring fingers to differentially elevate the medial, central, and lateral segments of the brow, respectively, into an aesthetically appropriate position. The brow is elevated only to an appropriate height and each upper lid is assessed for residual skin redundancy by determining the maximal amount of upper lid skin that can be grasped (with the patient's eyes closed) without causing lagophthalmos. This is done one lid at a time, so that the patient fully appreciates the relative contributions of brow ptosis and upper lid dermatochalasis in causing periorbital aging; this is a very useful sequence to help dispel the patient's misconception that the upper lid is the major source of the cosmetic deformity.

Once the general need for brow elevation has been satisfactorily demonstrated to the patient, the degree of involuntary frontalis contraction present is also illustrated. Indeed, Troilius[1] reported a 3-mm drop in brow position after upper blepharoplasty only (**Figure 4-3**). Flowers and coworkers[3] have

succinctly described the essence of this postoperative drop. Although patients may believe that upper eyelid skin resection has "pulled" the brow down, the beneficial effect of the skin resection (elimination of superior visual field impairment or excessive shadowing) allows the frontalis tone to decrease and the brow to fall farther (secondary to the intact brow depressor muscle tone). This can be demonstrated by first asking the patient to close his or her eyes gently. Again, with the visual field shadowing/field cut eliminated as a stimulus, the frontalis muscle will relax. The surgeon can observe the forehead skin become smoother and the brow slowly descend. Patients are asked to concentrate on breathing slowly to fully relax muscle tone. Some patients may benefit from the surgeon lightly stroking the forehead inferiorly to provide a light stimulus to further relax the frontalis muscle (**Figure 4-4**). Once the frontalis is maximally relaxed, the surgeon then holds firmly (but without further depressing) the brow and asks the patient to slowly open his or her eyes and look in a mirror; the true unelevated position of the brow is now visible to the patient.

Finally, specific features that will help determine the range of options available for brow rejuvenation are assessed. The position and density of the anterior and temporal (**Figure 4-5**) hairlines will help determine whether a trichophytic or a post-trichial

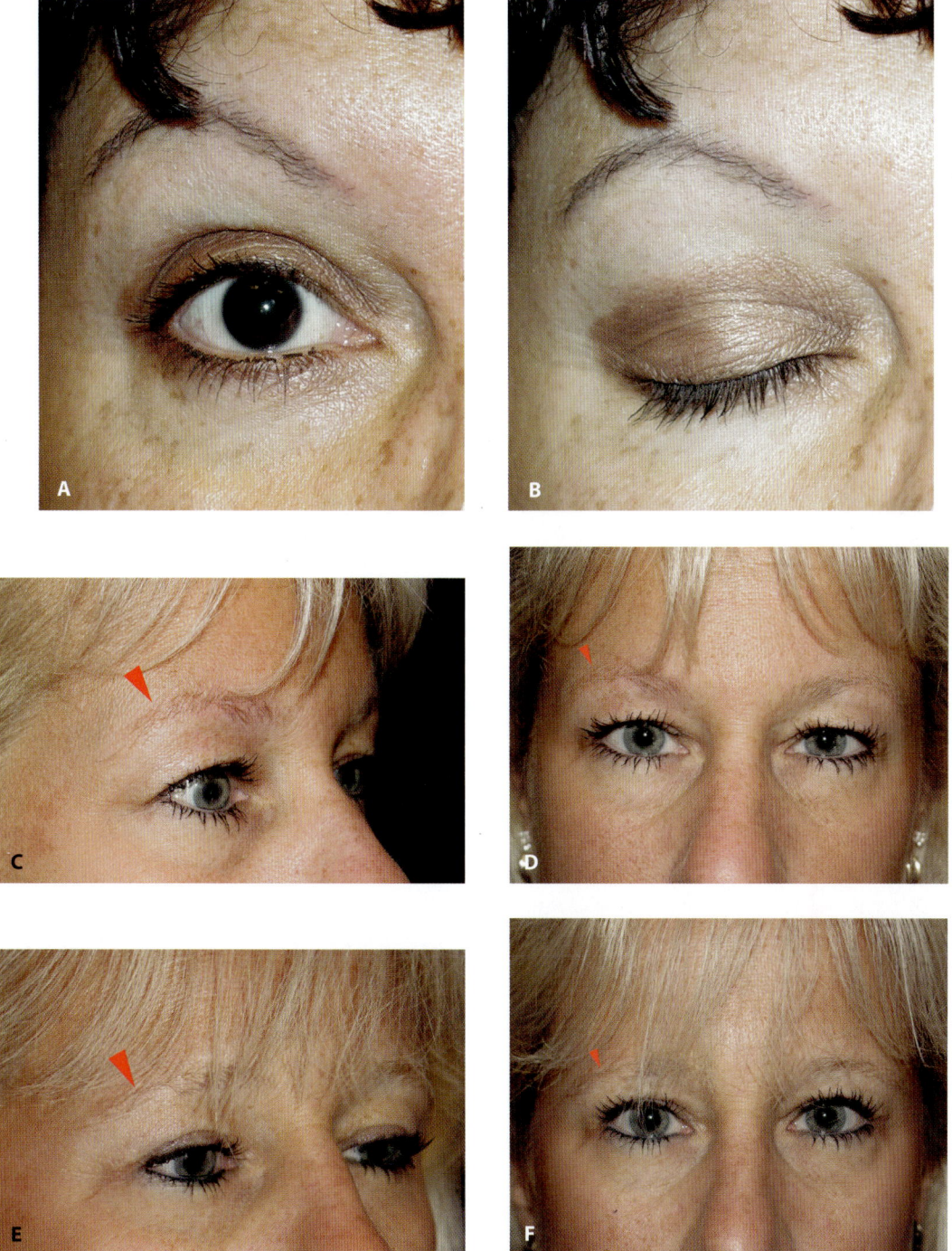

Figure 4-3. Patients are often unaware of the involuntary effect of frontalis contraction on brow position. (A) A patient with a high brow position with eyes open in repose. (B) Eyes closed in repose. Note the drop in the brow arch (relative to the lock of hair). With the brow gently stabilized manually, the patient is asked to slowly open her eyes and view the true, relaxed position of the brow. (C, D) Oblique and frontal views of another patient before upper blepharoplasty. This patient refused concurrent forehead lift. (E, F) Postoperative views of the same patient as in parts C and D. As seen from the oblique views, significant upper lid skin has been excised, but the postoperative result (especially seen on the frontal view) is compromised by failure to treat the brow. Note the lower postoperative position of the brows, obscuring some of the benefit of the blepharoplasty.

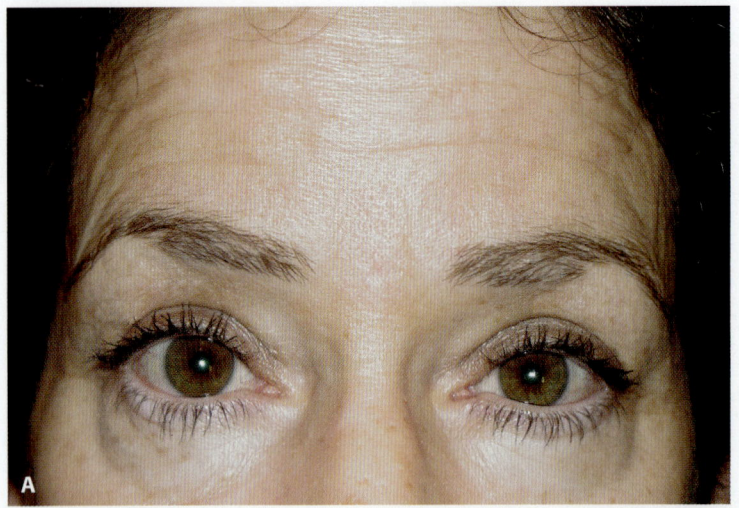

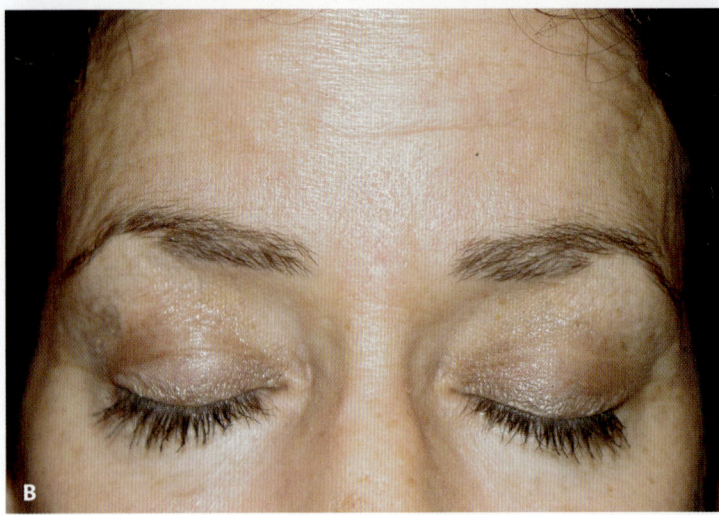

Figure 4-4. Evaluating brow position. (A) At first glance, this patient's brows may seem only slightly ptotic medially. (B) With eyes closed and the frontalis relaxed, note the descent of the brow position, especially temporally. The forehead is visibly smoother as the frontalis relaxes.

incision should be used. The appropriateness of a midforehead incision and the degree of frontalis myoplasty necessary are decided in great part based on the severity of active and resting central forehead rhytids. Glabellar horizontal and oblique rhytids and furrows will contribute to the decision to treat the medial brow depressor muscles.

Preoperative Determination of the Amount of Brow Elevation Necessary

Once the aesthetic needs of the brow have been established, the exact amount of brow elevation needed can be measured. With the patient's eyes closed and the forehead relaxed as described earlier, three marks are made at the superior limit of the brow: over the medial head of the brow, in the midpupillary line, and at the desired brow arch peak. The brow is manually elevated to the desired position, and the patient is asked to open her or his eyes and confirm this brow position as optimal (**Figure 4-6A**). The patient then closes her or his eyes, the point of the marker is held suspended over each mark in turn (**see Figure 4-6B**), and the brow is released and allowed to fully descend. The skin that has now descended under the marker tip in each of the three locations is marked, and the vertical distance between the resting and the elevated brow for each pair of marks is measured and recorded (**see Figure 4-6C**). It is important to consider each brow segment separately, because these three areas of the brow typically require different amounts of elevation.

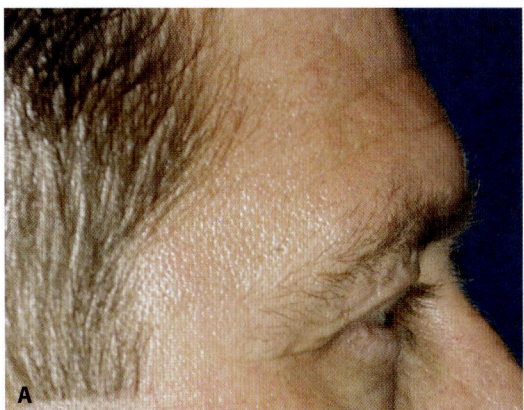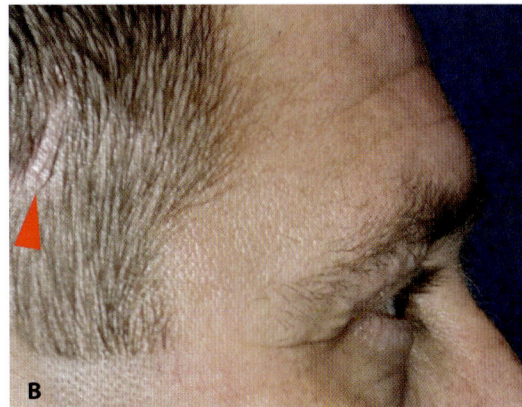

Figure 4-5. Hair density as well as hairline position should be noted and the effects of surgery on the hair should be anticipated. (A) This patient was counseled preoperatively that his thinning and short temporal hair would be insufficient (B) to maximally camouflage the temporal incision *(arrowhead)* of an endoscopic forehead lift.

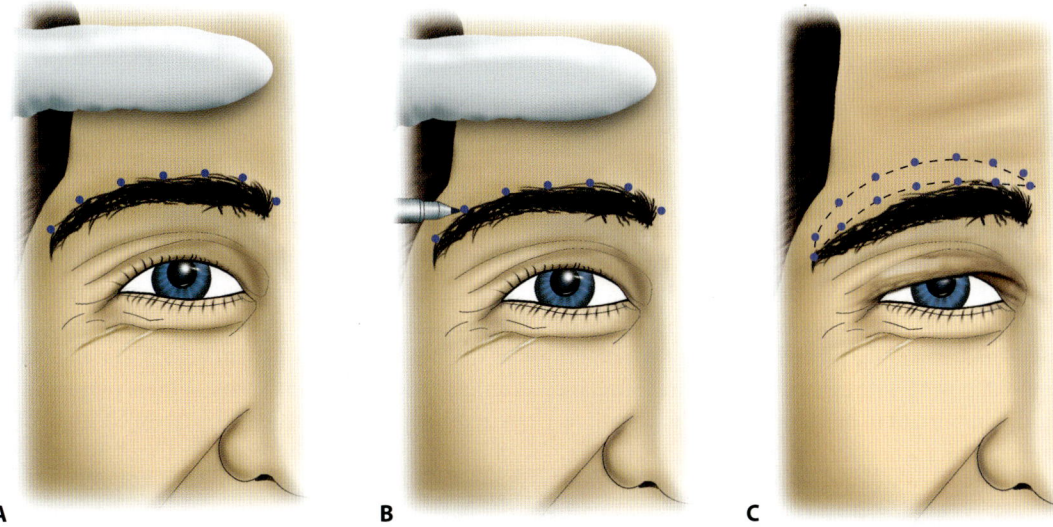

Figure 4-6. Determining the amount of brow elevation needed. (A) With the brow manually elevated to the most aesthetically pleasing position and shape, small dots are inked at the superior border of the brow over the lateral canthus, midpupil, and medial canthus. (B) Still holding the brow in its desired position, the marker is held in turn over each ink mark and the brow is released while the marker is held stationary. The skin that has descended underneath the marker tip is inked. (C) This step is repeated for the other two points, and the distance between the upper and the lower marks is measured as the amount of brow elevation desired in each location. Depending upon the preoperative brow shape and the result desired, measurements may vary significantly between the three sites.

Choosing the Correct Procedure

Once the patient has been evaluated, the surgeon must determine the procedure that best suits his or her aesthetic needs.[2,3,4] By assessing the relative degree of brow ptosis in each brow segment (**Table 4-1**) and the areas of forehead rhytids (**Table 4-2**), a limited list of appropriate procedures can be compiled. This list can be further refined by considering the severity of central forehead rhytids, hair density, and the height of the forehead[4,5] (**Table 4-3**). Ancillary procedures (e.g., upper blepharoplasty) are recommended if necessary (**Figures 4-7 to 4-9**).

The chosen procedure should then be explained in layman's terms to the patient. The brow position-

TABLE 4-1. Procedures for Brow Ptosis

Severity	Medial Brow	Central Brow	Temporal Brow
Mild to moderate	Soft tissue filler	Transpalpebral browpexy	Transpalpebral browpexy
	Botulinum toxin A	Soft tissue filler	Soft tissue filler
	Transpalpebral glabellar myoplasty	Botulinum toxin A	Botulinum toxin A
		Brow suture suspension	Brow suture suspension
Moderate to severe	Midforehead lift	Direct browlift	Direct browlift
	Coronal forehead lift	Midforehead lift	Coronal forehead lift
	Coronal forehead lift—trichophytic	Coronal forehead lift	Coronal forehead lift—trichophytic
	Endoscopic forehead lift	Coronal forehead lift—trichophytic	Endoscopic forehead lift
	Endoscopic forehead lift—trichophytic	Endoscopic forehead lift	Endoscopic forehead lift—trichophytic
		Endoscopic forehead lift—trichophytic	Transtemporal browlift
			Transtemporal browlift

ing sought should be demonstrated on the patient, who views this in a mirror, and this degree of improvement is agreed upon by the physician and the patient as an ideal goal. The basic surgical steps, risks, associated sequelae, and anticipated recovery period should be discussed.

The surgeon should answer all of the patient's questions about the procedure, and the patient should demonstrate a reasonable understanding. These questions will range from the obvious (e.g., length and risks of the procedure, type of anesthesia required, postoperative pain) to the more mundane but still important to the patient (how long until resumption of normal activities is allowed, when the patient can comfortably socialize [with and without cosmetics], and when healing is complete and improvement is maximal).

Surgical Coordination

Once the patient's questions have been answered, she or he again meets with the patient care coordinator. The patient care coordinator should be familiar with each technique, as well as the preoperative preparation and postoperative care of each procedure. The patient is provided with a breakdown of costs, including the surgeon's fee and facility and anesthesia costs. General availability of surgical time is discussed with the patient, as are any time constraints the patient may have. Unless prevented by circumstances, the patient is scheduled for a brief follow-up consultation between 1 and 3 weeks before consultation.

Before this second consultation, the patient is sent his or her preoperative packet. Included in

TABLE 4-2. Procedures for Forehead Rhytids

Glabella	Central Forehead	Lateral Hooding
Midforehead lift	Midforehead lift	Direct browlift
Coronal forehead lift	Coronal forehead lift	Coronal forehead lift
Coronal forehead lift—trichophytic	Coronal forehead lift—trichophytic	Coronal forehead lift—trichophytic
Endoscopic forehead lift	Endoscopic forehead lift	Endoscopic forehead lift
Endoscopic forehead lift—trichophytic	Endoscopic forehead lift—trichophytic	Endoscopic forehead lift—trichophytic
Transpalpebral glabellar myoplasty	Botulinum toxin A	Transpalpebral browpexy
Botulinum toxin A	Soft tissue filler	Transtemporal browlift
Soft tissue filler		Botulinum toxin A

TABLE 4-3. Special Circumstances for Forehead Procedures

	Avoid	*Consider*
Thinning hair	Coronal forehead lift	Coronal forehead lift—trichophytic
High/receding hairline (brow-hairline distance > 6 cm)	Coronal forehead lift	Coronal forehead lift—trichophytic
	Endoscopic forehead lift	Endoscopic forehead lift—trichophytic
Deep forehead rhytids		Midforehead lift
		Subcutaneous coronal forehead lift
Thick eyebrows		Direct browlift
Smoker	Subcutaneous coronal forehead lift	

this are a confirmed date of surgery, a summary of costs and deadlines for payment, and a date for the first postoperative visit. In addition, patients are provided with a procedure-specific, detailed surgical consent that, along with any surgical facility consents, should be signed and brought to the follow-up consult. This ensures that any questions the patient may have regarding finances can be addressed directly by the staff and any concerns about the procedure itself can be discussed with the physician. Also included in this mailing is a request for a general medical examination and all appropriate laboratory testing, as well as a list of over-the-counter (**Table 4-4**), and homeopathic medi-

cations[6] (**Table 4-4**) to avoid because these can have significant adverse effects in the perioperative period (**Table 4-5**). Patients without a history of cardiac or hepatic disease or bleeding disorders and who are not on anticoagulants are advised (but not required) to begin the use of *Arnica Montana* and bromelain 7 to 10 days before surgery (**Table 4-6**), because these may help minimize postoperative. bruising and swelling; these medications are continued for 10 days postoperatively. Patients undergoing any surgery involving the eyelids, either as a surgical approach or for blepharoplasty, should be considered for a routine general ophthalmologic evaluation preoperatively.

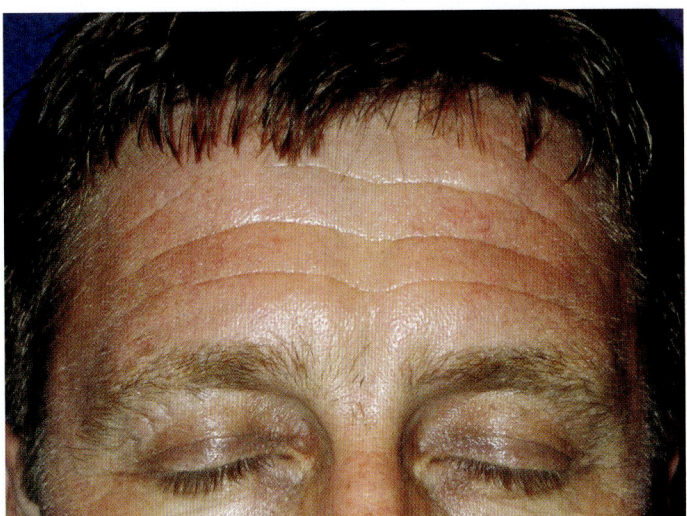
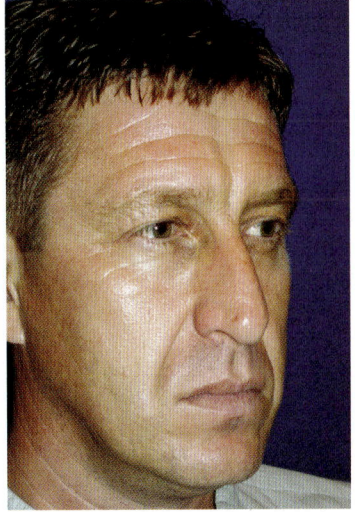

Figure 4-7. Male nonsmoker with moderately severe brow ptosis (medial, central, and temporal brow), moderately severe central forehead, and moderate glabellar rhytids with a borderline high forehead and thinning hair temporally and right brow scarring. Based on these criteria, the patient would be a candidate for a midforehead lift or an endoscopic forehead lift (possibly with a trichophytic incision). The patient refused the midforehead lift scar and opted for the endoscopic forehead lift, understanding that the temporal scar may be visible.

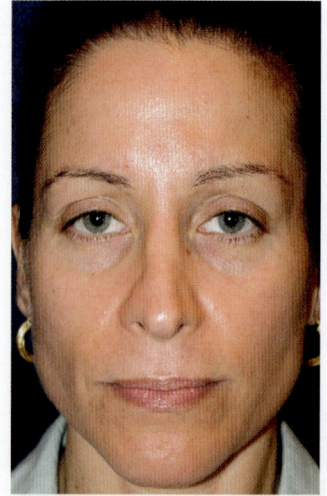
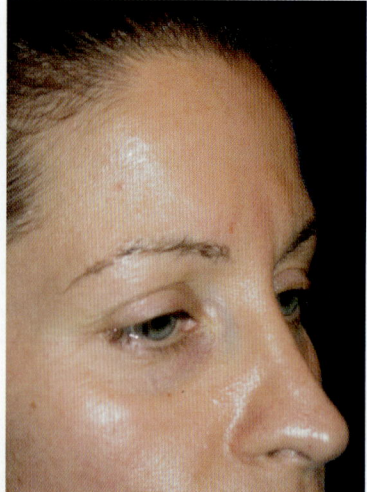
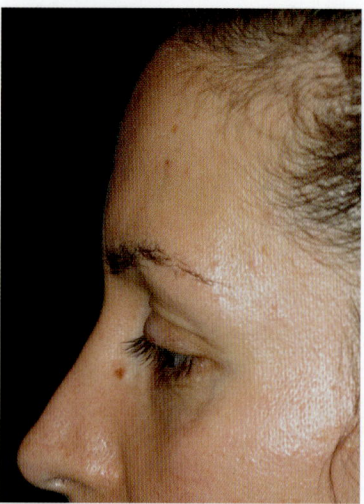

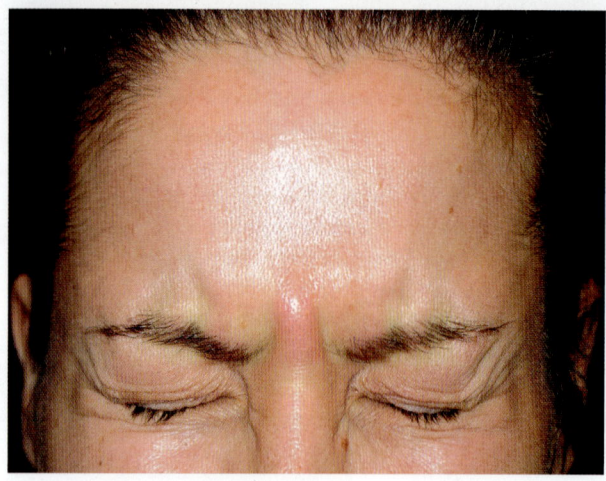

Figure 4-8. Young woman with moderate medial, mild central, and slight temporal brow ptosis, with significant glabellar muscular activity. Options for this patient would include soft tissue fillers, botulinum toxin A (BTX-A) treatment or transpalpebral glabellar myoplasty and transpalpebral browpexy. This patient ultimately opted for BTX-A only.

Follow-up Consultation

The follow-up consultation with the physician can be brief, typically lasting no more than 15 to 20 minutes. This allows the surgeon to review the salient features of the procedure and key postoperative instructions with the patient, as well as to directly address any patient concerns specifically related to the procedure itself. If not already done, the amount of elevation of each brow segment is measured and recorded. If the brow procedure chosen is based on reduction of depressor muscle tone, glabellar muscles can be treated with botulinum toxin A; if myotomy of the brow depressors is not entirely complete (by design or by accident), the botulinum will ensure elimination of depressor activity for 8 to 12 weeks, by which time, wound healing at the elevated position should be relatively complete. Finally, if not done already, preoperative photographs specific to the procedure are taken.

Photography

Pre- and postoperative photographs benefit the surgeon and the patient in ways besides standard documentation of the change in appearance. Preoperative photographs are used to demonstrate the initial pathology to patients (including brow ptosis, rhytids, scars, bleparoptosis, blepharochalasis, and preexisting asymmetries). In cases of extreme brow ptosis, third-party insurers may provide benefits after a review of the preoperative photographs and visual field obstruction documented by visual field testing. The surgeon will review these photographs in planning surgery and should always review pre- and postoperative photographs of each patient to continually refine her or his technique and to seek ways to improve this technique. Postoperatively, patients who question the efficacy of their procedure can be demonstrated the desired but often subtle changes by contrasting pre- and postoperative photographs.

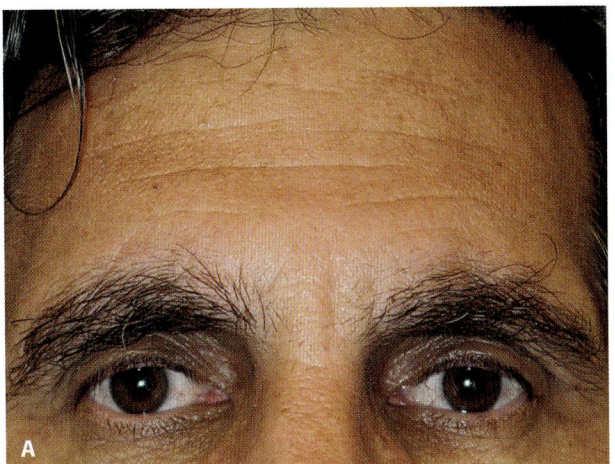

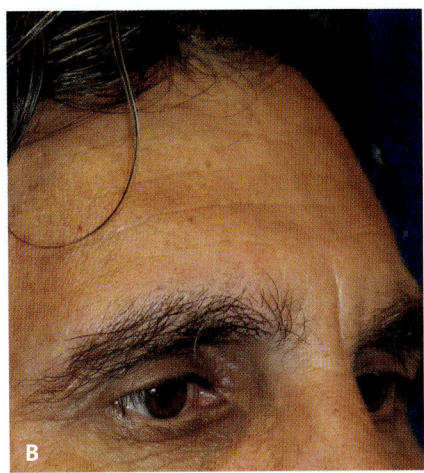

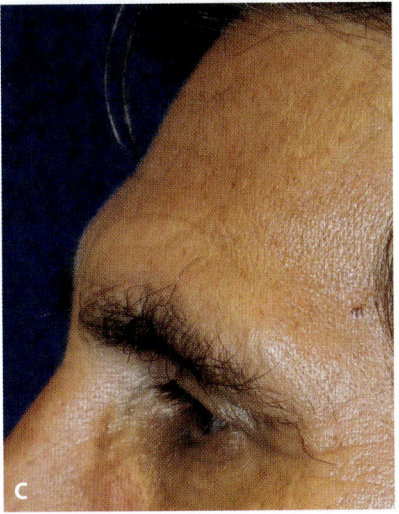

Figure 4-9. Male patient with posteriorly sloped forehead, dense hair, significant frontal ridge, and moderately severe medial and central and severe lateral brow ptosis. There are only mild central forehead rhytids. The best option for this patient would be an endoscopic or coronal forehead lift, especially if frontal bone osteoplasty is considered.

The question of "film versus digital" photography has been rendered somewhat irrelevant by the improvement in the sensors and optics of digital cameras. Relatively inexpensive digital cameras with resolutions of greater than 6 megapixels and reasonable optics are now available, and with some care to camera settings and lighting options, excellent photographs can be obtained easily, with significantly fewer storage issues than with 35-mm slides.

Lighting ideally consists of a camera-mounted master flash with overhead and side hard-wired "slave" flash units (**Figure 4-10**). These additional flashes help eliminate harsh shadows from a single illumination unit. Traditionally, a ceiling-mounted

TABLE 4-4.	Patients Using Any of the Following Should Notify the Physician Immediately
Type of Medication	*Examples*
NSAIDs	Advil, Alleve, Ansaid, Ibuprofen, Motrin
Aspirin, aspirin-containing preparations	Anacin, ASA, Ascriptin (any), Aspergum, Bayer (any), Bufferin, Ecotrin, Goody's pills, St. Joseph's
Ephedrine/pseudoephedrine	Dristan, Sine-Aid
Caffeine-containing preparations	Goody's pills, Sinutab, Sine-Aid, Midol

NSAIDs = nonsteroidal anti-inflammatory drugs.

TABLE 4-5.   Significant Effects of Homeopathic Medications

Name(s)	Effects
Ephedra (Ma Huang)	Stimulant; can induce seizures; can cause hypercoagulable state, myocardia infarction, arrhythmias, hypertension; can interact with anesthetic gases and cause hypotension.
Echinacea	Can cause immunosuppression, potentiate toxicity of barbiturates.
Omega-3 fatty acids (fish oils) (>3 g/day)	May increase surgical bleeding.
Garlic	Inhibits platelet aggregation and may prolong bleeding.
Ginger	Inhibits thromboxane synthetase and can cause prolonged bleeding, hyperglycemia.
Ginko biloba	Decreases seizure threshold and efficacy of anticonvulsants; inhibits thromboxane synthetase; can cause prolonged bleeding; can interact with barbiturates and cause prolonged sedation.
Ginseng	Inhibits platelet aggregation and may prolong bleeding; can cause tachycardia and hypertension.
Licorice	Inhibits platelet aggregation and may prolong bleeding; can cause hypertension and tachycardia.
St. John's wort	Can prolong postoperative sedation; long-term use has been associated with cardio-vascular collapse on induction of general anesthesia.
Vitamin E (>400 mg/day)	Inhibits platelet aggregation; antagonizes vitamin K–dependent clotting factors; may prolong bleeding.

TABLE 4-6.   Precautions for Prescribing/Allowing Use of Arnica Montana and Bromelain

Name	Dosage	Possible Adverse Effects	Avoid in Patients
Arnica Montana (wolf's bane)	30C, 5 pellets SL qid	Hypertension, cardiotoxicity	With hypertension, coronary artery disease, liver disease; taking anticoagulants; bleeding disorders
Bromelain (extract of pineapple core)	500 mg qid	Tachycardia; may enhance effects of anticoagulants	Taking anticoagulants; with bleeding disorders

SL = sublingually

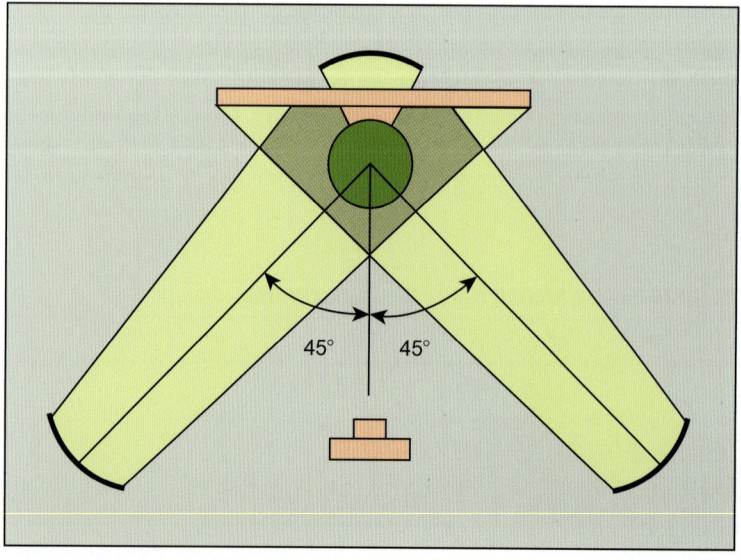

Figure 4-10. Overhead and side flashes (positioned 45° off center) help eliminate harsh shadows.

overhead slave flash and large umbrella flashes are used for this purpose, but smaller, infrared controlled slave units (e.g., Nikon Wireless Speedlight Systems, Nikon Corp., Tokyo, Japan) make such a system more compact and portable. Less preferably, positioning the patient directly below a strong overhead incandescent light, in front of a darker background (royal blue), and adding a light diffuser over the camera-mounted flash can reduce (not eliminate) shadowing. Above all, consistency of focal length, framing, lighting, and exposure is the most important step in obtaining valuable patient photographs.

By the end of the follow-up consult, the surgeon will have met with the patient twice and have had the opportunity to discuss each patient at least once with the patient care coordinator. Input should be solicited from all staff; patients often are on their "best behavior" with the physician and may act differently with or provide additional information to the staff. Support personnel can often provide valuable insight into a patient's motivation for surgery, and this information should be used in deciding whether the patient is an appropriate surgical candidate. By the end of the follow-up consultation, the surgeon should be comfortable that the patient is seeking surgery for the appropriate reasons, has reasonable and realistic expectations/goals, and fully understands the risks involved and the healing process. The patient should be able to articulate appropriate personal motivations and the results he or she desires; he or she should also comprehend and accept his or her responsibilities in the postoperative process and understand the recovery period required. If any of these standards is not met, it is essential that the surgeon address these issues more specifically with the patient preoperatively. Although the author does not use preoperative psychiatric screening tests routinely, patients who seem to be distressed by a physical feature out of proportion to its actual severity, believe surgery will make substantial improvements in interpersonal relations or who are unwilling or unable to agree to reasonable surgical goals may not be appropriate candidates for surgery. Consideration should be given to referring these patients for a formal psychiatric evaluation before agreeing to operate on them. Conversely, patients with well-managed (with or without medications) psychiatric disorders can be considered for surgery once cleared by their therapists. The treating mental health professional should always be made aware of the plan for sur-gery, because postoperative dysphoria may lead to transient but significant depression even in patients without preoperative psychiatric illness.

The Surgeon's Preparation

At the conclusion of the consultation, the surgeon should have mentally performed the procedure she or he is recommending and an impression of realistically achievable changes generated. Upon reviewing the patient's photographs in the next 2 to 3 days, this cognitive exercise should be repeated, and the potential complications and expected results anticipated; this is done again on the night before surgery. By the morning of surgery, the surgeon has mentally performed the exact procedure on that particular patient at least three times and is well prepared to perform it manually in the operating room. At each postoperative visit, the key points of the procedure are again mentally reviewed, allowing the physician to correlate these with the postoperative results and any possible complications. This exercise (and habit) keeps the surgeon "in the moment" at every encounter with the patient and helps in preparing for the surgery and critically evaluating results.

Choice of Anesthesia Methods

The choice of anesthetic method depends upon the needs of the patient and the surgeon. Most forehead and brow procedures could be performed comfortably under local anesthesia, but most patients and surgeons alike would benefit from at least some degree of mild anxiolysis for the patient. The anesthetic technique chosen should take into account the patient's anxiety about the procedure. The fear of pain and discomfort, awareness of mass tissue movements and general operating room processes may be severe enough to warrant general anesthesia; conversely, an informed and motivated patient may opt for intravenous sedation and faster recovery from a lighter anesthetic plane. Above all, the experience of the surgery, if not pleasant, should at least be nonthreatening, comfortable, and safe in the patient's mind. Few patients, even with the most outstanding surgical results, who have unpleasant anesthetic or operative experiences will willingly return to the surgeon for any treatment at a later date. As with all elements of the surgical process, ultimately all responsibility devolves to the surgeon.

Regardless of the systemic anesthetic technique chosen, patients benefit from competently performed locoregional anesthesia. The benefits to the sedated patient are obvious, but also patients under general anesthesia require less intravenous narcotics when local infiltration and regional nerve blocks are used adequately. Regional nerve blockade of the forehead can be accomplished with a few simple injections.[7] Chief among these are the supratrochlear and supraorbital nerve blocks. These two blocks (**Figure 4-11AB**) can provide anesthesia of the forehead from the midline to the temporal crest, from the brow to the crown. These nerves can be blocked with a single needlestick on each side. A 1½-inch 25-gauge needle is inserted through the skin and down to the orbital rim at the medial extent of the brow; the needle is then turned laterally and advanced along the inferior edge of the supraorbital rim to the midpupillary line. Approximately 2 mL of local anesthetic is then injected on needle withdrawal, focusing in particular at the midpupillary line and an area about 7 to 10 mm medial to that point. Anesthesia of the central forehead ensues rapidly, allowing painless, direct local infiltration of this area.

Posteriorly, the branches of the occipital nerves can be blocked with a subcutaneous infiltration of anesthetic at the far reaches of the supraorbital nerve distribution near the crown, because most forehead procedures rarely extend farther posteriorly. Laterally, the zygomaticotemporal nerve can be blocked by sliding a 1½-inch 25-gauge needle along the orbital wall just behind the lateral orbital rim to the level of the lateral canthus (**see Figure 4-11C**) and instilling 1 to 2 mL of anesthetic. By blocking the zygomaticotemporal nerve at its exit from the orbit, a fan-shaped area extending from the medial zygomatic arch posterosuperiorly to the temporal crest can be anesthetized. The auriculotemporal nerve can be blocked by infiltrating 2 to 3 mL of local anesthetic subcutaneously in a horizontal line just above the top of the helix. Once these basic nerve blocks are performed, the enclosed areas of forehead and temple can be further anesthetized using a more dilute solution (0.25–0.50% xylocaine with 1:400,000- 1:200,000 epinephrine) for hemostasis and additional anesthesia. By exercising particular attention to locoregional anesthesia, systemic analgesic dosages can be reduced and anesthetic recovery time shortened.

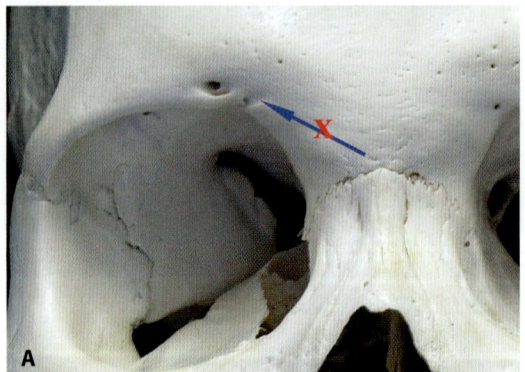

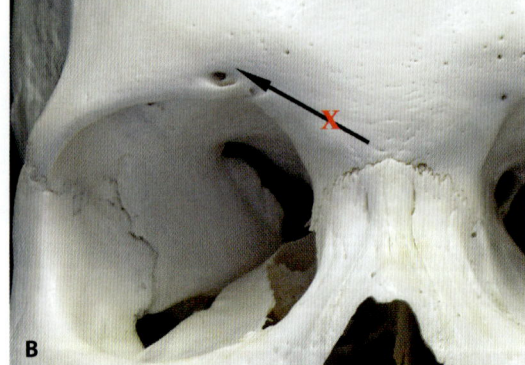

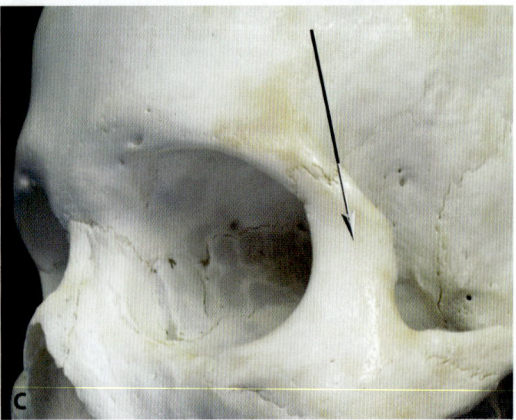

Figure 4-11. (A, B) Supratrochlear and supraorbital nerve blocks can be performed with a single needlestick using a $1^1/_2$-inch 25- or 27-gauge needle. The skin is entered *(red X)* just medial to the medial end of the brow and advanced down to the orbital rim, stopping just lateral to the midpupil. Anesthetic is then injected, focusing on the midpupillary line and a point approximately 7 to 10 mm medial to that point. (C) Blockade of the zygomaticotemporal nerve is performed by advancing a 25- or 27-gauge needle just behind the lateral orbital rim and infiltrating 1 to 2 mL of anesthetic at the level of the lateral canthus.

Conclusion

It bears frequent repetition that the ultimate responsibility rests entirely with the surgeon for guiding the patient through the entire operative experience. As "captain of the ship," the surgeon should periodically examine and evaluate each step of the process from both the patient's and the professional's perspective. All elements should flow smoothly and all physician team members should work together in a coordinated way. Processes and procedures should be designed to integrate well and afford a certain level of redundancy. Multiple steps should be included in the process to assess for key features and findings and enable the surgeon to provide the best care in the safest manner; key elements of the experience should be reiterated to the patient to ensure a complete understanding and full cooperation. Frequent sampling and interviewing of postoperative patients will allow the surgeon to fully assess his or her practice's procedures and permit him or her to continue to refine and improve his or her patients' experiences.

We delight in the beauty of the butterfly, but rarely admit the changes it has gone through to achieve that beauty.

Maya Angelou (1928)

Suggested Readings

1. Troilius C. A comparison between subgaleal and subperiosteal brow lifts. Plast Reconstr Surg 1999;104: 1079–1090A.
2. Withey S, Witherow H, Waterhouse N. One hundred cases of endoscopic brow lift. Br J Plast Surg 2002; 55:20–24.
3. Holcolmb JD, McCollough EG. Trichophytic incisional approaches to upper facial rejuvenation. Arch Facial Plast Surg 2001;3:48–53.
4. Matarasso A, Hutchinson OHZ. Evaluating rejuvenation of the forehead and brow: an algorithm for selecting the appropriate technique. Plast Reconstr Surg 2000;106:687–694.
5. Flowers RS, Caputy GG, Flowers SS. The biomechanics of brow and frontalis function and its effect on blepharoplasty. Clin Plast Surg 1993;20:255–268.
6. Broughton G, Crosby MA, Coleman J, Rohrich RJ. Use of herbal supplements and vitamins in plastic surgery: a practical review. Plast Reconstr Surg 2007;119:48e–66e.
7. Zide BM, Swift R. How to block and tackle the face. Plast Reconstr Surg 1998;101:840–851.

5

DIRECT BROWLIFT

The face is the mirror of the mind, and eyes without speaking confess the secrets of the heart.

Saint Jerome (AD 374–419)

Introduction

The direct browlift is, as the name implies, the most "direct" method to lift the eyebrow. Essentially a skin excision procedure (with modifications), the direct browlift alters brow position in a fairly direct relation to the amount of skin excised. Other forehead features, such as transverse forehead or horizontal or oblique glabellar rhytids, are not well treated with the direct brow lift. Conversely, the direct browlift is a simple, rapid, and easily performed procedure with a rapid recovery that, in carefully selected and managed patients, can yield exceptional results.

History

As with facelifting in the lower face, early forehead procedures were geared toward skin excision in remote areas designed to maximize scar camouflage. C. C. Miller (1924) described 10 patterns of hair-bearing scalp excision; the particular pattern chosen was based upon the paternal of upper forehead rhytids, lateral eyelid hooding, and the ideal vector for redraping of redundant and ptotic forehead and temple skin. Whereas Noel (1926), Joseph (1931), and Lexer (1931) all advocated excisions in the hair-bearing scalp, Passot first described the basic elements of the modern direct browlift in 1930. Unfortunately, the obvious scars dampened early enthusiasm for the direct browlift, and even Passot described an excision of hair-bearing scalp (performed with neurotomy of the temporal branch of the facial nerve) in 1933. Conversely, in carefully

selected patients, the direct browlift may be the most appropriate technique in brow management, even in the era of highly specific and reliable minimal incision techniques.

Rationale and Scientific Basis

The direct browlift specifically addresses the position of the eyebrow by resection of skin. The elliptical skin excision directly above the brow allows the surgeon to advance the hair-bearing brow skin superiorly, raising the brow position. In addition,

---

Direct Browlift

Indications: moderate to severe central and lateral brow ptosis; unilateral brow paralysis.
Contraindications: thin eyebrows; moderate to severe medial brow ptosis; history of poor wound healing and hypertrophic or keloid scars; patient unwilling to accept visible scar.
Ideal candidate: thick forehead skin, thick eyebrows, no significant medial brow ptosis.
Scientific basis: mechanical brow elevation by skin excision and suspension sutures.

Direct Browlift

Incisions: direct suprabrow.
Tissue modifications: skin excision.
Fixation: orbicularis-frontalis suspension sutures.
Wound closure: two-layer closure.
Complications: hematoma, neuralgias, paresthesias.

the upper fibers of the orbicularis are plicated superiorly to the frontalis muscle, aiding in the elevation of the brow. The brow is allowed to move superiorly, taking advantage of the mobility of the submuscular galeal glide plane. This plication also "unfurls" the upper orbicularis, reducing the depressor effect of its contraction. This procedure does not directly address forehead or glabellar rhytids,[1] but there is usually some improvement in transverse forehead rhytids, because full contraction of the frontalis muscle is no longer needed to raise the brow to a position that does not obstruct vision.

Advantages, Disadvantages, and Alternatives

The direct browlift is a quick and easily performed procedure that can be performed in the office with the patient under local anesthesia. This makes the procedure available to patients who are not candidates for or will not consent to more invasive procedures or deeper planes of anesthesia. Conversely, additional anxiolysis can supplement the local anesthesia for maximum comfort and, although not necessary, can be used for direct browlifting procedures. Positioning of the brow can be quite accurate; there is a nearly 1:1 relationship of skin excised–to–brow elevation,[2] because skin excision and not (the somewhat less direct and predictable) muscle modification is the primary modality of brow elevation. Described by Flowers and coworkers,[3] the direct browlift takes advantage of the "elastic band principle," whereby the elevation of the brow is maximized by proximity of the point of vertical pull; no other browlifting procedure has a point of elevation closer to the brow than does the direct browlift.[4]

Because the direct browlift is essentially a cutaneous procedure, the risk to the supraorbital, supratrochlear, and temporal branches of the facial nerve is minimized; subcutaneous dissection is fairly limited, with a low risk of hematoma formation. Recovery is fairly quick, typically allowing the patient to return to normal activities in 3 to 5 days.

Although infrequently performed today, the direct browlift is still a useful technique in selected patients. Patients with permanent unilateral facial paralysis (particularly those who are poor candidates for sedation or general anesthesia) are excellent candidates for the direct browlift. Patients with thick, bushy eyebrows, thick skin, and deep forehead rhytids also are preferred candidates for the direct browlift. Bald patients cannot benefit from any distant approach to the brows because there is no hair to camouflage the scars; in which case, the direct browlift is a relatively acceptable option.

The obvious disadvantage of the direct browlift is the visible scar above the brow, as well as to loss of a feathered superior brow margin. These are changes the patient and surgeon must acknowledge and be willing to accept. Both the patient and the physician must also acknowledge that the direct browlift is limited in its ability to elevate the medial brow[5] and does fairly little to alleviate transverse forehead rhytids and little to improve glabellar lines and furrows.

Alternatives to the direct browlift obviously include most other forehead and browlift procedures, but these are generally associated with larger incisions, more dissection, a steeper learning curve, more specifically designed instrumentation, and longer recovery times. Transtemporal or transblepharoplasty approaches have similarly small (but better camouflaged) scars and are likewise suitable for predominantly central and lateral brow elevation. However, the reproducibility and direct relationship of surgical excision of tissue to brow elevation are significantly better with the direct browlift.

Indications and Contraindication

The direct browlift is indicated for cases of moderate to severe central and lateral brow ptosis, especially in patients with thick, bushy eyebrows and thick skin (**Figure 5-1**). The direct browlift is most commonly used for treatment of unilateral brow paralysis and ptosis, but can be used for cosmetic reasons, and is especially helpful in cases of severe brow asymmetry.

The direct browlift is absolutely contraindicated in patients unwilling to accept a visible scar. Thin eyebrows or severe medial brow ptosis are also contraindications to the direct browlift, as is a history of poor wound healing or hypertrophic or keloid scars.

Range of Anesthesia

As mentioned earlier, the direct browlift can be easily performed under local anesthesia. After all incisions are planned and marked on the forehead, a solution of 1% xylocaine with 1:200,000 epinephrine can be injected under the medial two thirds of the brow from medial to lateral, blocking the supratrochlear and supraorbital nerves with a single needle skin penetration. Lesser amounts of the anesthetic

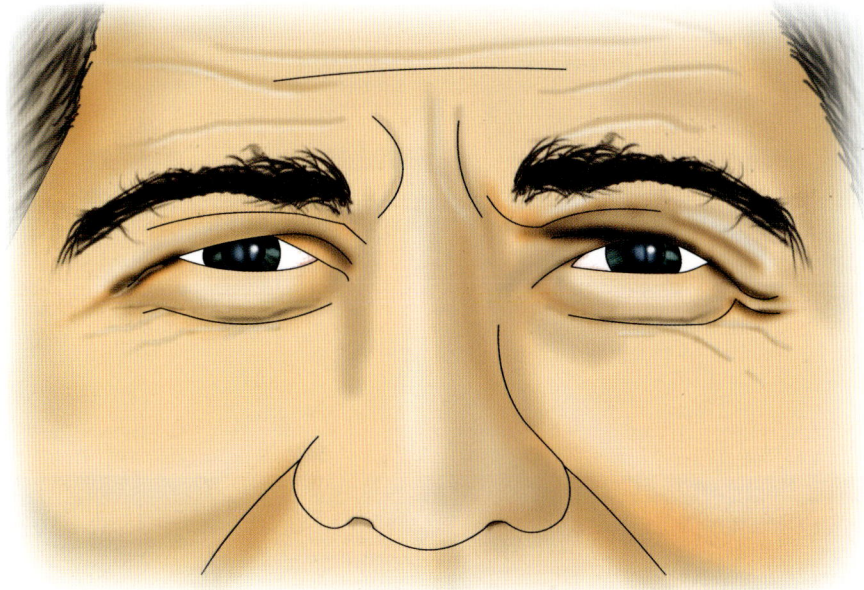

Figure 5-1. The ideal patient for direct browlift has thick, bushy eyebrows, thick skin, and deep forehead creases.

are also injected subcutaneously under the planned skin excision outlined on the skin, carefully avoiding tissue distortion. With proper gentle technique, local anesthesia alone can suffice for a direct browlift and allows the surgeon to most easily sit the patient upright during the procedure to assess adequacy of brow elevation and symmetry. Alternatively, intravenous sedation or general anesthesia can be used in the medically stable, apprehensive patient, but it should be recognized that local anesthesia alone can provide sufficient analgesia during a direct browlift.

Equipment

No specialized equipment is needed for the direct browlift. Fine-toothed forceps, skin hooks, and a #15 blade are used for the majority of the procedure. Excellent hemostasis is paramount and ideally is provided with an ophthalmic-size bipolar cautery, although judicious use of a monopolar cautery with a fine-needle tip is also acceptable.

Operating Room Setup

As with any forehead or brow procedure, complete and unhindered access to the entire head is essential. The patient's face is prepared into the field and the head is draped. A Mayo stand with the essen-

tial instruments should be positioned off the side of the head, close enough to provide easy access to all instruments but still allow the surgeon to approach the forehead and brow from the sides as well as above. The surgeon generally is seated above the patient's head but needs frequent access to the side of the patient's head to assess brow contour and position.

Incisions

The incisions are planned and mapped before any infiltration of local anesthetic solution. The patient is placed in a seated upright position, the surgeon positions the patient's head in a Frankfort horizontal position, and the patient is asked to maintain a neutral gaze. The lower margin of the crescentic skin excision is marked along the highest row of brow hair follicles. These hairs are typically directed downward in the lateral three quarters of the brow; more medially, the hairs extend more superolaterally and superiorly. This row is usually fairly well defined, although medially and laterally, the upper brow border becomes less distinct; the surgeon should choose the most superior contiguous row of hairs as the lower margin of the skin excision. The lateral extent of the incision stops at the end of the dense brow hairs, whereas medially, the incision ends

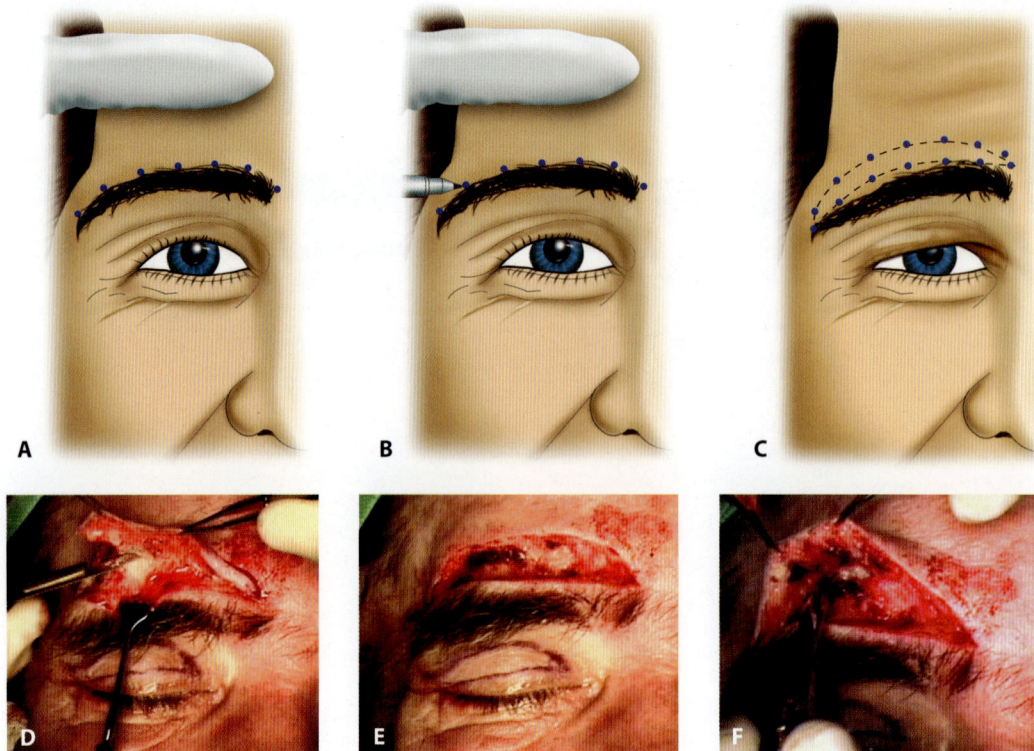

Figure 5-2. (A) Preoperative marking for the direct browlift. The brow is marked along its superior border, with particular attention paid to the brow directly above the lateral and medial canthi and the midpupil. (B) The brow is manually elevated to the appropriate height, and the pen is held over each mark in turn. (C) After the brow is released, the skin that has descended below the point of the pen is marked, outlining the upper border of the required skin resection. (D) The ellipse is then carefully excised, with dissection just above the orbicularis oculi and frontalis muscles. (E) Excision of the skin ellipse is performed more superficially at the medial end of the brow to maximally preserve branches of the supraorbital and supratrochlear nerves. (F) The superior edge of skin is undermined approximately 10 mm to better expose the frontalis muscle.

just lateral to the medial end of the brow clubhead (**Figure 5-2A**). Once this is marked, the brow is elevated with the nondominant hand (palm flat on the upper forehead and the thumb elevating brow skin just above the brow margin marking). With the brow held at the desired height and shape, the marking pen is placed directly over the first line and the brow elevation released; a skin marking is now placed on the forehead skin under the pen (**see Figure 5-2B**). This is repeated at multiple points along the length of the brow, marking the new desired upper brow border and completing the design of the crescentic skin excision (**see Figure 5-2C**). When both sides are marked, symmetry of the planned result is assessed by manually elevating both brows simultaneously. Skin excisions may differ from side to side if there is preoperative brow asymmetry.

Plane of Dissection

The marked skin crescent is incised with a #15 blade (**see Figure 5-2D**). Laterally, the dissection is taken down through skin and subcutaneous fat until fibers of the orbicularis oculi and frontalis muscles are seen; medially, the incision penetrates to subcutaneous fat. Near the brow tail, the deeper plane is safe, because the deep division of the supraorbital nerve is deep to the deep galeal fascia, and the skin excision is inferior to the temporal branches of the facial nerve. Dissection should become more superficial more medially in order to protect the branches of the superficial division of the supraorbital and the supratrochlear nerves, as they run over the frontalis muscle, thereby reducing the risk of postoperative sensory disturbance[6] (**see Figure 5-2E**). This limits the exposure of the brow depressor muscles, so that adequate myoplasty is difficult to impossible with the direct browlift. Bames[7] did describe corrugator and procerus removal with this approach, but because of the anticipated significant sensory morbidity, this is not recommended. The superior edge of the excision is undermined approximately 10 mm in a pre–frontalis muscle plane to allow for superior fixation and tissue edge eversion (**see Figure 5-2F**). Meticulous hemostasis should be ensured while avoiding excessive cautery.

Tissue Modifications

The lateral and mid frontalis and orbicularis muscles are now evident at the base of the wound (**Figure 5-3A**). Inferiorly, the fibers of the orbicularis can be seen intermingling with the deep surface of the dermis. Multiple 3-0 braided polyester sutures (Mersilene, Ethicon, Inc., Piscataway, NJ) or other permanent sutures are placed in this confluence, and a horizontal mattress suture is placed into the frontalis muscle (if possible, the more medial sutures also penetrate the frontalis and grab the postmuscular fascia and the periosteum) (**see Figure 5-3B**, **C**) under the superior wound edge (**Figure 5-4**). This advancement should bring the skin edges together neatly. Multiple mattress sutures are placed to maintain this elevation. The suture ends are clamped until all sutures are placed and then are tied sequentially from medial to lateral. Again, the wound is inspected, and once again, exquisite hemostasis is ensured with the cautery because no drain will be placed.

In 1957, Bames[7] described additionally dissecting in the subcutaneous plane superiorly to the hairline, resecting corrugator muscle and avulsing procerus muscle through this suprabrow approach. However, this substantially increases the risk of hematoma, skin slough (particularly in smokers), and forehead sensory disturbances. Also, exposure of the corrugator and procerus muscles is limited through this approach and is generally not recommended.

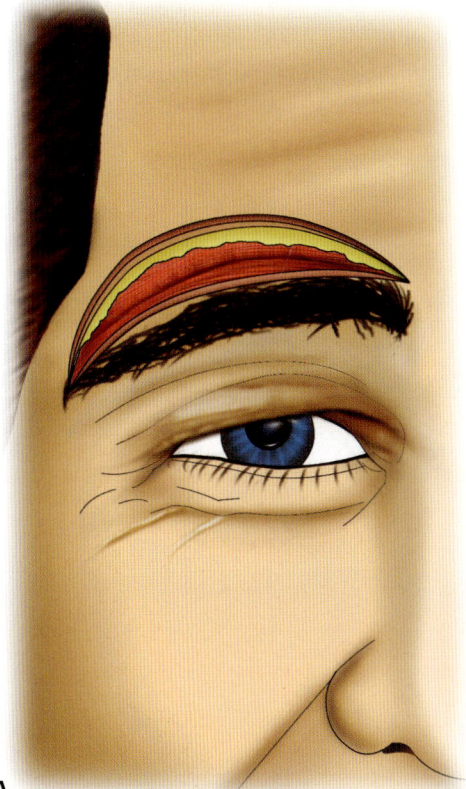
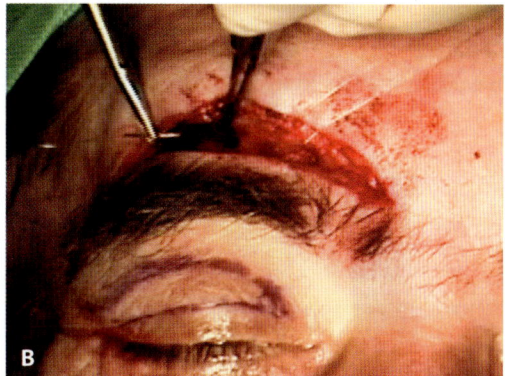
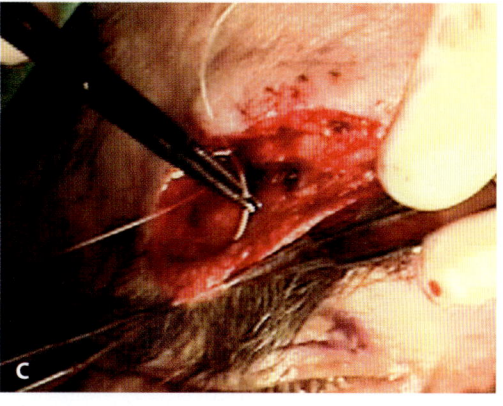

Figure 5-3. (A) Circular fibers of the orbicularis oculi muscle (inferiorly) and vertical frontalis muscle (superiorly) can be seen. (B, C) Braided permanent sutures are placed between the frontalis muscle and galea (B) and the dermis and orbicularis oculi muscle (C) inferiorly.

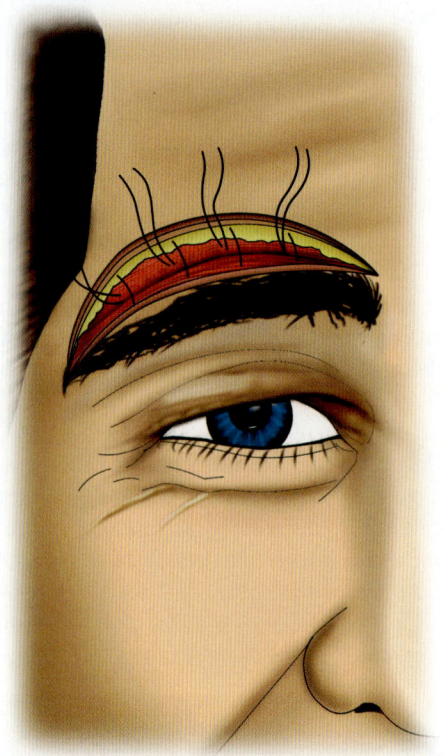

Figure 5-4. Superior sutures are anchored to the frontalis muscle slightly above the superior skin edge.

Wound Closure

Alignment of the skin edges should be fairly well done by the placement of the muscle plication sutures. The skin edges are then closed with multiple 5-0 polyglactin 910 sutures (Vicryl, Ethicon, Inc., Piscataway, NJ), dermal sutures, and 6-0 polypropylene (Prolene, Ethicon, Inc., Piscataway, NJ) sutures either in an interrupted fashion or as a carefully placed running cuticular suture (**Figure 5-5**). Sutures are then coated with bacitracin ophthalmic ointment.

Postoperative Management

Postoperatively, ice compresses are applied intermittently to the forehead and eyes. The patient is kept in a quiet room with his or her head elevated. When stable, the patient is discharged home and told to continue head elevation and ice compresses for 24 hours; when not contraindicated, the patient is kept on oral corticosteroids (dexamethasone, 0.75 mg every 12 hr) for 3 days. Ophthalmic-grade bacitracin is applied to the sutures three times daily and as needed. If the patient began his or her use of *Arnica Montana* and bromelain at least 72 hours

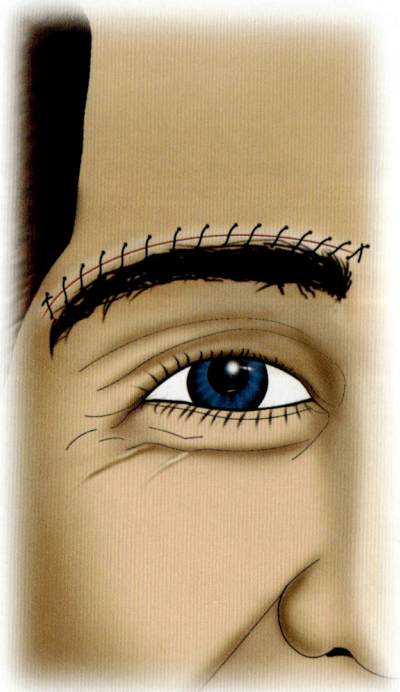

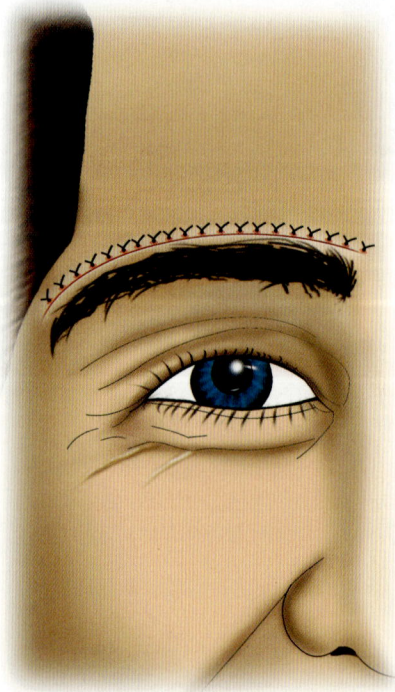

Figure 5-5. The wound is closed in layers with either running or interrupted skin sutures. Note the somewhat abrupt superior border of the brow.

before surgery, he or she is maintained on these homeopathic supplements for 7 days. The patient is contacted by telephone on the night of surgery, and again the following day, and is seen in the office on postoperative day 7 for suture removal. Over the course of the first week, there is typically moderate brow and upper eyelid edema that gradually resolves. Mild hypesthesia of the forehead generally resolves within 2 to 3 weeks.

Results

Figure 5-6 shows the use of the direct browlift for the treatment of unilateral brow paralysis. The patient underwent Mohs micrographic excision of a large basal cell carcinoma of the temple. An immediate ipsilateral brow elevator paralysis was evident. The defect was repaired with opposing advancement-rotation flaps; in the forehead, flap incisions

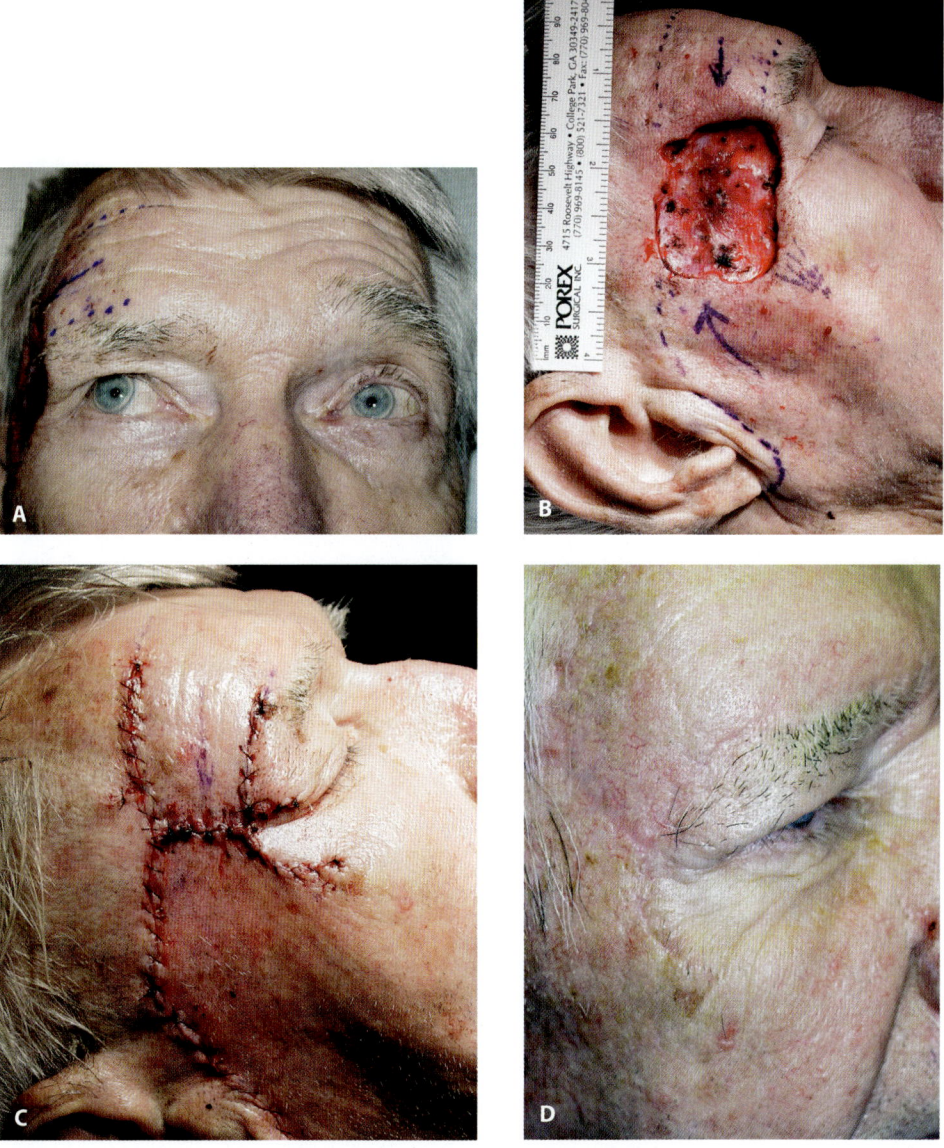

Figure 5-6. Direct brow lift. (A, B) Patient with a neglected basal cell carcinoma of the temple who underwent Mohs excision. Resection included the temporal branch of the facial nerve with resultant ipsilateral forehead paralysis. (C) The wound was closed with a forehead advancement and a lateral facial advancement-rotation flap. Whereas the wounds healed well (D), the brow paralysis and brow ptosis persisted. *(Continued)*

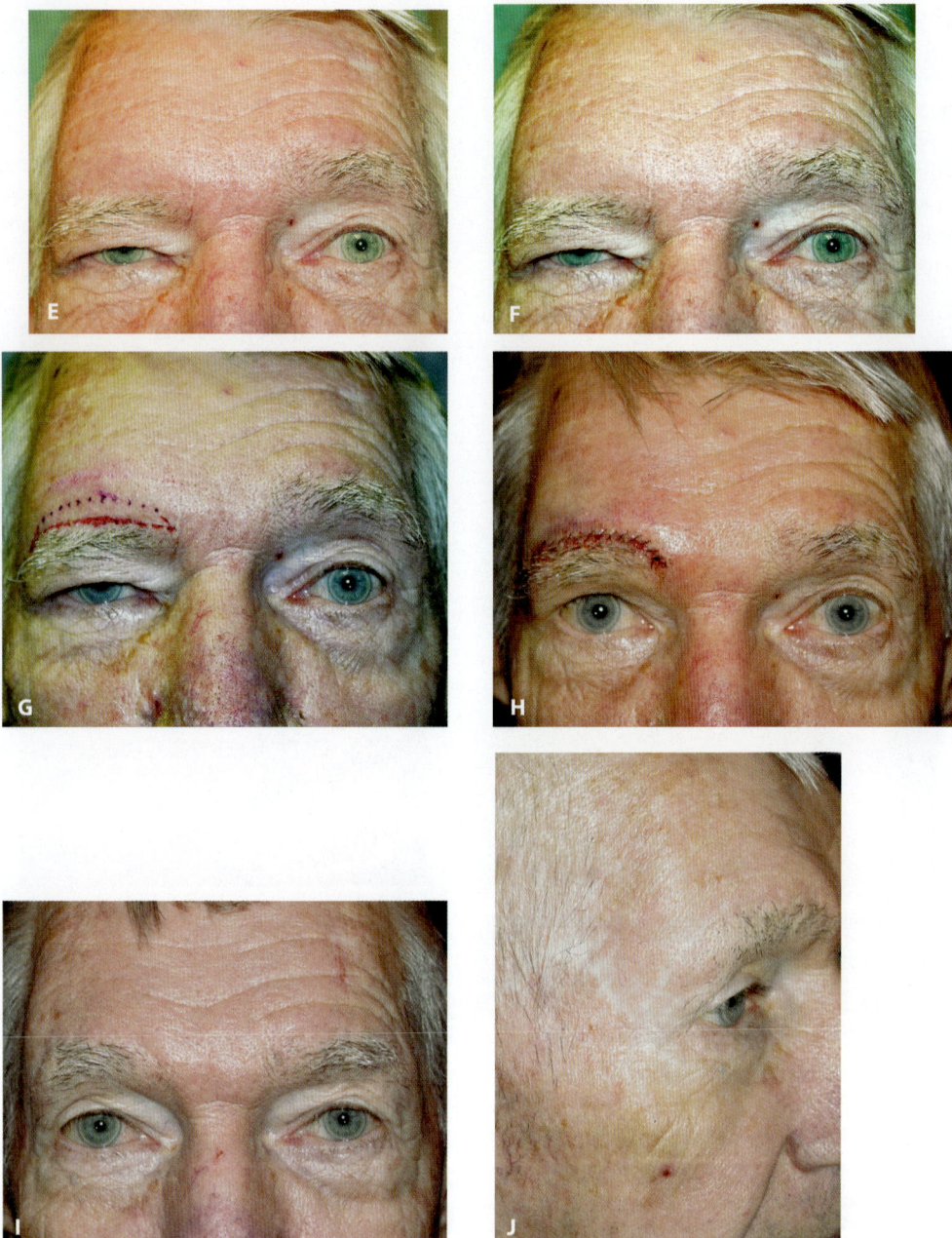

Figure 5-6. *(Continued)* (E), with no improvement by 6 months postoperatively. (F) Owing to significant superior temporal visual field impairment, the patient opted for a direct browlift under local anesthesia. (G) Elliptical skin incision is outlined. (H) Immediately after completion of the direct browlift. (I, J) Good brow symmetry is maintained at the 1-year follow-up.

were brought along the brow margin inferiorly and in a deep preexisting rhytid superiorly. The patient was observed for spontaneous nerve recovery and the severity of the disability from the brow ptosis for 6 months, but the patient requested treatment because of significant ipsilateral visual field impairment. A direct browlift was performed in the office under local anesthesia without any sedation. Postoperatively, the patient healed well with good positioning of his brow.

Complications: Incidence, Management, and Avoidance

If appropriate technique is followed, complications of the direct browlift should be rare. Dissection should stay superficial to the frontalis; at the level of the superior margin of the eyebrow, most supraorbital and supratrochlear branches are either within or deep to the frontalis. However, care should be taken during dissection to preserve these vertically oriented nerve fibers (if seen overlying the frontalis muscle) in order to avoid postoperative neuralgia and paresthesias. Hematomas should be uncommon if careful attention is paid to achieving hemostasis before wound closure. Avoiding significant subcutaneous dissection and blunt avulsion of the corrugator supercilii and procerus muscles should decrease the risk of hematoma as well. Paralysis of branches of the temporal branch of the facial nerve is unlikely (even if desired), as the branches to the corrugator enter the deep surface of the muscle in its lateral third and should be deep to the plane of dissection; also, the motor branches to the frontalis muscle run significantly higher above the tail and midportion of the eyebrow when entering the muscle.

The most significant drawback to the direct browlift is the uncamouflaged scar. Whereas it cannot be completely concealed, several steps can minimize its appearance. The incision should be placed just at the level of the most superior brow hair follicles and should follow that line in an undulating fashion, ensuring that the scalpel blade is held at all times parallel to the hair shafts. Whereas excellent hemostasis is essential, care should be taken to minimize cautery injury to hair follicles. The ends of the dermal sutures should be cut short and buried to avoid postoperative suture spitting. Sufficient dermal sutures should be placed to prevent excessive tension on the skin sutures. Skin sutures should merely appose the skin edges, not strangulate the tissue; allowance should be made for postoperative edema. Postoperative scar erythema is observed for spontaneous resolution, but can be treated with 1064-nm neodymium:yttrium-aluminum-garnet (Nd:YAG) laser for quicker resolution. Patients are counseled to observe strict sun precautions for at least 3 months, and early and aggressive skin lightening is instituted if hyperpigmentation is noted.

Conclusions

The direct browlift, although infrequently used today, is an excellent, powerful, and simple method to rehabilitate the ptotic brow. In light of the visible scar, the direct browlift is generally reserved for older patients with brow paralysis, especially those who cannot tolerate deeper levels of sedation. However, when properly applied, the direct browlift can be an excellent procedure in the setting of central and lateral brow ptosis.

All action is of the mind and the mirror of the mind is the face, its index the eyes.

Marcus Tullius Cicero (106–43 BC)

Suggested Readings

1. Adamson PA, Cormier R, McGraw BL. The coronal forehead lift—modifications and results. J Otolaryngol 1992;21:25–29.
2. McKinney P, Celetti S, Sweis I. An accurate technique for fixation in endoscopic brow lift. Plast Reconstr Surg 1996;97:824–827.
3. Flowers RS, Caputy GG, Flowers SS. The biomechanics of brow and frontalis function and its effect on blepharoplasty. Clin Plast Surg 1993;20:255–268.
4. Arneja JS, Larson DL, Gosain AK. Aesthetic and reconstructive brow lift: current techniques, indications, and applications. Ophthalmic Plast Surg 2005;21:405–411.
5. Cook TA, Brownrigg PJ, Wang TD, Quatela VC. The versatile midforehead browlift. Arch Otolaryngol Head Neck Surg 1989;115:163–168.
6. Booth AJ, Murray A, Tyers AG. The direct brow lift: efficacy, complications, and patient satisfaction. Br J Ophthalmol 2004;88:688–691.
7. Bames HO. Frown disfigurement and ptosis of eyebrows. Plast Reconstr Surg 1957;19:337–340.

6

MIDFOREHEAD LIFT

To get back my youth I would do anything in the world, except take exercise, get up early, or be respectable.
Oscar Wilde (1854–1900), *The Picture of Dorian Gray*

Introduction

The midforehead lift is an open forehead procedure designed primarily to elevate the central and medial brow while reducing deep transverse forehead rhytids. It is similar to the direct browlift in that the point of elevation is relatively close to the eyebrow. However, whereas the direct browlift incision is camouflaged in the junction between the superior brow and the forehead skin, the midforehead lift incision is in plain sight and, hence, clearly visible. The scar is obvious until it has completely matured and only if it has healed precisely. Conversely, the midforehead lift is truly a forehead lift procedure, because in addition to raising the brow, this procedure allows smoothing of the central forehead and glabella.

Visually, the central forehead scar is designed to fall into preexisting transverse forehead rhytids in as random a way as possible. Once healed, the scar should ideally mimic the natural textural lines and fine rhytids of the forehead. Although dissection can be performed completely in the subcutaneous plane, it is advantageous to transition to the subgaleal plane, which allows modification and repositioning of the forehead and mediocentral brow musculature and preserves a more vascular flap.

History

The origins of the modern midforehead lift are somewhat obscure. Early 20th-century surgeons clearly described excision of ellipses of skin from the central forehead, strategically placed in preexisting forehead creases. This type of procedure developed on a course parallel to the direct browlift and, initially, was designed to allow cutaneous brow advancement and elevation. Whereas the direct browlift camouflaged its scar at a natural facial subunit boundary (superior brow border), the midforehead excision rendered its scar less noticeable by utilizing preexisting forehead creases. The relatively smoother midline forehead

---

Midforehead Lift

Indications: heavily creased forehead, mostly medial and central brow ptosis in patients with an unfavorable hairline.
Contraindications: history of hypertrophic or keloid scarring, severe lateral brow ptosis, smoker (relative contraindication).
Ideal candidate: male, deep transverse rhytid creases, thin skin, little temporal brow ptosis, severely thinning hair or receding hairline.
Scientific basis: interruption of cutaneous tethering to the frontalis muscle, elimination of medial brow depressor muscle action, forehead skin resection, and superior skin advancement.

Midforehead Lift

Incisions: irregular central forehead incision in a central forehead rhytid(s).
Tissue modifications: central frontalis/galea incision and elevation with advancement and resection, myotomies of corrugator supercilii and procerus muscles.
Fixation: frontalis/galea closure.
Wound closure: two-layered skin closure.
Complications: forehead paresthesias (temporary), skin slough (rare), hematoma (3%).

skin provides less camouflage than the more heavily creased lateral skin, making a continuous transverse forehead scar more visible.

The "indirect browlift" was an approach similar to the direct browlift, although the incisions were placed in asymmetrical lower forehead creases. As described by Castanares,[1] the indirect browlift was accomplished by excising crescents of skin in the lateral aspect of the lower forehead, designed so that the upper limb of each crescent fell exactly into the second-lowest transverse rhytids. Ideally, the two sides were at different heights to maximize scar camouflage. Through these access points, the forehead skin would be dissected off of and elevated from the frontalis muscle up to the anterior hairline and the wound closed in layers, elevating the brows. In addition, oblique incisions within the medial end of each brow and a vertical glabellar incision were made to provide access for sectioning of the corrugator supercilii and procerus muscles. In what was probably a tacit admission that complete corrugator resection is difficult and often incomplete through this approach, Castanares[1] also advocated selective neurotomy of the temporal branches of the facial nerve for more complete ablation of corrugator function.

Rafferty[2] described a similar technique that utilized skin excisions based on the first crease above the brow, followed by subcutaneous dissection to the top of the eyebrow. The brow dermis was then elevated by suturing the brow dermis superiorly to the frontalis muscle and periosteum, followed by layered skin closure. Rafferty advocated 1 to 2 mm of overcorrection and did acknowledge recurrent brow ptosis postoperatively. Rafferty's procedure relied on skin excision and permanent sutures for brow elevation but did not address the chronic downward pull of the brow depressor musculature that was the likely cause of the brow ptosis recurrence.

Whereas separate lateral forehead incisions could be placed at different levels and the discontinuity of these scars used to aid in providing camouflage, access to brow muscles was still limited. A more complete approach to the brow depressors could be obtained by making a continuous transforehead incision such as in the midforehead lift. This, however, requires incision across the smoother (compared with the lateral forehead skin) medial suprabrow and glabella, which would produce more scarring and a greater potential for postoperative neuralgia and hypesthesia. Also, the frequent asymmetry of forehead and suprabrow rhytids makes blending a continuous, single forehead scar more difficult.

A straight-line forehead scar also increases the difficulty of creating an imperceptible scar. However, by connecting the two separate lateral forehead skin incisions with a Z-plasty across the smoother midline forehead, the surgeon gains vastly improved access to the various tissue levels of the lower forehead all the way to the orbital rim.

The midforehead lift, therefore, is effective in releasing cutaneous attachments to the frontalis muscle associated with deep rhytids, allows elevation of the brow through muscular manipulation and skin excision, and provides safe access to the brow depressors to reduce glabellar and medial brow rhytids.

Rationale and Scientific Basis

The modern midforehead lift smoothes lower forehead rhytids by separating the skin from the underlying, tonically contracted frontalis muscle. After the skin is redraped, contraction of the frontalis muscle is less effectively transferred to the forehead skin, as the fibrous tethering of the skin to the muscle is rendered less dense. Also, the sectioning of the corrugator supercilii and procerus muscles eliminates most of the tonic depressor strain on brow position. With less brow depressor pull, the need for the brow elevator (frontalis muscle) to contract in order to maintain the brow in a nonvisual field–obstructing position is considerably reduced.

Second, the midforehead brow lift reduces the appearance of glabellar rhytids directly because of the sectioning of the corrugator supercilii and procerus muscles. The removal of contractile forces on the medial and central brow and glabellar skin by the corrugator and procerus muscles, respectively, eliminates the folding of this skin and reduces rhytids in these areas. If these muscles are adequately resected, the chance of significant rhytid recurrence in the glabella is minimal.

Finally, brow position is changed by a number of tissue alterations. First, the lower forehead skin is excised and the entire lower forehead skin flap is elevated and sutured at a higher level. Second, the frontalis muscle is elevated, resected, and resutured, raising the brow position through tension on the cutaneous attachments to the lower frontalis and orbicularis oculi muscles. The same is true for the plication of the superior orbicularis muscle: raising the upper fibers of this muscle also causes "unfurling" of the contracted orbicularis, thereby raising the brow. Lastly, by resecting the medial brow depressors, the chronic downward muscle pull on the brow is eliminated, allowing the compensatory, chronic frontalis muscle contraction, now unopposed, to raise the brow to a more neutral position. By performing brow depressor myotomies, in addition to elevating the brow elevator muscle, there is both a dynamic as well as a static mechanism leading to a stable brow elevation.

Indications and Contraindications

The midforehead lift is indicated for moderate to severe brow ptosis in patients with deep forehead rhytids, especially those with severe frontal hairline recession or thinning. The midforehead lift is contraindicated in patients with a history of poor wound healing or keloid scars and in patients who will not accept a visible scar.

Advantages, Disadvantages, and Alternatives

The midforehead lift elevates and allows for contouring of the eyebrows as well as for smoothing the central forehead. In addition to the fixed effect on brow position of skin excision, the midforehead lift also incorporates a more functional and physiologic approach by reducing/eliminating the action of the brow depressor musculature. The incision placed in the midforehead provides a more direct exposure of the lower brow musculature for myoplasty. The obvious disadvantage of the midforehead lift is the scar extending across the forehead. This scar, once healed, can be quite imperceptible; however, it may take several months to fully mature. The ideal patient for the midforehead lift is a male patient with thin, fair skin with deep forehead transverse creases and severe (current or anticipated) frontal hairline recession who is completely realistic and willing to accept the permanent forehead scar in exchange for reduced forehead rhytids and correction of brow ptosis.[3,4,5] Although the scar can ultimately heal quite well, the midforehead lift commits the patient with severe frontal rhytids and brow ptosis to, at best, a more relaxed, neutral brow position and a smooth forehead with a residual transverse crease (the scar). In light of the prominent position of the scar, adequate preoperative counseling is crucial to surgical success.

Although any of a number of brow procedures can serve as an alternative to the midforehead lift, in the highly selected patient described earlier, few

of the alternative brow/forehead procedures can match the midforehead lift in result achieved and a scar as well camouflaged. The patient with a heavily creased forehead and an unfavorable hairline can be treated with a direct browlift[6] or a combination of transpalpebral depressor muscle sectioning with a transtemporal browlift. The former enables the surgeon to reposition the central and lateral thirds of the brow while camouflaging the scar along the superior margin of the brow but does not address central forehead or glabellar rhytids, whereas the latter combination does allow recontouring of the entire brow and depressor myoplasty through an upper eyelid incision. The combination of temporal and upper lid incisions in this approach is generally well hidden (unless the patient is totally bald, there is generally sufficient temporal hair density to camouflage the temporal incision), but as noted by Walden and coworkers,[7] myotomy of the corrugator muscle through the transpalpebral approach is frequently difficult and incomplete. In addition, heavily creased foreheads are better addressed by the skin flap elevation of the midforehead lift.

Range of Anesthesia

Adequate anesthesia of the forehead can be achieved with supraorbital and supratrochlear nerve blockade. However, because of the extent of the dissection, the multiple planes developed, and the myotomies required, patients generally benefit from intravenous sedation. Because active patient participation is not needed to assess brow position intraoperatively, general anesthesia is an acceptable alternative.

Equipment

A good, basic assortment of plastic surgical instruments is adequate for the midforehead lift, and no specialized equipment is mandatory. Sharp double hooks and fresh #15 and #10 blades and a Stevens tenotomy scissors are useful in dissecting forehead skin from frontalis muscle. Metzenbaum scissors, a Freer elevator, and Senn retractors assist in elevating the frontalis muscle and deep galeal fascia. Longer right-angle retractors and a headlight or a lighted fiberoptic retractor aid in performing myotomies of the brow depressor muscles while protecting the supratrochlear and supraorbital neurovascular bundles. Bipolar or needle-point monopolar cautery should be used to achieve meticulous pinpoint hemostasis.

Operating Room Setup

Adequate visualization during the midforehead lift requires an angled view under the skin and muscle flaps. The surgeon should be seated at the head of the table, with full access to both sides of the patient's head. A Mayo stand with selected instruments can be positioned at the side of the patient's head on one side, while an assistant is positioned opposite, on the side of the dominant hand.

Incisions

The meticulous execution of the design, incision/excision, and closure of the midforehead incision is probably the skin treatment most critical to the success of any forehead procedure. By choosing an incision directly across the midforehead, the surgeon does not have the benefit of the scalp hair or hair/forehead transition to aid in camouflaging the scar, but rather must rely on skin-oriented facial scar camouflage techniques (**Figure 6-1**). The midforehead lift is best performed in patients with thin, heavily creased forehead skin. This is especially true for those patients, typically but not exclusively male, with thinning and/or receding hairline (**Figure 6-2**), in which low hair density would make a trichophytic or coronal incision difficult to cover with hair.

The midforehead lift skin excision is planned so that the upper limb of the ellipse falls into a preexisting horizontal midforehead rhytid. Ideally, this incision is planned to utilize rhytids at two different heights in order to maximize scar camouflage (**Figure 6-3**). Close inspection of the forehead will demonstrate brow asymmetry in more than 80% of patients, usually associated with asymmetrical

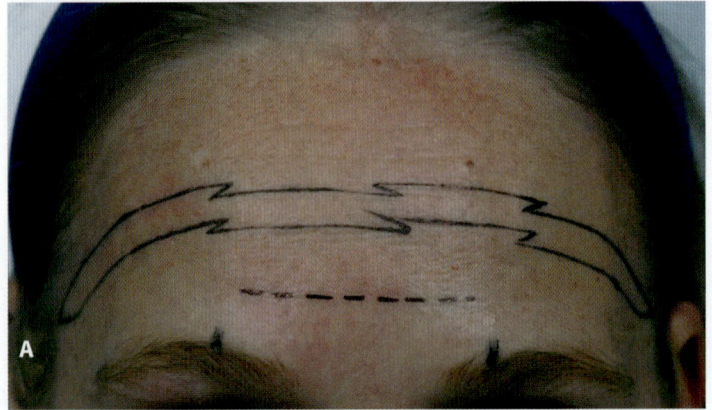

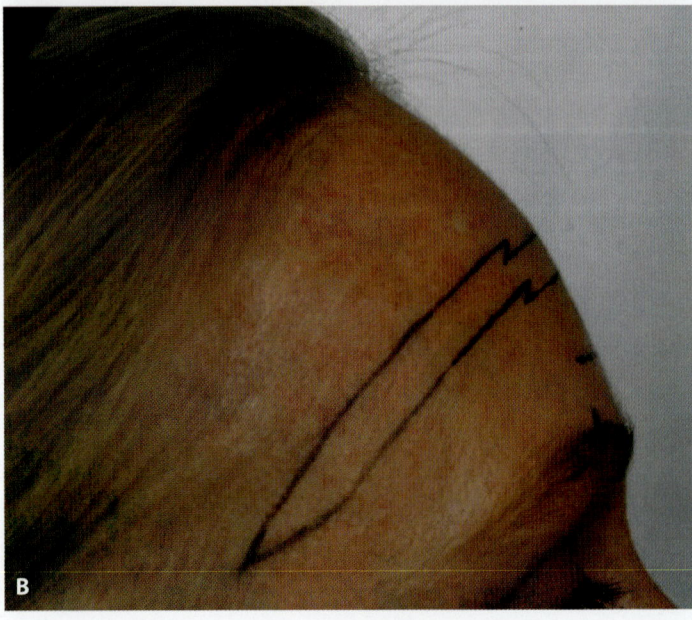

Figure 6-1. (A, B) Midforehead lift incision, as modified by Calvin M. Johnson, Jr., MD. (Photos courtesy of Calvin M. Johnson, Jr., MD).

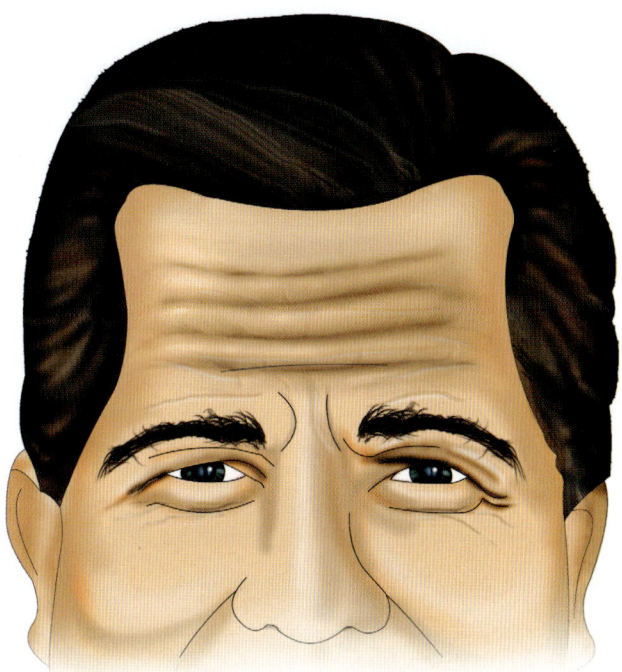

Figure 6-2. In patients with thick skin and deep rhytids, the midforehead lift can produce excellent access to the brows in patients with high hairlines.

rhytids. By taking advantage of this asymmetry, the surgeon designs an incision from the rhytids on the left to those on the right, with an irregularity in the generally smoother central forehead, to allow better camouflage of the central scar as well as to transition the scar from the higher to the lower rhytid.[8] The incision should be made no more superiorly than the midforehead in order to protect the branches of the supraorbital and supratrochlear nerves, because these nerve fibers pierce the frontalis muscle to run on its superficial surface over the upper half of the muscle.

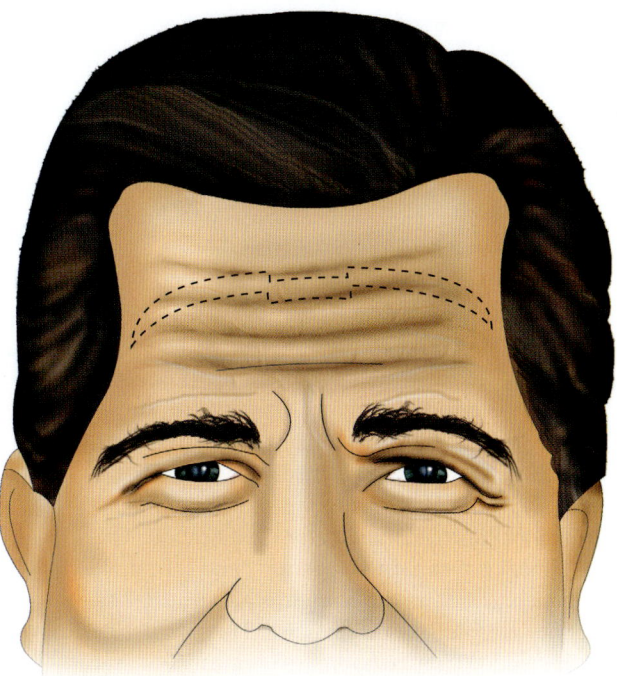

Figure 6-3. The midforehead lift incision is planned to allow the upper limb to fall within an existing horizontal rhytid. By staggering the central incision, rhytids at two different heights can be used to maximize scar camouflage.

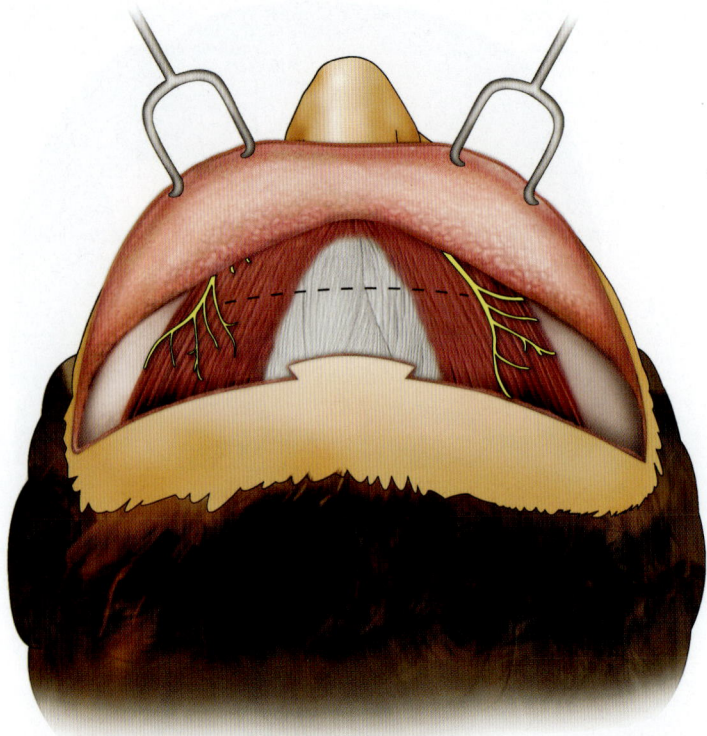

Figure 6-4. A skin flap is raised inferiorly to the orbital rim. Minor oozing from the frontalis muscle or the elevated dermis should be controlled carefully with cautery. Care should be taken to protect the branches of the supraorbital nerve. The frontalis muscle is then incised medial to the supraorbital nerves *(dotted line)*.

Planes of Dissection

The midforehead lift is a biplanar procedure,[8] initially, as the skin flap is raised over the lower forehead (**Figure 6-4**). This requires that the attachments between the frontalis muscle and the skin be sharply incised with a #10 scalpel blade or sharp scissors, down to the level of the upper brow. Because the skin incision is placed in the midforehead, the branches of the supraorbital nerve are located deep to or within the frontalis muscle under the skin flap, and only cutaneous branches of the supratrochlear nerves are divided along with an occasional branch of the supraorbital nerve that supplies the skin of the lateral brow and lower forehead. After the skin flap is raised, an incision is made through the frontalis muscle (**Figure 6-5**) in between the medial-most branches of the supraorbital nerves, and a dissection plane is developed *below the deep galeal fascia,* bluntly with a Freer elevator or scissor-spreading dissection. This plane is carried down to the supraorbital rim centrally, exposing both procerus and corrugator supercilii muscles for modification. The instrument is then turned superiorly and subgaleal[8] dissection to the anterior hairline is performed. The superior subgaleal dissection upward to the anterior hairline is thus deep to both the supratrochlear and

the superficial branches of the supraorbital nerves. Although this subgaleal plane is fairly avascular, the skin elevation often divides cutaneous perforating vessels and time must be devoted to careful control of these small vessels with bipolar forceps or precise use of a needle-tipped monopolar cautery. Obviously, the need for hemostasis should not compromise skin flap viability.

Tissue Modifications

Once separate skin and frontalis muscle flaps have been developed, vertical spreading with Metzenbaum scissors in the subgaleal plane progressively stretches and separates the corrugator supercilii muscle from the surrounding soft tissue near the superomedial orbital rim, before the muscle enters the galeal fat pad. Once the muscle is adequately exposed, a 5-mm segment near the origin is excised and the muscle stumps cauterized with the bipolar cautery (**Figure 6-6**). Further dissection to the nasal root exposes the procerus muscle, which is divided with the cautery. In heavily creased foreheads, the undersurface of the frontalis muscle can be lightly scored to further decrease postoperative folding of the overlying skin. (This last maneuver decreases the degree of functional brow position modification,

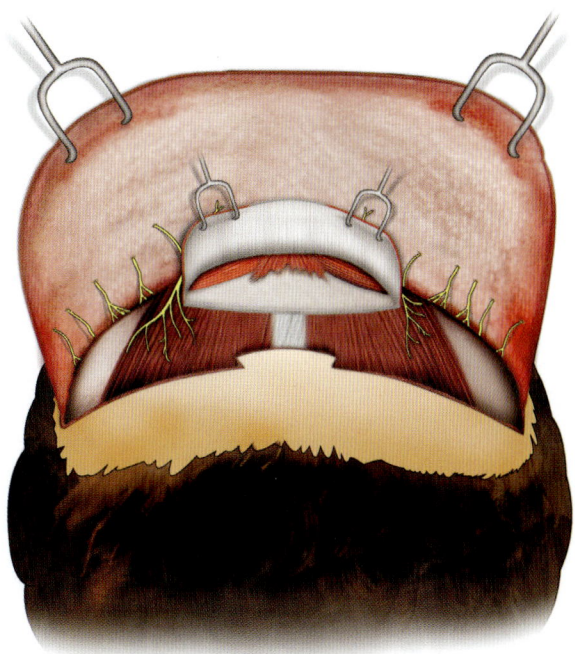

Figure 6-5. The frontalis muscle is incised between the supraorbital nerve branches and elevated above the periosteum to the orbital rim, exposing the brow depressor muscles.

because it would necessarily decrease the amount of lift of brow position generated by the frontalis. This step is likely to increase the need of upper frontalis mobilization and skin excision.)[8]

Next, the frontalis and attached deep galea are mobilized superiorly, excess is resected (**Figure 6-7**),

and the edges of the muscle are resutured with 3-0 nylon or other permanent sutures. The upper orbicularis, overlying the inferior frontalis, is then plicated superiorly with the same permanent sutures to the frontalis muscle and underlying fascia. The lower forehead skin is then redraped superiorly.

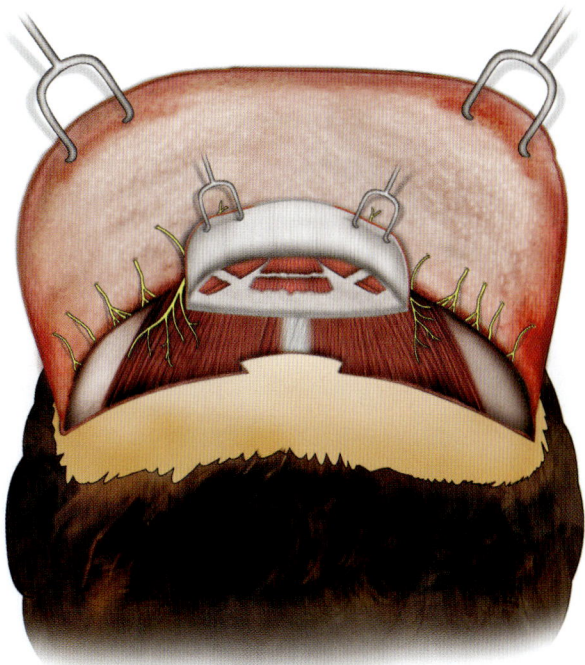

Figure 6-6. Five-millimeter segments of the corrugator supercilii muscle are excised and the stumps are cauterized. Further inferior dissection is performed in the midline, so that the procerus muscle can be divided with cautery.

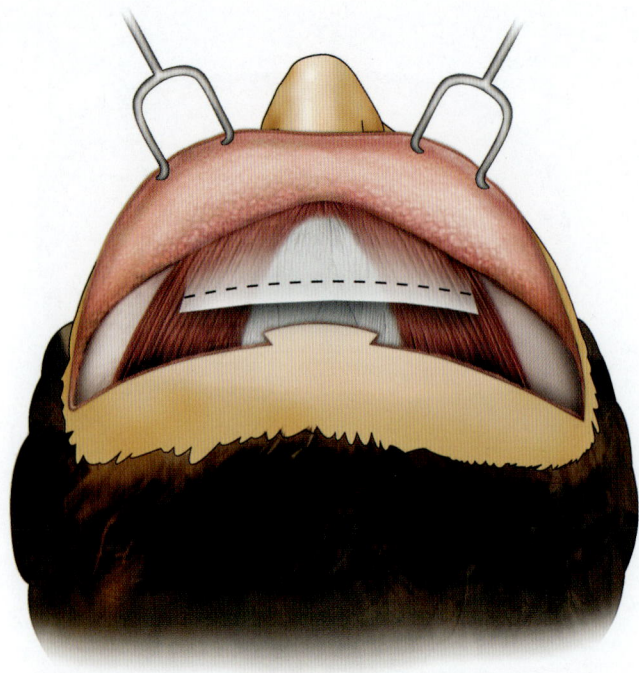

Figure 6-7. Elevated frontalis muscle–deep galeal flap is advanced superiorly. The muscle extending beyond the original cut *(dotted line)* is excised and the muscle/fascial flap repaired with permanent sutures. The upper border of the orbicularis oculi muscle (not shown for clarity) can be plicated superiorly to the frontalis muscle for additional elevation.

Excess skin is marked and excised exactly parallel to the upper edge of the skin excision (**Figure 6-8**). Typically, the amount of skin advanced and excised is twice the amount of brow elevation desired,[9] following the general rule of increasing need for elevation as the distance from the brow to the point of fixation increases. By comparison, most authors recommend resecting 2.5 to 5 times the desired amount of brow elevation during a coronal forehead lift.

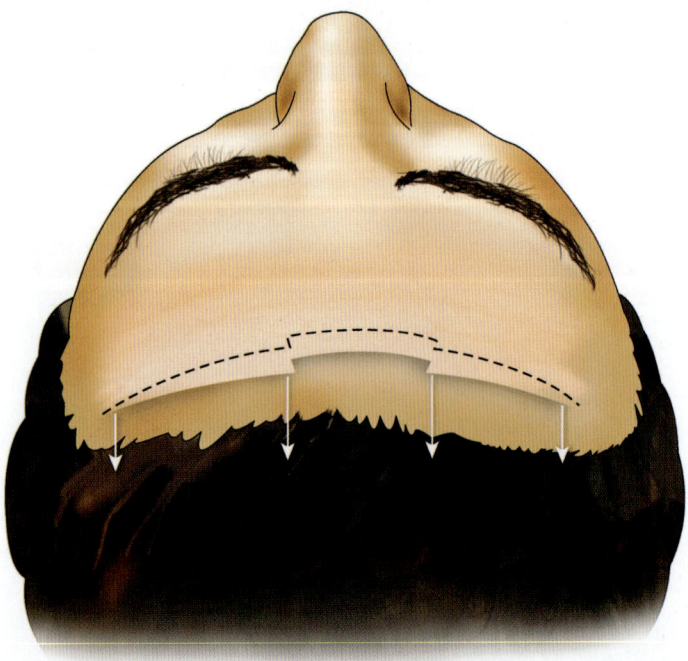

Figure 6-8. The skin flap is redraped and redundant skin is excised.

Wound Closure

The wound should be thoroughly inspected for bleeding points, which should be meticulously controlled with electrocautery, because no drain is placed. Because some brow elevation after a midforehead lift is due to skin excision and elevation, a layered closure is imperative to reduce the risk of a widened scar. 4-0 Vicryl or Monocryl sutures are placed to reapproximate the dermis, and running 5-0 Prolene sutures are used to evert the skin edges during skin closure (**Figure 6-9**).

Postoperative Management

A lightly compressive dressing is placed over the forehead, and postoperatively, ice compresses are applied intermittently to the forehead and eyes. The patient is kept in a quiet room with her or his head elevated. When stable, the patient is discharged home and told to continue head elevation and ice compresses for 24 hours; when not contraindicated, the patient is kept on oral corticosteroids (dexamethasone, 0.75 mg every 12 hours) for 3 days. If the patient began her or his use of *Arnica Montana* and bromelain at least 72 hours before surgery, she or he is maintained on these homeopathic supplements for 7 days. The patient is contacted by telephone on the night of surgery; the patient should be questioned for any symptoms of active bleeding, including severe pain. The patient is seen in the office on the day after surgery, when the dressing is removed. Mupirocin (Bactroban) ointment should be applied to the sutures two to three times daily, and the patient seen in the office again on postoperative day 7 for suture removal. Over the course of the first week, there is typically moderately severe forehead, brow, and upper eyelid edema that gradually resolves. Patients should be counseled to expect periorbital ecchymosis lasting 7 to 10 days. Postoperative forehead anesthesia generally extends from the brow to the crown, and may take 12 to 14 weeks to fully resolve. Intermittent pruritus over the forehead typically develops in week 3 or 4 and usually resolves by the 8th to 10th week after surgery. As mentioned earlier, the midforehead scar may take several months to fully mature; consideration should be given to scar dermabrasion at 8 to 10 weeks after surgery. Generally, scars are observed for 3 to 4 months to allow for spontaneous resolution of erythema, but can be treated with the 1064-nm neodymium:yttrium-aluminum-garnet (Nd:YAG) laser for quicker resolution. Patients are counseled to observe strict sun precautions for at least 3 to 4 months, and early and aggressive skin lightening is instituted if hyperpigmentation is noted.

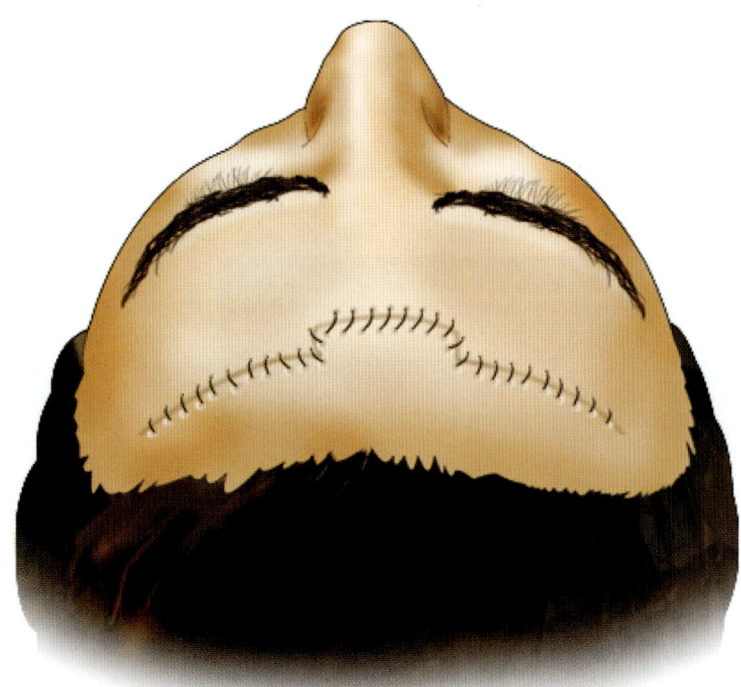

Figure 6-9. Meticulous two-layered closure of the incision is performed. As the skin between the midforehead lift incision and the brow is trimmed and the brow rises, the distance from the brow to the wound shortens. The distance from the wound to the hairline is unchanged.

Complications: Incidence, Management, and Avoidance

The midforehead lift is typically a well-tolerated procedure with a fairly rapid recovery. Bruising and edema, as stated, generally resolve in 7 to 10 days, and significant pain is unusual. Pruritus and numbness are common but generally not problematic. Incisions are placed so as to prevent supraorbital nerve injury by incising through the frontalis muscle and galea only between the major supraorbital nerve branches and above the main trunks of the supratrochlear nerves. Long-term or problematic forehead or scalp numbness should be rare.

The most feared complications of the midforehead lift are skin slough and hematoma. Cook and colleagues[6] reported a 3% incidence of hematoma in a series of patients undergoing midforehead lift. Meticulous attention must be paid to elevation of the lower forehead skin flap off of the frontalis muscle. The surgeon must dissect fibers of the frontalis muscle from the skin flap without compromising the subdermal plexus. After flap elevation, the frontalis muscle surface should be carefully, thoroughly, and meticulously inspected for bleeding, and hemostasis ensured with the bipolar cautery. Likewise, the undersurface of the skin flap should be evaluated and any bleeding sites judiciously cauterized. Postoperatively, hematomas should be diagnosed and treated promptly, whether by aspiration or open evacuation; the patient should be placed on systemic antibiotics and followed closely.

Skin slough, although rare, can be catastrophic. Careful dissection respecting the subdermal vascular plexus, thorough hemostasis, and layered skin closure with minimal tension are mandatory steps in the midforehead lift necessary to reduce the chance of skin slough. Patients should refrain from tobacco use for a minimum of 6 weeks before and 3 weeks after surgery. If an area of skin slough develops, the wound should be managed carefully but cautiously, débriding only obviously necrotic skin. Although unlikely, for large areas of slough, consideration can

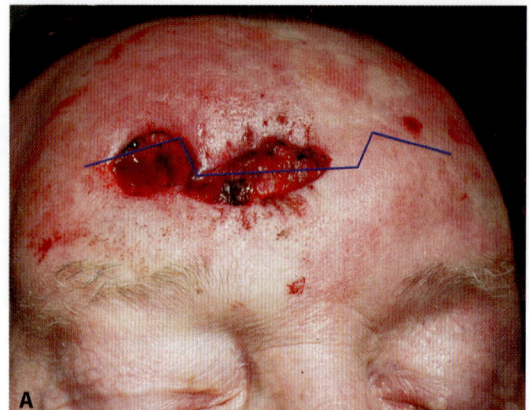
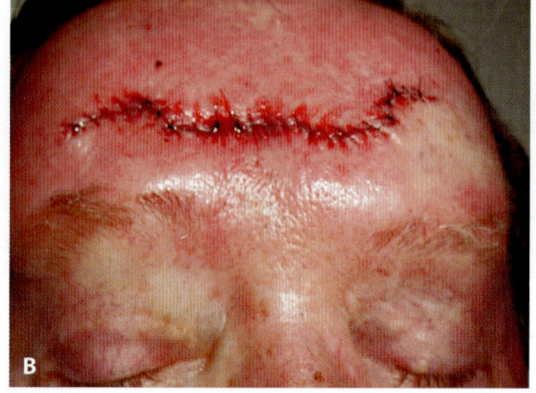
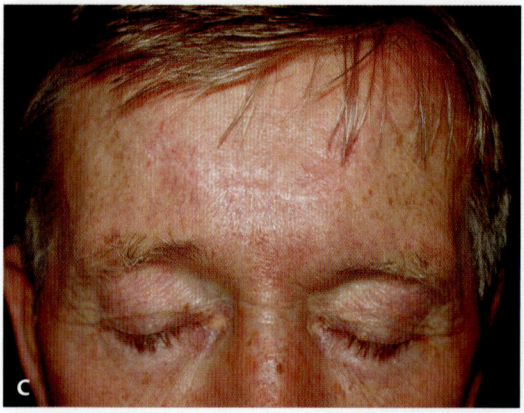

Figure 6-10. (A–C) Patient with thin hair and a high hairline. A Mohs excision of a basal cell carcinoma and wide excision of a melanoma. (B A) midforehead lift approach under local anesthesia was used, camouflaging the closure into asymmetrical central forehead rhytids. (C) One year later, brow position is adequate and the scar is imperceptible.

be given to hyperbaric oxygen treatments. During this time, patient concerns and expectations should be anticipated and managed, while at the same time, the patient should be prepared for any required scar revision procedures.

Conclusion

The midforehead lift is an excellent procedure in carefully selected patients for treatment of moderate to severe brow ptosis and central forehead rhytids. Although less frequently performed than in the past, the midforehead lift is a well-tolerated and effective foreheadplasty technique in specific patients, and every facial plastic surgeon should be familiar with this procedure (**Figure 6-10**).

The scars of others should teach us caution.
St. Jerome (AD 374–419)

Acknowledgments

The author would like to thank Calvin M. Johnson, Jr., MD for the patient illustrations used in the chapter.

Suggested Readings

1. Castanares S. Forehead wrinkles, glabellar frown and ptosis of the eyebrows. Plast Reconstr Surg 1964;34: 406–413.
2. Rafferty FM, Goode RL, Abrumson NR. The brow-lift operation in a man. Arch Otolaryngol 1978; 104: 69–71.
3. Arneja JS, Larson DL, Gosain AK. Aesthetic and reconstructive brow lift: current techniques, indications, and applications. Ophthal Plast Surg 2005;21:405–411.
4. Adamson PA. The forehead lift: refinements in technique. J Otolaryngol 1986;15:89–93.
5. Brennan HG, Rafaty M. Midforehead incisions in treatment of the aging face. Arch Otolaryngol 1982;108: 732–734.
6. Cook TA, Brownrigg PJ, Wang TD, Quatela VC. The versatile midforehead browlift. Arch Otolaryngol Head Neck Surg 1989;115:163–168.
7. Walden JL, Brown CC, Klapper AJ, Chia CT, Aston SJ. An anatomical comparison of transpalpebral, endoscopic, and coronal approaches to demonstrate exposure and extent of brow depressor muscle resection. Plast Reconstr Surg 2005;166:1479–1487.
8. Johnson CM, Waldman SR. Midforehead lift. Arch Otolaryngol 1983;109:155–159.
9. McKinney P, Mossie RD, Zukowski ML. Criteria for the forehead lift. Aesthetic Plast Surg 1991;15: 141–147.

7

CORONAL FOREHEAD LIFT

Wear a smile and have friends, wear a scowl and have wrinkles.

George Elliot (1819–1880)

Introduction

The coronal forehead lift has long been considered the gold standard procedure for brow and forehead rejuvenation, and many surgeons still consider it the most reliable and effective treatment of the aging upper third of the face. Approaching the forehead and brow through an incision at or behind the frontal hairline, the coronal forehead lift can achieve the four major goals of aesthetic forehead surgery: raise the eyebrows and increase the eyebrow-to-eyelash distance, smooth the central forehead by eliminating or effacing transverse forehead rhytids, eliminate glabellar rhytids by decreasing or eliminating tonic glabellar depressor muscle contraction, and (when necessary) use a trichophytic incision to shorten a long forehead and restore the frontal hairline to a more neutral and aesthetic position.

The most significant drawback of the coronal forehead lift is the lengthy scar, extending from one temple to the other and either running (in one pattern or another) within the hair-bearing skin or detouring along the frontal hairline between the temporal hair troughs. The proper healing of this scar is imperative, because any imperfections can render it more difficult to camouflage or frankly obvious and negate many of the benefits of the procedure. Scar widening or pericicatricial alopecia of the hair-bearing portion of the scar may commit the patient to a lifetime of hairstyling restrictions. Widening of or telangiectasias around the frontal hairline scar or *regularization* of the normally random frontal hairline fringe will also require the patient to style his or her hair with bangs to maximize camouflage of these imperfections. Careful consideration should be made before choosing the coronal forehead lift for any patient with current or anticipated male pattern alopecia; in patients with female pattern alopecia, progression of the condition will render a well-executed coronal forehead

---

Coronal Forehead Lift

Indications: deep central rhytids; medial, central, and/or lateral brow ptosis.
Contraindications: bald or severely thinning hair, high hairline or unwilling to accept hairline scar.
Ideal candidate: normal hairline and hair density, mild to severe brow ptosis and forehead and glabellar rhytids.
Scientific basis: reduction of skin contraction caused by frontalis muscle contraction, elimination of medial brow depressors, mechanical elevation, and suspension of the brow.

Coronal Forehead Lift

Incisions: coronal (paralleling frontal hairline), trichophytic, or pretrichial.
Tissue modifications: subgaleal and subtemporoparietal fascial elevation; corrugator myectomy; procerus and frontalis myotomies.
Fixation: galea/frontalis closure.
Wound closure: two-layered skin closure.
Complications: incisional alopecia (2–3%); widened scar (up to 10–15%); permanent neuralgias (2–5%); permanent hypesthesias (1–8%); hematoma (0.6–2%); facial nerve injury (temporary: 0.1–0.6%; permanent: rare); revision rate (0–20%).

lift obvious as time progresses. However, in properly selected patients, the coronal forehead lift is an outstanding tool in the surgeon's repertoire for rejuvenation of the senescent forehead and brow.

History

As with all modern aesthetic procedures of the forehead, the coronal forehead lift developed as an extension of forehead skin excision procedures described in the early 20th century. In 1926, Hunt and Noel both described coronal incisions in the hair-bearing scalp, and in the same year, Hunt also described the anterior hairline incision later advocated by Joseph and Lexer in 1931. In 1933, Passot combined a posthairline skin excision to lift the central brow and bilateral neurotomies of the temporal branch of the facial nerve to smooth the forehead.

The modern coronal forehead lift was first elaborated by Gonzalez-Ulloa in 1962,[1] and the definitive description of the procedure was succinctly outlined by Vinas and coworkers in 1976.[2] They described forehead rejuvenation through a bicoronal incision that ran through hair-bearing skin in the central forehead (patients with low or normal hairlines) or a trichophytic incision running along the fringe of the frontal hairline (patients with elevated hairlines). This incision was taken down to the subgaleal level (centrally) and below the superficial temporal fascia (temporally) and followed down to the orbital rims. Forehead myoplasty consisted of corrugator supercilii division and excision[3,4-6] as well as excision of a horizontal strip of frontalis muscle 3 to 4 cm above the level of the brows. Deactivation of the frontalis muscle was commonly advocated[7] and, in the 1970s and 1980s, could take the form of muscle strip excision,[8] horizontal scoring distributed along the height of the muscle[9] or limited to just below the deepest rhytids,[10,11] or horizontal and vertical scoring to form a frontalis muscle "checkerboard[12,13]." As our understanding of brow and forehead physiology has expanded through several outstanding anatomic dissections and clinical experience with surgical procedures and with functional treatments such as botulinum toxin, myoplasty procedures have become more conservative;[14] however, Vinas and coworkers' description[2] still incorporates the mainstream of thought on the modern coronal forehead lift.

Variations in technique chiefly are related to the plane of dissection and forehead muscle management, as well as incision placement (which is discussed elsewhere). Proponents of a complete subperiosteal dissection cite the anatomic argument of enhanced skin flap vascularity and enhanced ability to protect the supraorbital nerve. Moreover, subperiosteal advocates cite the inelasticity of the periosteum as providing more effective traction in brow elevation than the galea-frontalis complex. Less common, subcutaneous dissection through a coronal approach provides the surgeon with the ability to smooth deep forehead rhytids by separating skin from the underlying contracted frontalis muscle.

Treatment of the forehead muscles likewise has been varied. Early coronal approaches such as those described by Hunt, Joseph, Lexer, and Passot lacked muscle modifications and relied solely on skin excision to elevate the brow. The desire to further improve results led to more extensive dissections at deeper planes (subgaleal and subperiosteal). With this more extensive exposure came a greater opportunity to modify forehead musculature. Most authors have agreed that the corrugator supercilii muscle should at least be transected and possibly be segmentally resected. Implicit in this dissection and myoplasty near the origin of the corrugator supercilii muscle is division of the depressor supercilii muscle as well. In addition, the procerus muscle is generally incised horizontally. The frontalis muscle has seen the greatest variety of treatments. Early authors advocated interruption of frontalis function by excising a horizontal strip of muscle; subsequently, frontalis myoplasty became limited to horizontal myotomy below deep transverse rhytids. A few others have advocated horizontal and vertical incisions, creating a checkerboard pattern and individual muscle squares. However, most surgeons now agree that muscle treatment in the coronal forehead lift should consist of conservative horizontal incision of the deep galea and frontalis muscle to assist in effacing a deep transverse rhytids while maintaining the frontalis as a functional brow elevator.

Rationale and Scientific Basis

The coronal forehead lift, when properly performed, can completely rehabilitate the aging forehead and brow with a predictable recovery and limited risk. The coronal forehead lift blends skin excision with functional muscle modification to produce brow elevation. As mentioned earlier, the modern coronal forehead lift incorporates glabellar myoplasty by either transecting or resecting a portion of the proximal corrugator muscle and midprocerus muscle. This effectively releases the depressor action of these muscles and allows the brow to rise to a more neutral position. Horizontal myotomy(ies) of the frontalis muscle, although allowing effacement of deep transverse forehead furrows, decreases the brow elevation from static frontalis contraction. In addition, frontalis muscle incisions through this approach by definition will section the deep galea. Traction applied to the superior edge of the flap during elevation is thus less effectively transferred to the brow, because the deep galea and frontalis muscle will "gape" open and allow the more flimsy and elastic overlying structures (superficial galea, subcutaneous fat and skin) to stretch. Because of this less efficient transfer of force from the galea closure to the brow, significantly more scalp must be resected than brow elevation desired, with recommended ratios of 2.5:1 to 5:1. Because the brow elevation is provided chiefly by skin excision and galeal resection, these layers must be closed under tension, and a layered closure is mandatory to avoid scar widening due to flap recoil.

Advantages, Disadvantages, and Alternatives

The coronal forehead lift provides unparalleled exposure of all pertinent bony, muscular, and fascial structures necessary to fully contour the forehead and brow. Complete modification of these muscles by scoring or resection can be performed under direct vision. A study by Walden and colleagues[15] noted incomplete division of the corrugator supercilii muscle through a translid approach as compared with either an endoscopic or a coronal approach. The full breadth of the frontalis muscle is exposed for myoplasty as deemed necessary. The coronal forehead lift also facilitates a complete release at the orbital rim; complete release is an essential step to enable full superior mobilization of the forehead flap and the brow. The coronal forehead lift is an excellent procedure in appropriately selected patients for repositioning of the eyebrows and secondarily smoothing the forehead. In addition, in the rare patient with significant frontal bossing or prominent supraorbital rims, the coronal forehead lift provides excellent exposure for bony forehead reduction with a high speed bur.

Whereas the coronal forehead lift is a powerful technique for upper facial rejuvenation, it does have clear and distinct disadvantages. The coronal forehead lift requires extensive dissection and undermining, with an attendant increased risk of hematoma and risk of injury to the temporal branch of the facial nerve. As mentioned previously, elevation of the brow is done at a distance, and the amount of skin excision is based on the surgeon's experience and judgment. Although this may vary from 2.5 to 5 times the amount of brow elevation desired, most patients generally require 10 to 16 mm of skin excision. Whereas the experienced surgeon can obtain predictable results with the coronal forehead lift, there is a learning curve in relating the thoroughness of myoplasty with the skin excision and flap necessary to produce aesthetic brow elevation. Finally, the classic coronal incision will invariably raise the frontal hairline and may not be appropriate in patients with severe male pattern alopecia or high hairlines. Even in appropriately selected patients, the long coronal scar can be a challenge to hide and requires that the scar heal well without any hypertrophy and that there be no significant hair loss around the scar. Ideally, hair should grow through the cutaneous scar for maximal camouflage. The coronal incision transects superficial branches of the supraorbital nerve; if the incision is made anterior to the crown, the patient may have a variably wide zone of permanent crown anesthesia. There is generally a period of temporary paresthesias, itching, and numbness postoperatively, which can be disturbing to patients and occasionally be permanent. If the temporal dissection plane is too superficial, injury (temporary or permanent) to the temporal branch of the facial nerve can occur, whereas too deep a dissection can enter the superficial temporal fat pad and lead to fat pad atrophy and postoperative temporal wasting. The most substantial disadvantage (and occasional advantage) of the coronal forehead lift is that it can elevate the frontal hairline. In patients with a low or normal hairline, this is generally not problematic, but those with existing high hairlines are not candidates for a camouflaged hair-bearing scalp central incision. In these cases, a trichophytic incision can be used to maintain or lower the hairline, but this approach requires meticulous wound closure and wound management, and the scar will be variably visible as it matures, similar to but less dramatic than the scar associated with the midforehead lift.

For the patient requiring complete elevation and/or recontouring of the brow and moderate smoothing of central forehead rhytids, the coronal forehead lift is an excellent option. Alternatives to the coronal forehead lift for patients objecting to the scar or recovery or who are poor candidates because of hairline issues are the endoscopic forehead lift or the combination of transtemporal and transpalpebral limited incision approaches. Whereas a direct brow lift will reposition the central and lateral eyebrows, it is limited in its treatment of the nasal end of the brow and does not smooth the forehead or glabella significantly. Alternatively, the midforehead lift can treat glabellar and severe forehead rhytids and reposition the brow, but it is generally reserved for patients with thin, fair skin and deep forehead rhytids that can be used to camouflage the scar.

Indications and Contraindications

The coronal forehead lift is indicated in patients with moderate to severe brow ptosis with or without glabellar and forehead rhytids. Contraindications to the coronal forehead lift include thinning hair and current or anticipated male pattern baldness, severely elevated frontal hairline, or history of hypertrophic scarring. The extensive nature of the coronal scar requires sufficient hair for camouflage, and it is essential to angle the incision parallel to hair follicles to preserve hair density along the scar. Even a well-placed and well-healed coronal scar may be visible through severely thinning hair, and male pattern baldness and hairline recession may reveal the coronal scar if not placed posteriorly enough. Coronal forehead lifting using an incision through hair-bearing skin is contraindicated in patients with a high hairline (generally considered as brow-to-hairline distance ≥ 5 cm, but must be considered in the context of facial and forehead shape).[16,17] These patients already have an elevated hairline and further elevating the hairline with a posthairline skin excision will give an unnatural and displeasing appearance to the face. A pretrichial incision can be used during a coronal forehead lift to avoid further elevation of the hairline.

Range of Anesthesia

The forehead and scalp are remarkable for the highly consistent nature of its innervation. This consistency provides the opportunity for excellent regional anesthesia with selected nerve blocks. By injecting local anesthetic across the supraorbital rim (supraorbital and supratrochlear nerves), along the lateral aspect of the lateral orbital wall (zygomaticotemporal nerve), and across the crown (occipital nerves), sufficient anesthesia can be obtained for the coronal forehead lift. However, patients may be apprehensive during the procedure (especially as the coronal flap is reflected down over the face); sufficient anxiolysis is necessary to adequately perform the procedure and monitored intravenous sedation is generally minimally required. General anesthesia, especially when combining the coronal forehead lift with other procedures, can also safely provide patient comfort.

Equipment

The equipment required for the coronal forehead lift is similar to that for a midforehead lift, and most complete plastic surgical trays contain sufficient instrumentation. Rainey clips can be helpful in expediting elevation of the forehead flap by rapidly controlling bleeding from the portion of the scalp (anterior wound edge) that will ultimately be excised. A bipolar cautery is useful to obtain hemostasis from the posterior edge of the incision and is also helpful in safely sectioning the glabellar muscles. Sharp double hooks, wide rakes, and right-angle retractors can aid in progressively elevating the forehead flap. Centrally, the flap can easily be elevated with a Freer elevator or Metzenbaum scissors to within 2 cm of the orbital rim. Temporally, the plane of elevation is below the temporoparietal fascia, which elevates quite easily with a #10 scalpel or a Freer or Cottle elevator. Allis, towel, or D'Assumpcao clamps are used to grasp the end of the forehead flap when advancing it posteriorly before excision and fixation.

Operating Room Setup

During the coronal forehead lift, the surgeon will need access to the entire forehead and scalp up to the crown. The surgeon is seated at the head of the operating table; it is important that the patient's head be placed so that the upper occiput rests on the end of the table, and the vertex and crown actually extend beyond the end of the surgical table. This provides unencumbered access to the forehead from the crown. An assistant stands on the side of the surgeon's dominant hand and the scrub nurse stands opposite. A Mayo stand is positioned over the patient's chest, providing the surgeon with complete access to three sides of the patient's head.

Once the incisions are planned and marked (see "Incisions"), a 1- to 2-cm strip of scalp anterior to the marking is trimmed. Ideally, the hair is left long enough to demonstrate the natural slant of the hair. The remainder of the hair is parted, taped,

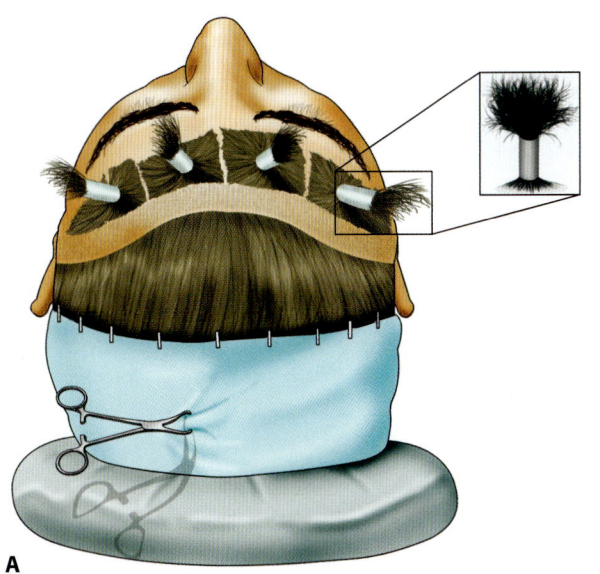

A

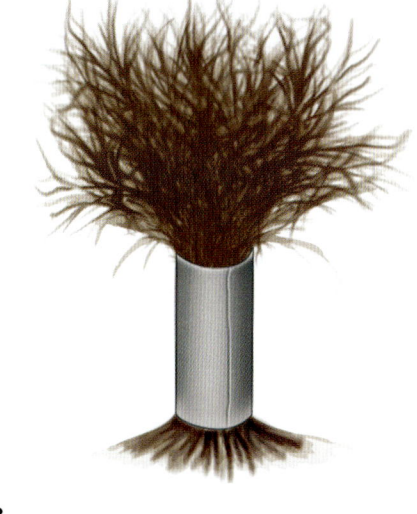

B

Figure 7-1. (A) Patient's hair is appropriately parted, tied, taped, and draped. The hair along a 1- to 2-cm strip anterior to the planned incision is trimmed to facilitate surgery. The hair should be left long enough to demonstrate the natural slant of the hairs. (B) Anteriorly, the hair can be parted, gently twisted, and secured with paper tape or bands. (C) A modified head drape can be secured to the scalp with skin staples to ensure that posterior hair does not drift into the wound.

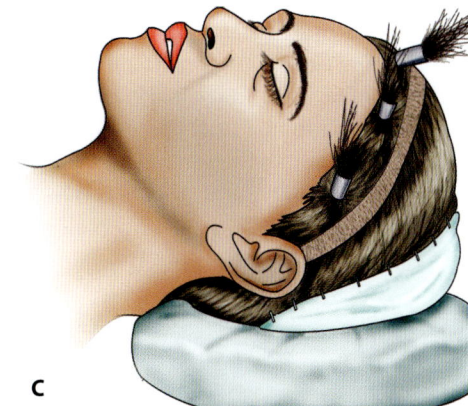

C

and covered to facilitate dissection and maximize sterility (**Figure 7-1**).

Incisions

The choice of incision for the coronal forehead lift is a critical decision that will affect the patient's recovery time and the ultimate success of the procedure. Retrotrichial incisions are obviously easier to camouflage in the early postoperative period, but the decision to choose a coronal or an anterior hairline incision should be based on the needs of the forehead vis-à-vis the anterior hairline.

McKinney and associates[18] have defined the maximal aesthetically acceptable distance between the brow and the anterior hairline to be 5 cm. It should be recognized that a coronal incision will advance the anterior hairline posteriorly as the forehead "un-

furls," thus increasing the brow-to-hairline length. Most authors advocate a 2:1 to 5:1 overcorrection for the coronal forehead lift, so elevating the brow as little as 5 mm may shift the hairline 1 to 3 cm posteriorly. Conversely, anterior hairline incisions will maintain the hairline position while elevating the brow, thus shortening the brow-to-hairline distance. The correct choice for the central incision is imperative to appropriately manage the anterior hairline.

Before beginning the procedure, the incision is planned and the hair should be appropriately prepared. The temporal aspect of the coronal incision is marked, beginning 1 cm above the superior aspect of the helix and extending upward toward the crown. Upon reaching the temporal crest, the incision can either follow the frontal hairline from temporal trough to temporal trough (trichophytic) or cross the frontoparietal junction (classic coronal) and traverse the hair-bearing scalp. If the latter is chosen, ideally it should cross the scalp posterior to the terminal ends of the supraorbital nerve; this would require an incision across the crown, which may run 7 to 8 cm posterior to the hairline. Although this is possible, it generates a long flap that is more difficult to turn down. If the hairline (and any anticipated androgenetic hair loss) allows, the incision can curve anteriorly and parallel the frontal hairline while remaining 2 to 3 cm posterior to it. This can considerably shorten the length of the flap and avoid a long, straight scar that would be more prone to contracture.

The classic central coronal incision is located posterior to the hairline. Prior authors have varied in the appropriate distance the central coronal incision should be from the hairline, varying from 3 to 8 cm. Ramirez[3] has described the incision lying behind a biauricular line. There is a mechanical advantage to a more anterior incision, but at the price of a potentially more visible scar and transaction of terminal branches of the supraorbital nerve. More posterior sloping foreheads make elevation and exposure of the orbital rim easier; in these cases, it is both easier and more important to position the central coronal incision more posterior. However, in patients with high hairlines, a trichophytic or pretrichial incision should be used centrally to avoid an unnaturally posterior hairline.[19] This incision should follow the natural undulation of the frontal hairline with gentle irregularities to minimize the visibility of the scar. Temporally, this incision curves posteriorly at the temporal trough to continue down to just above the ear (**Figure 7-2**). To additionally maximize scar camouflage, the incision should be beveled anteriorly, leaving some hair follicles, but not the overlying epidermis, in the posterior skin edge. When the flap skin is resected at the conclusion of the procedure, the skin is cut in a parallel bevel. Once the scar heals, hairs will grow through the scar from posterior (deep) to anterior (superficial) to the scar (**Figure 7-3**).

The central portion of the incision, whether at or behind the hairline, continues laterally to the area of the temporal crest, where the incision turns and runs inferiorly down to the top of the helix. This extension of the incision down to the ears allows the surgeon to reflect the forehead flap inferiorly on itself, assisting in exposure of the inferior forehead as well as providing a vector for posterolateral elevation of the tail of the brow.

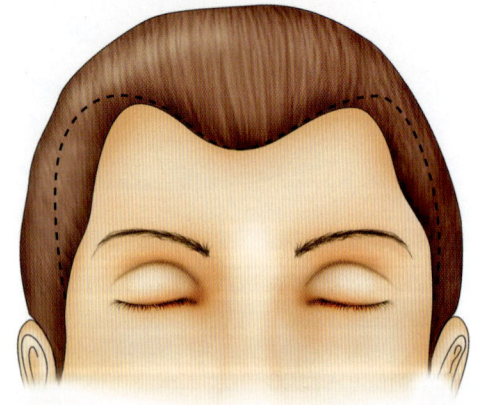

A

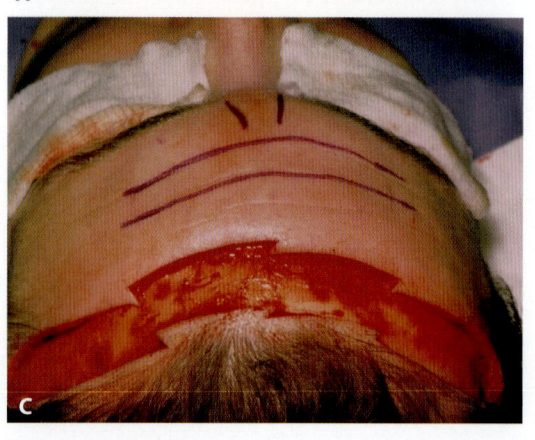

C

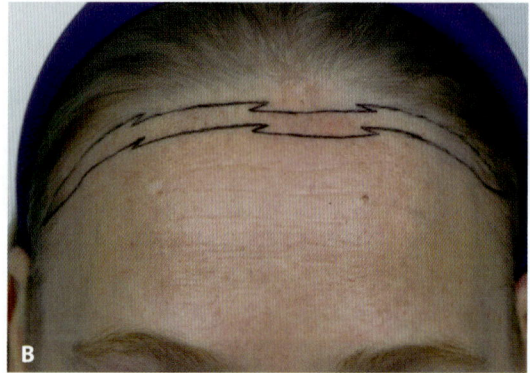

B

Figure 7-2. (A) A trichophytic incision in patients with high hairlines can provide sufficient access for the coronal forehead lift and can also shorten the forehead height. The incision runs along the anterior central frontal hairline, then courses back into the temporal hair beginning at the temporal troughs. (B) Modified pretrichial forehead lift incision. (C) Modified pretrichial forehead lift incision. Redundant skin is measured and excised before elevation of the forehead skin in the subgaleal plane. (B, C Photos courtesy of Calvin M. Johnson, Jr., MD.)

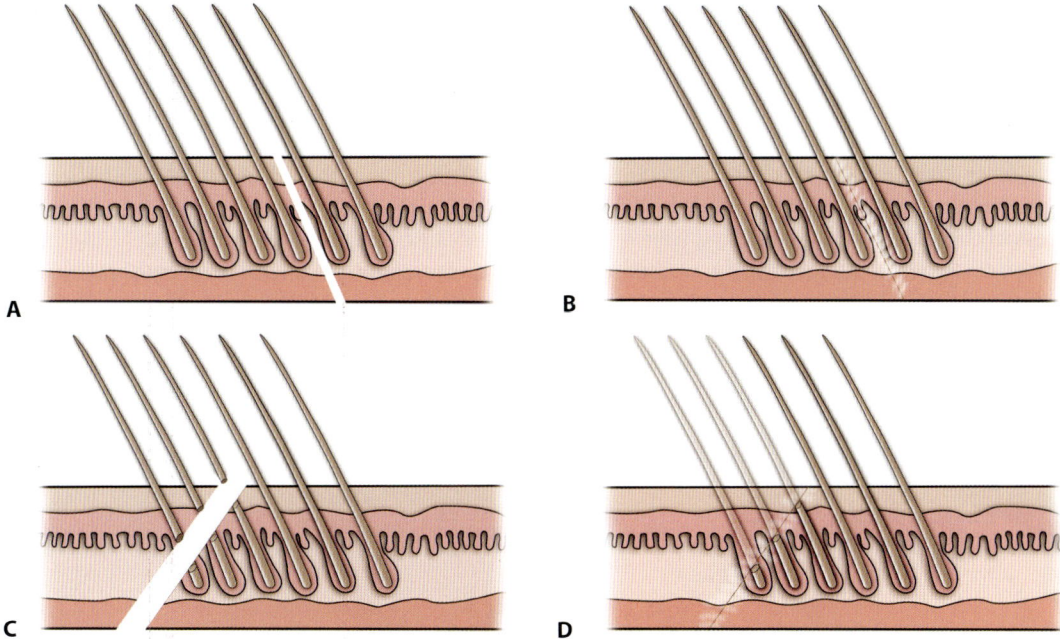

Figure 7-3. Care must be taken to preserve hair follicles along the incision. (A) Beveling the incision *parallel* to the hair follicles allows development of a thin scar (B) easily camouflaged by surrounding hair. If the skin incision is made at an angle to the hair shafts (C), the scar is no longer bordered by hair-bearing skin (D). E As the scar tissue develops around the hair follicles, new hair growth may not penetrate this fibrosis, leaving the scar easily visible.

Plane of Dissection

The majority of authors perform the coronal forehead lift centrally in the subgaleal plane—that is, between the deep galeal fascia on the undersurface of the frontalis muscle and the periosteum.[20] This plane is easily identified and dissected. Gentle inferior retraction and elevation of the forehead flap after skin incision demonstrates the loose connections between these two layers, which are easily divided with scissors or a scalpel (**Figure 7-4**). Laterally, the flap is elevated in the loose plane in between the temporoparietal fascia and the superficial layer of the deep temporal fascia. The

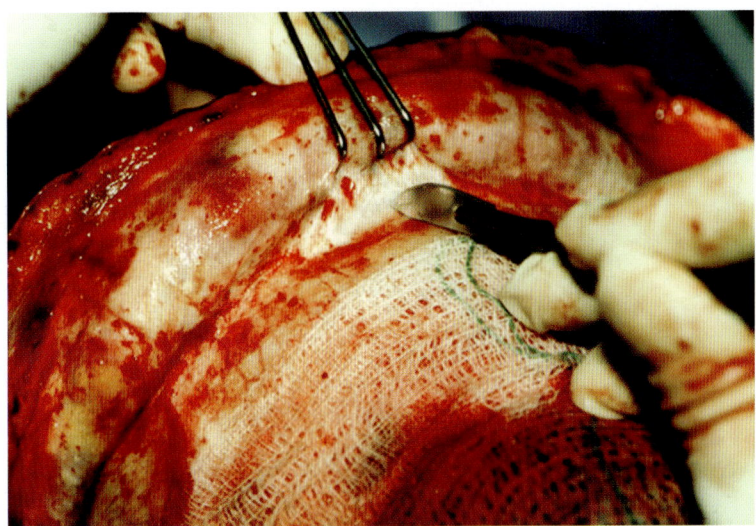

Figure 7-4. Trichophytic forehead lift. Elevation in the subgaleal (supraperiosteal) plane in the midline at the glabella. (Photo courtesy of Peter A. Adamson, MD.)

temporoparietal fascia is densely adherent to the subdermis whereas there is a natural glide plane between the temporoparietal fascia and the superficial layer of the deep temporal fascia. With traction on the anterior edge of the wound, this glide plane is readily apparent and is easily developed with spreading scissors or a Freer elevator. This plane is easily dissected superiorly until the temporal crest and zone of fixation are encountered. In this area, the various layers of temporal fascia (temporoparietal fascia, superficial and deep layers of the deep temporal fascia) and the galea and the periosteum are bound tightly to

bone. Although the galea is the continuation of the temporoparietal fascia, the area of the zone of fixation must be sharply incised to complete the elevation. This plane is continued inferiorly at least to the zygoma (**Figure 7-5**).

At this point, the galea or periosteum becomes more rigidly attached to frontal bone and the surgeon can either continue to dissect in this plane[21] or transition to the subperiosteal plane inferiorly to the orbital rim. Continuing with a preperiosteal plane allows access to the medial brow musculature without entering the periorbita, perhaps limiting

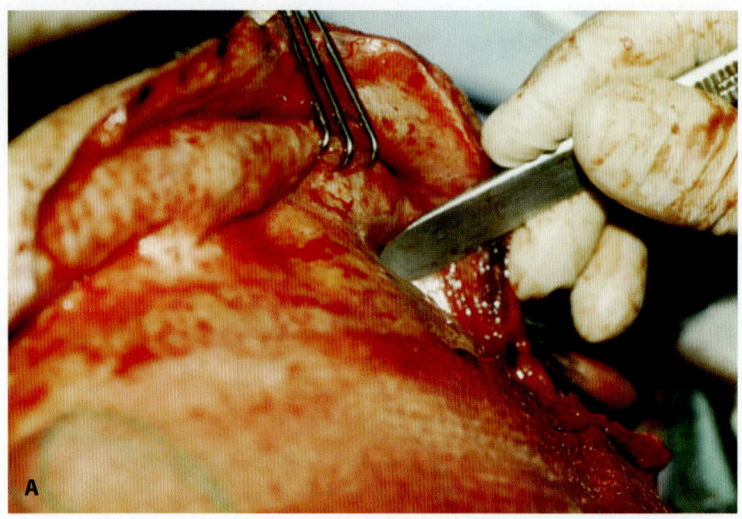

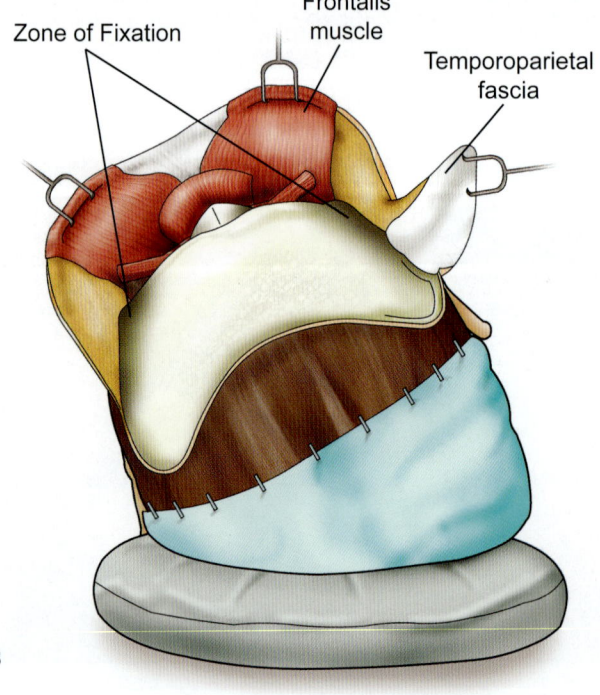

Figure 7-5. (A) Trichophytic forehead lift. Elevation in the subgaleal plane continuing laterally superficial to the superficial layer of the deep temporal fascia, down to the zygoma. (B) The coronal flap is raised below the temporoparietal fascia (superficial to the superficial layer of the deep temporal fascia) laterally and between the deep galea and periosteum centrally. Dense fixation at the zone of fixation near the temporal crest requires sharp lysis. (Photo courtesy of Peter A. Adamson, MD.)

postoperative chemosis and ecchymosis. Conversely, incising the periosteum and transitioning to the subperiosteal plane protects the proximal supraorbital nerves from injury. Also, the corrugator and depressor supercilii and procerus muscles can be treated by myotomy or myectomy closer to their origin.[10] Lastly, and probably most significantly, subperiosteal dissection enhances release of the retaining structures (orbital ligament, arcus marginalis) of the brow.

Ramirez[3] has argued that the subperiosteal plane is appropriate for the entire central dissection; this is then connected to the subtemporoparietal fascia dissection at the temporal crest. He reasoned that not only is the vascular supply to the flap heartier (a view also endorsed by Knize[22]) but also the inelastic periosteum provides a better platform to transfer the forces of elevation from the coronal closure to the level of the brow. Compared with the galea, the periosteum is considerably more rigid and less elastic, and hence there is less "stretch-back" of the elevated brow than when elevation relies primarily on the galea. Conversely, Nassif and coworkers[21] found less wound tension was required the elevate the brow at the galeal versus the periosteal level.

Tissue Modifications

The key component of the coronal forehead lift in terms of providing reliable, long-lasting brow elevation is a complete release of the forehead tissues at the superior orbital rim between both lateral canthi. Brennan[12] emphasized the importance of a complete release at the supraorbital rim and nasal root, but Ramirez[3] believed that periosteal release within 1 to 2 mm of the arcus marginalis is sufficient. When the flap is elevated down to the orbital rim, it is important to ensure this dissection extends laterally past the frontozygomatic suture, ensuring release of the orbital ligament. This release does not alter lateral canthal position. More medially, the flap elevation can continue to the arcus marginalis, elevating it from the orbital rim. Alternatively, a subperiosteal dissection can be performed to the arcus, where the periosteum is again incised and a supraperiosteal plane established and dissected over the arcus marginalis.

Historically, the central forehead lift achieved brow elevation by creation of a large forehead skin-muscle flap, advancing it posteriorly, resecting excess skin, and closing the wound in layers with significant tension applied to the galeal closure. Treatment of the forehead muscles was reserved for effacing deep

transverse rhytids or oblique brow rhytids. Segments of corrugator and procerus muscles were resected primarily to smooth the central glabella and have generally remained a constant feature of the coronal forehead lift. However, treatment of the frontalis muscle was initially relatively simple and conservative but became increasingly complex as the procedure matured. Ultimately, as our understanding of brow dynamics has evolved, treatment of the frontalis muscle has returned to its more conservative roots. Vinas and coworkers[2] advocated removal of a horizontal strip of frontalis muscle during the coronal forehead lift; other authors have recommended single or multiple horizontal muscle scoring, partial strip excision, "checkerboard" incisions, or complete muscle excision. Extensive frontalis incisions may lead to irregular muscular activity and produce unwanted forehead deformities, prompting Flowers and colleagues[23] to advise against excessive frontalis muscle modification. Most surgeons today will make one or two parallel horizontal incisions through the galea/frontalis complex directly below the deepest transverse rhytids(s) in the central forehead to allow the skin in this area to stretch with elevation and efface these rhytids. Fine needles can be passed through the rhytids of interest and the needle exit sites noted on the undersurface of the flap and marked. The needles are then removed. With the surgeon holding the flap with the nondominant hand and the third and fourth fingertips on the rhytids of interest and everting the flap, a cut is carefully made through the galea and frontalis muscle with either a scalpel or monopolar cautery along the marked area. The incision stops once subcutaneous fat is noted. The temporal branches of the facial nerve and branches of the supraorbital nerves are protected by making these transverse cuts extend no farther than the midpupillary line (**Figure 7-6**).

Brow depressor myoplasty has been much more uniform over the years, with some type of incision or excision being performed as close to the muscle origin as possible. Kaye[24] recommended that a 5- to 10-mm segment of corrugator muscle be excised; Adamson[10] also recommends a 10-mm segment of corrugator be excised in order to eliminate oblique glabellar furrows. A fine hemostat can be used to dissect out a segment of muscle in between the branches of the supratrochlear and the superficial division of the supraorbital nerves, and the intervening muscle block excised and the stumps carefully cauterized with a bipolar cautery (**Figure 7-7**). Simple incision may lead to recurrence of the

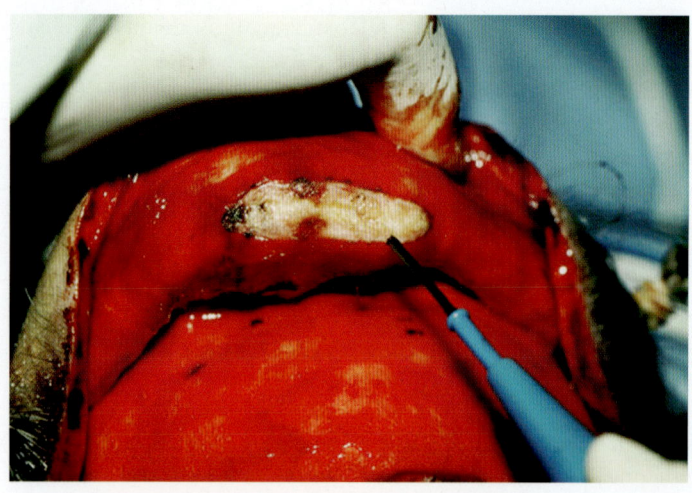

Figure 7-6. Trichophytic forehead lift. Unipolar cautery is used to incise the deep galea and frontalis muscle just into the subcutaneous tissue, between the pupils, deep to the forehead rhytids. (Photo courtesy of Peter A. Adamson, MD.)

rhytids if the muscle edges heal together sufficiently, so a substantial length of muscle is generally excised. However, this may lead to a visible depression postoperatively, and fat grafting can be performed prophylactically if this is a concern. A substantial excision near the origin of the corrugator will also interrupt the depressor supercilii, which lies intimately on the deep aspect of the corrugator muscle. The procerus muscle can either be disinserted or, similar to the corrugator muscle, be treated with

a 10-mm square excision (**Figure 7-8**). Again, free fat grafts can be placed to prevent any postoperative skin depression in this area.

At this point, the forehead skin-muscle flap has been fully elevated, the depressor muscles sectioned, the frontalis muscle divided underneath the deepest forehead rhytids, and the flap periosteum released along the supraorbital rims. The flap is now freely mobile and can be advanced posterior enough to position the brow at an attractive position.

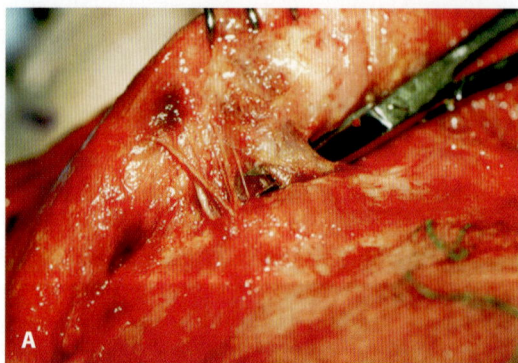

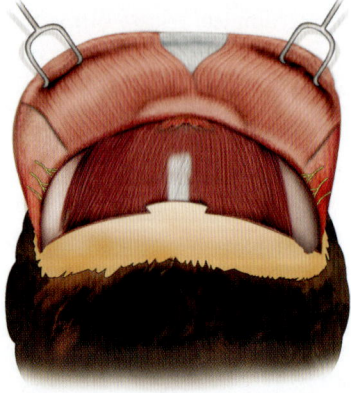

B

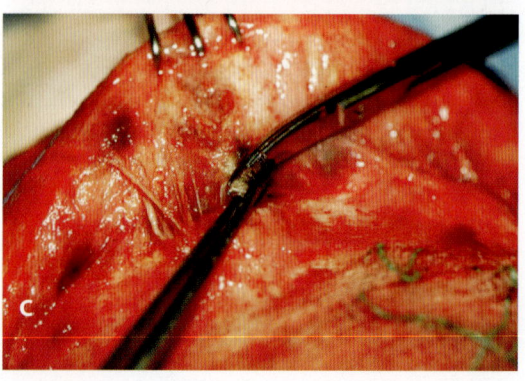

Figure 7-7. (A) Trichophytic forehead lift. Identification and preservation of the supraorbital neurovascular bundle and blunt scissors dissection of the corrugator supercilii muscle. (B) A hemostat is used to dissect a segment of corrugator muscle between the branches of the supratrochlear and the supraorbital nerves. A 10-mm segment of muscle is resected and the muscle stumps are cauterized. (C) Trichophytic forehead lift. Bipolar cautery and scissors resection of the central portion of the corrugator supercilii muscle. (A, C Photos courtesy of Peter A. Adamson, MD.)

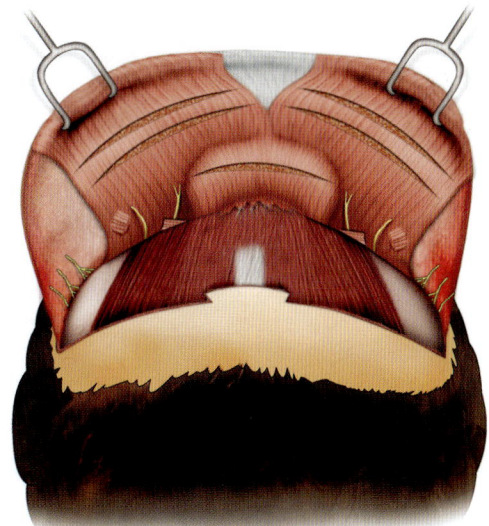

Figure 7-8. An incision can be made through the procerus muscle to decrease medial brow depressor forces. One or two incisions through the frontalis muscle can be made directly below deep transverse forehead rhytids.

Compared with the direct browlift and the midforehead lift, the point of fixation in the coronal forehead lift is farther away from the brow, and hence, a greater correction factor is needed to elevate the brow than in those other, more proximate, procedures. Ratios of skin excision required to brow elevation desired that have been recommended in the past have ranged from a low of 1:1 to as high as 5:1. Most authors[2,5], however, generally recommend a 2.5:1 to 3:1 ratio. Ramirez[3] noted that significantly less overcorrection was needed if the coronal forehead lift dissection is done completely in a subperiosteal level rather than a subgaleal plane.

The forehead flap is retracted and redraped posteriorly with Allis or D'Assumpcao clamps, excess skin is marked (**Figure 7-9**), and the requisite amount resected. The tissue should be cut at a

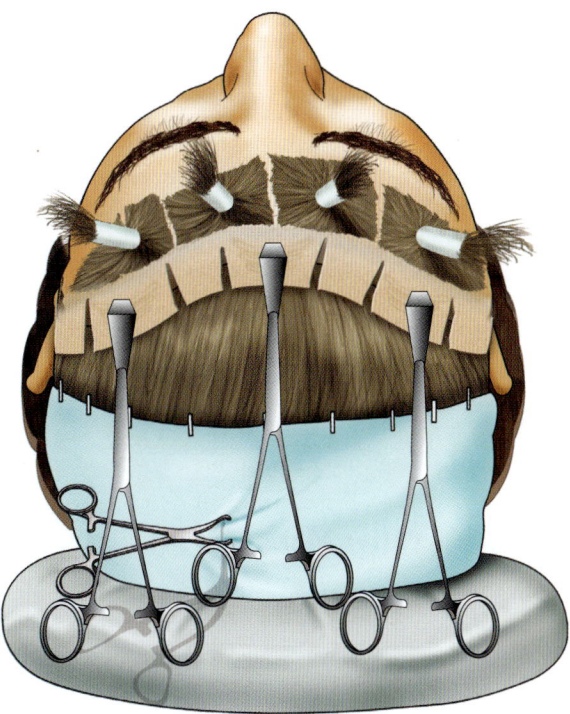

Figure 7-9. The coronal flap is redraped and elevated appropriately. Redundant skin can then be excised.

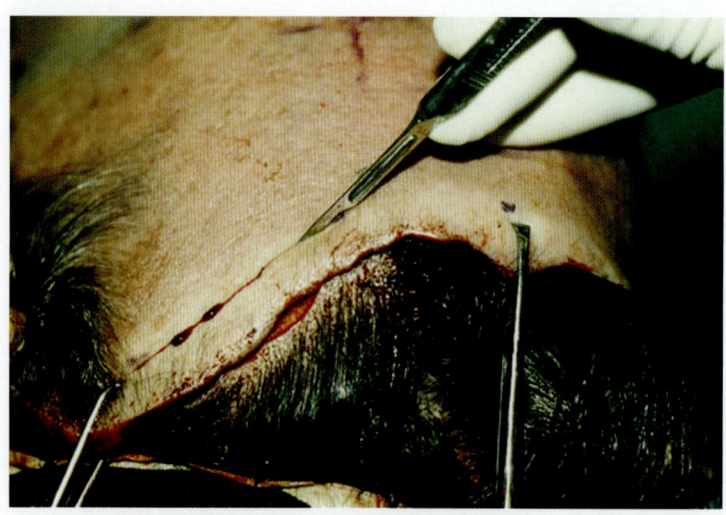

Figure 7-10. Trichophytic forehead lift. Excision of redundant skin with an irregularly irregular incision parallel to the trichophytic incision centrally. (Photo courtesy of Peter A. Adamson, MD.)

bevel identical to that made when making the initial incision (**Figure 7-10**). The galea (centrally) and the temporoparietal fascia (temporally) are then reapproximated with 3-0 polydiaxanone or other long-lasting resorbable sutures. It bears repeating that special caution is exercised in determining the amount of skin excision, especially in patients with borderline xerophthalmia or who have had prior blepharoplasty. If a concurrent upper blepharoplasty is planned, it generally should be performed *after* the forehead procedure, so that any lagophthalmos can be avoided.

Wound Closure

Before complete closure, a suction drain is placed under the flap and run along the supraorbital rims. The galea is then closed, followed by skin staples or a running 4-0 nylon suture. Care should be taken to ensure that minimal wound tension exists at the skin level. The skin edges should be everted, especially when using staples for skin closure (**Figure 7-11**). If a trichophytic or pretrichial central incision is used (**Figure 7-12**), again the flap is retraced and the excess skin excised at an appropriate angle. The galea is reapproximated and the skin closed with a running 5-0 polypropylene suture.

Postoperative Management

A mildly compressive dressing is placed over the forehead and ice compresses are placed over the forehead and eyes intermittently for the next 24 hours. The patient can be discharged home on the day of surgery; however, because a postoperative visit is required the following day, the patient may opt to stay in a nearby hotel to facilitate follow-up care. The head should be kept elevated, and the patient is discharged with a mild narcotic pain medication and (if not contraindicated) oral steroids (dexamethasone, 0.75 mg every 12 hours for 3 days). Although not required, patients are encouraged to take the homeopathic supplements *Arnica Montana* and bromelain beginning 3 weeks before the surgery, and those that do opt to take these supplements are maintained on them for 7 days postoperatively.

On the first postoperative day, the forehead is undressed and the drain can generally be removed as well. Typically, there is fairly substantial forehead and periorbital edema, which decreases over the first 5 to 7 days but may take up to 10 to 14 days to substantially decrease. The patient is instructed to apply topical antibiotic ointment three or four times per day to all sutures/staples. Beginning on postoperative day 2, the patient is allowed to shower, but because there will be fairly dense anesthesia of the forehead and scalp up to the crown for as long as 12 to 14 weeks, patients should be cautioned to wash with lukewarm water. If a hairdryer is used, it should be placed on the low heat setting and the patient's hand should be placed within the hair below the dryer to ensure that any excessive heat is recognized immediately.

Sutures and staples can be removed on postoperative day 7. Postoperative ecchymosis generally is limited to the upper eyelid and suborbital groove, and patients are allowed to use makeup

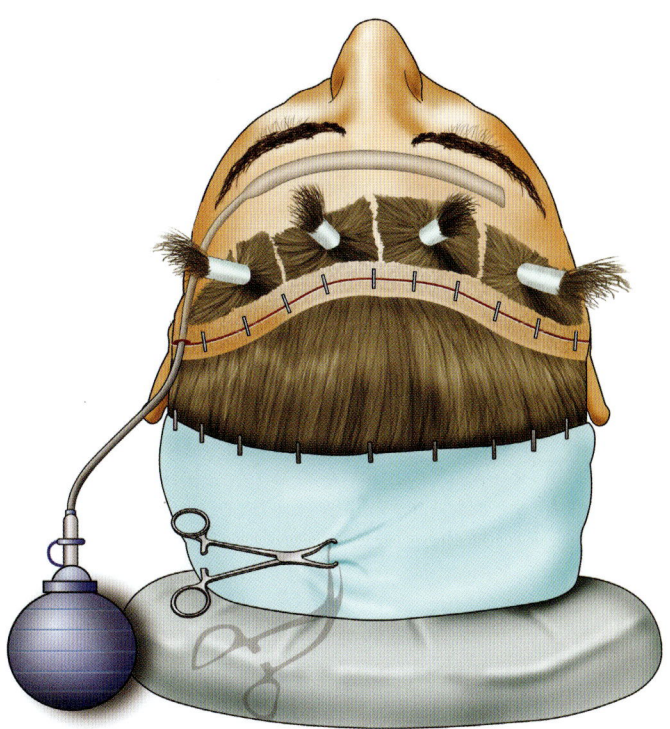

Figure 7-11. A suction drain is placed over the forehead and the wound closed is in two layers.

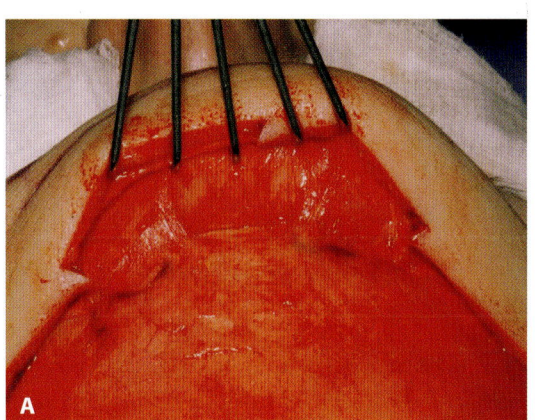

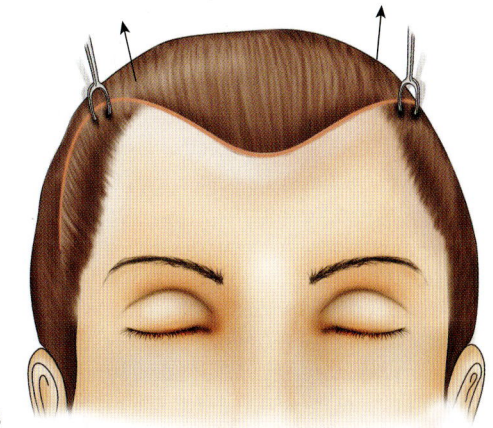

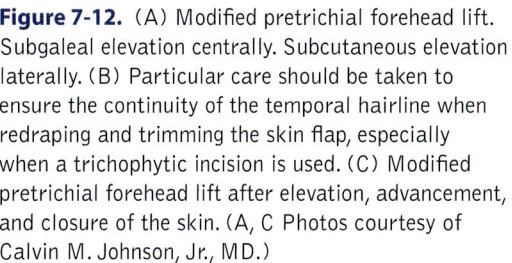

Figure 7-12. (A) Modified pretrichial forehead lift. Subgaleal elevation centrally. Subcutaneous elevation laterally. (B) Particular care should be taken to ensure the continuity of the temporal hairline when redraping and trimming the skin flap, especially when a trichophytic incision is used. (C) Modified pretrichial forehead lift after elevation, advancement, and closure of the skin. (A, C Photos courtesy of Calvin M. Johnson, Jr., MD.)

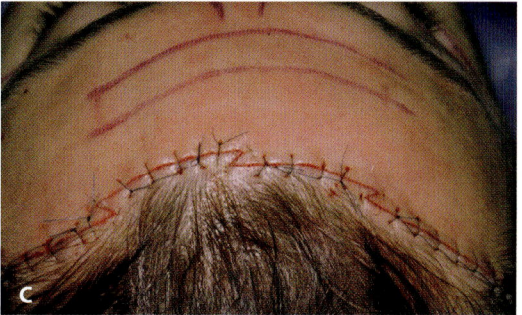

to camouflage this immediately. If a trichophytic incision is used, cosmetics can be applied 1 day after suture removal. Generally this incision, once mature, is well tolerated; however, in the early postoperative period (and occasionally beyond), patients are better served to choose a hairstyle that allows the frontal hair to drape downward over the scar.

Complications: Incidence, Management, and Avoidance

The coronal forehead lift is a proven workhorse procedure for improving the appearance of the forehead and brows. There are well-defined complications to the coronal forehead lift that should be discussed with the patient preoperatively, as with any other procedure. Because the most obvious disadvantage of the coronal forehead lift relates to the extensive scar, any event that adversely affects the quality or ability to camouflage that scar is a significant complication. Hair loss around the scar, although generally temporary, is not uncommon and can significantly compromise the final result of surgery. Pericicatricial alopecia has been reported in 0.2% to 33% of patients undergoing a coronal forehead lift. Temporary hair loss, telogen effluvium, is not uncommon after many other procedures and most likely represents a stress response to the surgery. However, even temporary hair loss can be significant to the patient and require a conscious effort by the patient to adequately style the hair to sufficiently camouflage the scar. Permanent hair loss occurs much less frequently and is on the order of 2.5% to 5%, although Adamson, Johnson, et al.[20] noted an 8% incidence of permanent temporal alopecia; with careful avoidance of excessive skin resection and ensuring minimal wound tension, this has been reduced to about 3% (P. Adamson, personal communication). Consideration should be given to excision of the area of alopecia or microfollicular hair transplantation if the hair fails to regrow. Ramirez attributed postoperative alopecia to excessive wound closure tension, the use of monopolar cautery, the use of "key" tension sutures during the closure, delayed suture removal, and the length of time the forehead flap is folded on itself (with possible vascular compromise, especially at the distal tip of the flap).

Similarly, a widening of the scar will make it more visible. Connell and coworkers[26] reported only 5 widened scars in 500 cases, and in a survey of plastic surgeons performing forehead procedures, unacceptable scarring was noted in 0.8% of coronal forehead lifts. However, Roberts et al.[27] and Adamson et al.[11] reported 15.3% and 12% incidences of widened scars. What defines a clinically significant widened scar is highly subjective, but it would seem reasonable to define such a scar as one that requires additional patient effort to camouflage; these appear to occur in 10% to 15% of patients. Again, scar excision (serial partial excision if excessively wide) or microfollicular hair transplantation can be performed if treatment is considered necessary. Avoiding excessive wound closure tension and ensuring that incisions are performed parallel to the follicles are the most important steps the surgeon can take to avoid this complication.

More problematic is the occurrence of postoperative neuralgias over the forehead and scalp; these can occasionally be permanent. The incidence of this complication ranges from 2% to 23% of cases, but generally resolves over a few months. However, it can be permanent in 2% to 5% of patients. Patients may describe "shooting pains," "electric shocks," or "burning sensation," all of which are presumably related to irritation of the supraorbital and supratrochlear nerves. Dissection, especially during treatment of the corrugator supercilii muscles, should carefully protect the multiple branches of these nerves. Permanent numbness is probably related to disruption of the terminal fibers of the supraorbital and supratrochlear nerves and has been reported in 1% to 8% of cases. Typically, this occurs in a relatively small region of the scalp and is generally well tolerated by patients, as long as they have been advised of this possibility preoperatively. Pruritus of the scalp is not uncommon and can be permanent. Even when temporary, pruritus may persist 3 to 9 months postoperatively. It has been reported to occur (at least temporarily) in 28% to 58% of coronal forehead lift patients, and Adamson and colleagues[20] reported a 10% incidence of permanent pruritus. The etiology of this is not clear but may be related to nerve injury as well.

Hematomas are uncommon after the coronal forehead lift, occurring in 0.6% to 2% of cases. Most dissection during the coronal forehead lift is done in relatively avascular planes, and bleeding should be minimal except from the edges of the skin incision. Before wound closure, the surgeon should ensure excellent hemostasis of all areas (including the skin edges), and either an active or a passive drain is generally sufficient. Hematomas, when present, are generally small and isolated and can frequently be managed by aspiration.

More significantly, temporary paralysis of the frontalis muscle due to injury to the temporal branch of the facial nerve is much more uncommon, occurring in 0.1% to 0.6% of patients, and permanent paralysis, although possible, is even less common. Mechanisms for nerve injury include use of monopolar cautery during the temporal dissection and stretching of the nerve while folding the flap on itself to access the supraorbital muscles; hence, careful and judicious use of bipolar cautery, especially during the temporal dissection, is essential; limiting traction on the flap, especially in the temple, will also help limit neuropraxia.

Conclusion

In appropriately selected and carefully prepared patients, the success rate of the coronal forehead lift is quite high (**Figures 7–13 and 7–14**). Connell and coworkers[26] reported that once treated, glabellar rhytids rarely recurred; however, they noted that 20% of patients treated for brow ptosis required revision surgery. The mechanism for maintenance of brow correction is probably multifactorial, and the best way of ensuring the longevity of brow ptosis correction is a complete release at the orbital rim and glabella and secure fixation at the galeal/periosteal layer. Roberts and Ellis[27] noted an 88% patient satisfaction rate after the coronal forehead lift, although only 65% of patients noted very good or excellent reduction in forehead wrinkles, and only 65% of patients would choose to undergo the procedure again. It is, however, a reliable and potent weapon to rejuvenate the upper third of the face.

Addendum: Coronal Subcutaneous Forehead Lift

The coronal subcutaneous forehead lift is the most extreme extension of the cutaneous scalp and forehead excision procedures of the early 20th century. It has been successfully advocated for patients with severely wrinkled foreheads and pronounced brow ptosis. Edwards[28] described a subcutaneous forehead lift with corrugator muscle excision, bitemporal neurotomies, and skin resection and advancement. More recently, Wolfe and Baird,[29] Vogel and Hoopes,[30] deBenito,[31] and Ullmann and Levy[32] all

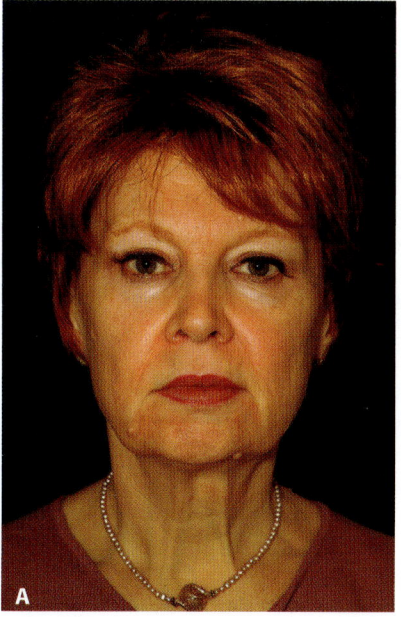 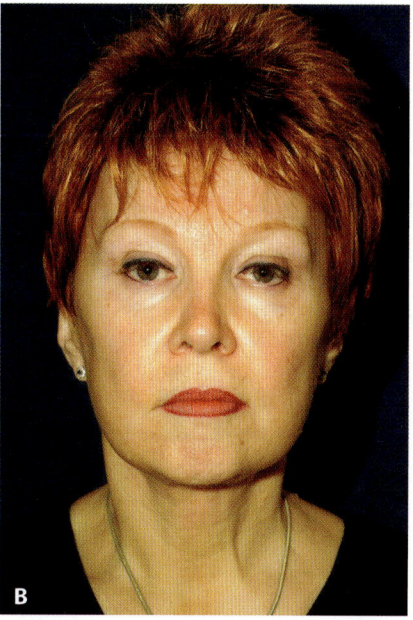

Figure 7-13. (A) A 58-year-old female with a chief complaint of "looking old." (B) Six months after coronal forehead lift, deep plane face and neck lift and shave excision of facial moles. (A, B Photos courtesy of Peter A. Adamson, MD.)

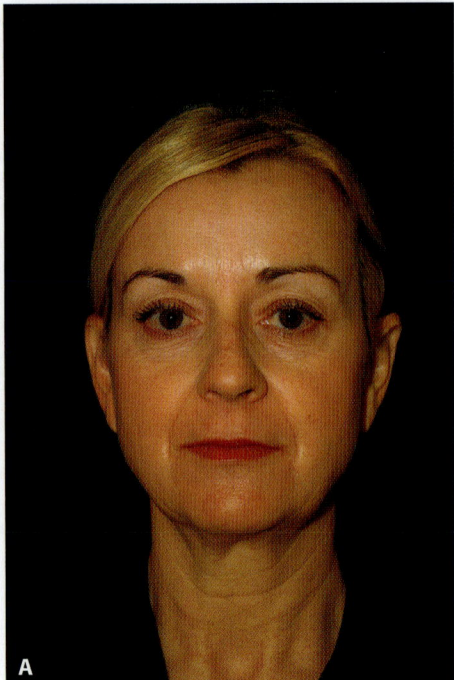
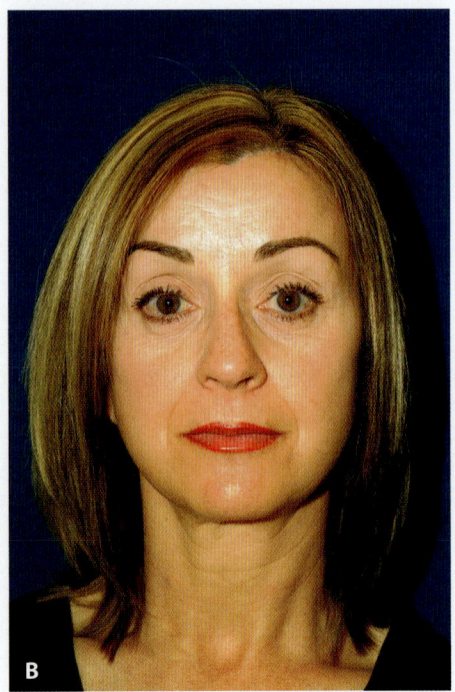

Figure 7-14. (A) A 51-year-old female with a chief complaint of "heavy" upper eyelids. (B) Fifteen months after trichophytic forehead lift and upper and lower blepharoplasties, and 12 months after deep plane face and neck lift and dermal filler injection for upper lip rhytids. (A, B Photo courtesy of Peter A. Adamson, MD.)

have been proponents of this procedure (without the neurotomies) in carefully selected patients with ptotic brows and severely creased central foreheads. This procedure also improves heavily hooded crows' feet.

A post-trichial or trichophytic incision is made through skin only. The subcutaneous tissue is then sharply dissected from the frontalis muscle down to the orbital rims. Portions of the corrugator muscles are directly excised. The skin is now dedraped superiorly, excess is excised, and the wound is closed in two layers. During dissection, great care must be taken to preserve the branches of the supratrochlear and supraorbital nerves.

The procedure, being skin-based, may have a relatively short period of effectiveness and up to one third of patients will have persistent hypesthesias/paresthesias postoperatively. In addition, great care must be taken in ensuring excellent hemostasis, because there is no well-developed surgical plane between the frontalis muscle and the dermis. Skin necrosis is a distinct possibility, especially in smokers or where significant tension on the wound closure exists.

One brow wrinkle is the result of 200,000 frowns.
Snapple bottle top, "real fact" #168, Snapple Beverage Corp., Rye Brook, NY

Acknowledgments

The author would like to thank Peter A. Adamson, MD, for assistance in the preparation of this chapter and Dr. Adamson and Calvin M. Johnson, Jr., MD, for the patient illustrations used in the chapter.

Suggested Readings

1. Gonzalez-Ulloa M. Facial wrinkles. Integral elimination. Plast Reconstr Surg 1962;29:658–673.
2. Vinas JC, Caviglia C, Cortinas JL. Forehead rhytidoplasty and brow lifting. Plast Reconstr Surg 1976;57:445–454.
3a. Ramirez OM. The anchor subperiosteal forehead lift. Plast Reconstr Surg 1995;95:993–1003.
3b. Ramirez OM. Anchor subperiosteal forehead lift: from open to endoscopic. Plast Reconstr Surg 2001;107:868–871.

4. Pitanguy I. Indications for and treatment of frontal and glabellar wrinkles in an analysis of 3,404 consecutive cases of rhytidectomy. Plast Reconstr Surg 1981;67:157–168.

5. Pitanguy I. Section of the frontalis-procerus corrugator aponeurosis in the correction of frontal and glabellar wrinkles. Ann Plast Surg 1979;5:422–427.

6. Toledo GA, Tate JL. Coronal approach for rejuvenation of the eyes and forehead. Arch Otolaryngol Head Neck Surg 1986;112:738–744.

7. Brennan HG. The frontal lift. Arch Otolarngol 1978; 104:26–30.

8. Wojtanowski MH. Bicoronal forehead lift. Aesthetic Plast Surg 1994;18:33–39.

9. Dayan SH, Perkins SW, Vartanian AJ, Wiesman IM. The forehead lift: endoscopic versus coronal approaches. Aesthetic Plast Surg 2001;25:35–39.

10. Adamson PA. The forehead lift: refinements in technique. J Otolaryngol 1986;15:89–93.

11. Adamson PA, Johnson CM, Anderson JR, Dupin CL. The forehead lift. A review. Arch Otolaryngol 1985; 111:325–329.

12. Brennan HG. The forehead lift. Otolaryngol Clin North Am 1980;13:209–223.

13. Uchida J-I. A method of frontal rhytidectomy. Plast Reconstr Surg 1965;35:218–222.

14. Paul MD. The evolution of the brow lift in aesthetic plastic surgery. Plast Reconstr Surg 2001;108: 1409–1424.

15. Walden JL, Brown CC, Klapper AJ, Chia CT, Aston SJ. An anatomical comparision of transpalpebral, endoscopic, and coronal approaches to demonstrate exposure and extent of brow depressor muscle resection, Plcx Reunstr Surg 2005; 116:1479–1487.

16. Fleming RW, Mayer TG. Hairline aesthetics and styling in hair replacement surgery. Head Neck Surg 1985;7:286–302.

17. Fleming RW, Mayer TG. Scalp flaps—reconstruction of the unfavorable result in hair replacement surgery. Head Neck Surg 1985;7:315–331.

18. Holcomb JD, McCollough EG. Trichophytic incisional approaches to upper facial rejuvenation. Arch Facial Plast Surg 2001;3:48–53.

19. Adamson PA, Cormier R, McGraw BL. The coronal forehead lift—modifications and results. J Otolaryngol 1992;21:25–29.

20. Connell BF, Lambros VS, Neurohr GH. The forehead lift: techniques to avoid complications and produce optimal results. Aesthetic Plast Surg 1989;13: 217–237.

21. Nassif PS, Kokoska MS, Homan S, et al. Comparison of subperiosteal vs subgaleal elevation techniques used in forehead lifts. Arch Otolaryngol Head Neck Surg 1998;124:1209–1215.

22. Knize DM. Reassessment of the coronal incision and subgaleal dissection for foreheadplasty. Plast Reconstr Surg 1998;102:478–489.

23. Flowers RS, Caputy GG, Flowers SS. The biomechanics of brow and frontalis function and its effect on blepharoplasty. Clin Plast Surg 1993;20: 255–268.

24. Kaye BL. The forehead lift: a useful adjunct to face lift and blephaoplasty. Plast Reconstr Surg 1977;60: 161–171.

25. Friedland JA, Jacobsen WM, TerKinda S. Safety and efficacy of combined upper blepharoplasties and open coronal browlift: a consecutive series of 600 patients. Aesthetic Plast Surg 1996;20:453–462.

26. Roberts TL, Ellis LB. In pursuit of optimal rejuvenation of the forehead: endoscopic brow lift with simultaneous carbon dioxide laser resurfacing. Plast Reconstr Surg 1998;101:1075–1084.

27. McKinney P, Mossie RD, Zukowski ML. Criteria for the forehead lift. Aesthetic Plast Surg 1991;15: 141–147.

28. Edwards BF. Bilateral temporal neurotomy for frontalis hypermotility. Case report. Plast Reconstr Surg 1957;19:341–345.

29. Wolfe AS, Baird WL. The subcutaneous forehead lift. Plast Reconstr Surg 1989;83:251–256.

30. Vogel JE, Hoopes JE. The subcutaneous forehead lift with an anterior hairline incision. Ann Plast Surg 1992;28:257–265.

31. deBenito J. Aesthetic incision in the subcutaneous forehead lift. Aesthetic Plast Surg 1993;17: 239–242.

32. Ullmann Y, Levy Y. In favor of the subcutaneous forehead lift using the anterior hairline incision. Aesthetic Plast Surg 1998;22:332–337.

8

Limited Incision Approaches for Brow and Forehead Rejuvenation Procedures

The greatest pleasure I know, is to do a good action by stealth, and to have it found out by accident.
Charles Lamb (1775–1834)

Introduction

Patients who express dissatisfaction with their appearance and who are candidates for periorbital rejuvenation often assume the only or most effective corrective procedure is a blepharoplasty. They will often stress that they wish to avoid a "hollowed-out" or "surprised" appearance and desire only conservative lid changes. The most astute and sophisticated patients often overlook the significant effect that brow position has upon upper eyelid appearance. Even mild brow ptosis will affect the overall appearance of the eyes in such a way that the upper blepharoplasty cannot correct. Moreover, upper lid blepharoplasty has been shown to result in up to a 3-mm drop in the height of the eyebrow postoperatively. Most likely, there is a reflexive contraction of the frontalis muscle preoperatively, which would assist in mitigating the effect of lateral brow ptosis on the patient's visual field. With the excision of an appropriate amount of upper lid skin, the visual field cut is improved, reducing the need for this frontalis activity, resulting in a subtle drop in brow position as frontalis tone decreases.

Patients, however, may not require a complete forehead lift, whereas blepharoplasty alone leaves them undercorrected. Alternatively, some patients who would benefit from a complete brow and forehead lift may be suboptimal candidates or refuse a standard open or endoscopic approach. A number of procedures have been described that can adjust specific or global brow and forehead issues. By carefully examining and analyzing the patient-specific needs, the surgeon may find that brow and forehead aesthetics can be addressed and improved with procedures that limit incisions and dissections and, in turn, ecchymosis, edema, and/or recovery time for the patient.

Transtemporal Limited Incision Approaches

Indications: mild, lateral brow ptosis with only minimal central or medial brow ptosis or glabellar furrows.
Contraindications: severe medial and central brow ptosis; bald or preexisting high temporal hairline.
Ideal candidate: thick temporal hair tuft; isolated lateral brow ptosis (mild to moderate).
Scientific basis: varies by specific procedure: most rely on release of fascial attachments at the temporal crest and/or orbital ligament.

History

The history of limited incision brow and forehead rejuvenation is relatively short. As noted in previous chapters, early work in forehead and brow surgery was limited to large and more obvious incisional approaches, from the direct suprabrow to midforehead incisions/excisions and finally to the coronal incision in the 1970s. These approaches, as initially developed, relied on skin excision for brow elevation, but the desire for a more long-lasting correction led to the more stable and reliable fixation methods in the deeper tissue planes of muscle, fascia, and periosteum. One of the earliest attempts to modify brow position in a minimally invasive way was described by Parkes and Kamer in 1976.[1] These authors used loops of permanent sutures through the brow soft tissue and fixated superiorly to the superficial galea in the post-trichial forehead. This approach was overshadowed by the subsequent popularization of the coronal forehead lift, which ruled supreme for most of the next decade and a half. However, dissatisfaction with the long scar, extensive dissection, and often prolonged recovery associated with the coronal approach prompted development of less invasive treatments of the brow and forehead. Today, we primarily think of the endoscopic browlift when considering minimally invasive options. There are, however, a number of other nonendoscopic, limited incision procedures designed to provide focused improvements in the appearance of the brow and forehead. Unfortunately, the small, often distant incisions utilized in these procedures frequently limit the degree of permanence of successful rejuvenation of the brow. However, when these procedures are intelligently selected and carefully applied in the correct circumstances, they can achieve significant aesthetic improvements with small, well-hidden incisions and limited recovery.

These procedures may include temporal fascia and galeal elevation, release of the orbital-retaining ligament, and suspension performed through temporal incisions[2], often combined with paramedian[3] or upper lid supratarsal crease incisions.[4,5] Alternatively, solely transpalpebral approaches have been advocated, primarily for brow sculpting and glabellar myoplasties,[4,5-9] although some brow elevation does occur. Finally, isolated forehead approaches have been described.[10,11]

Although a surgeon may not choose to include all of these procedures in his or her repertoire, familiarity with and evaluation of each, coupled with an appreciation of brow physiology, provide the reader with a better understanding of the degree of change possible with various surgical maneuvers and interventions. This understanding will also be useful in evaluating nonsurgical treatments of the brow, such as botulinum toxin and injectable soft tissue fillers.

Rationale and Scientific Basis

The scientific basis of limited incision forehead procedures is difficult to describe, because these techniques attempt to exploit a variety of tissue planes and structures to enhance the appearance of the forehead and brow. Early limited incision procedures such as the suture suspension simply raised the brow by elevating the brow along the glide plane space and fixating it in position with dermal sutures at a higher level mechanically. Subsequent procedures incorporated a wider plane of dissection, usually at a subperiosteal level, to provide fixation through a wider scar bed in addition to fixation sutures or implants. This deeper plane of dissection also provided a greater *release,* thus reducing the tension required to mobilize and stabilize the position of the brow.

Procedures performed through a blepharoplasty incision provide access to the orbital rim, where the deep brow tissues can be fixed directly to the frontal bone in an elevated position. In addition, the transpalpebral approach enables the surgeon to perform brow depressor myotomies, decreasing the downward muscular pull that the corrugator and depressor supercilii and procerus muscles exert on the brow as well as sculpt brow fat

Physiologically, elevating the forehead tissues, removing/reducing the inferiorly directed forces acting on the brow, and fixating the brow at a higher position leaves the frontalis activity unopposed. The involuntary contraction of the frontalis muscle subsequently decreases because the brow has been surgically elevated into a position that does not obstruct vision. The lack of depressor muscle activity smoothes the glabella, whereas the decreased frontalis contraction smoothes the forehead. The chief issues of concern regarding these limited incision approaches are the degree of elevation possible and the longevity of that correction.

Advantages, Disadvantages, and Alternatives

The main advantage of limited incision surgical approaches to the brow is obvious—smaller incisions with less extensive dissection, generally with less morbidity, and a faster recovery. Several small incisions are more easily and more thoroughly camouflaged than a long coronal incision. Patients with advanced alopecia may be inappropriate candidates for coronal or endoscopic browlift. Depending upon the specific limited incision approach taken, different areas (central brow and forehead, lateral brow and temple, glabella) will be better accessed and addressed; combining approaches may provide adequate access to multiple areas of interest.

It should be obvious from the previous discussion that an accurate and complete preoperative evaluation and analysis of aesthetic needs is critical if a limited incision procedure is chosen, because full access to all subunits of the brow and forehead is not always possible with most limited approaches performed singly. Transtemporal approaches can be useful in elevating the tail and central brow and can provide some smoothing of the forehead. Lateral forehead incisions are limited in the access they provide to the central brow (unless combined with a central forehead incision and forehead dissection), but can be used successfully to elevate the tail of the brow. Transpalpebral approaches can elevate the lateral brow, address glabellar musculature, smooth the forehead, and allow soft tissue "sculpting" of brow tissue. Finally, all of these procedures can be performed without specialized or endoscopic equipment.

Conversely, limited incisions provide limited access to some areas and adequate exposure and treatment may require multiple approaches. Transtemporal approaches alone cannot adequately treat the glabellar muscles or medial brow. Transpalpebral approaches are hindered laterally by the zone of fixation just medial to the temporal crest (see Chapter 2) and (partially) by the supraorbital neurovascular pedicle medially. Additional medial palpebral dissection is required to access medial brow depressor musculature. With limited dissections, the amount of brow elevation feasible is less than with an open or endoscopic approach: this is not only due to more limited dissection in general but, as only certain portions of the brow are being targeted, significant focal brow elevation may create an "unbalanced," "unpleasant," "quizzical," or "surprised" appearance.

Alternatives to the limited incision techniques include more extensive procedures, such as the endoscopic forehead lift. The endoscopic forehead lift incorporated the temporal approach, the glabellar dissection, and myotomies performed in trans-

palpebral approaches and the central and lateral forehead dissection and elevation. Each of these can be performed independently as a limited incision procedure. In addition, brow and forehead lifts can be performed with an open approach such as the coronal forehead lift.

Indications and Contraindications

The indications for a limited incision surgical procedure for brow and forehead rejuvenation vary by the approach. In general, limited incision procedures typically can be used to smoothly elevate the brow 3 to 4 mm and can be especially beneficial in balding patients.

Temporal Approaches

Limited incision approaches through the temple generally can elevate the tail of the brow 3 to 5mm. In addition to the lateral brow elevation, the midbrow generally also elevates, but to a lesser degree; there may be effacement of forehead creases due to relaxation of frontalis muscle contraction in patients who reflexively elevate moderate to severe lateral brow ptosis.

A limited incision temporal approach is, therefore, indicated for mild degrees of lateral brow ptosis with only minimal central brow ptosis or glabellar furrows. A temporal approach alone is relatively contraindicated in the presence of severe central and medial brow ptosis, because principally elevating the brow tail will produce an unpleasant appearance; however, combining a transtemporal approach with a transpalpebral treatment of the brow depressors can avoid this unwanted result. Temporal approaches are also relatively contraindicated in patients with preexisting high temporal hairlines.

Transpalpebral Approaches

Transpalpebral approaches provide access to both the brow depressor muscles as well as the central and lateral brows. In addition, a translid approach also exposes the brow fat and allows for contouring lipectomy in patients with prominent and/or ptotic brow fat pads.[12] In patients undergoing concurrent upper blepharoplasty, no additional incisions are required, a major benefit of this approach. However, stabilization of the elevated brow through this approach can be more limited compared with the transtemporal approach, and a cadaver study by Walden and coworkers[13] demonstrated myotomies

---

Transpalpebral Limited Incision Approaches

Indications: moderate brow ptosis; mild glabellar rhytids in patient with high hairline or male pattern alopecia.
Contraindications: prior periorbital trauma; active eye disease; severe brow ptosis or furrows.
Ideal candidate: mild brow ptosis and glabellar furrows; concurrent upper blepharoplasty.
Scientific basis: varies by procedure: most rely on subperiosteal elevation and release, superiorly-directed fixation.

---

performed through a transpalpebral approach were less complete than those performed through either a coronal or an endoscopic approach. Transpalpebral myotomies of the corrugator and depressor supercilii and procerus muscles will allow for a modest degree (2–4 mm) of medial brow elevation.

The transpalpebral approach to browlifting is thus indicated for moderate (3–4 mm) lateral brow ptosis, mild (2–4 mm) medial brow ptosis, mild to moderate glabellar or midforehead rhytids, or for patients with heavy brow fat herniating below the orbital rim. Also, patients with male pattern baldness, very high hairlines, prior frontal hair transplantation, or highly convex foreheads should be considered for this approach. This approach is relatively contraindicated in patients with prior periorbital trauma, eye disease, or severe brow ptosis or glabellar furrows.

Forehead Approaches

A lateral forehead approach, typically through small trichophytic incisions, can also moderately elevate the lateral brow, but it sacrifices access to the medial brow muscles. An incision and approach medial to the supraorbital and supratrochlear nerves is additionally required if complete forehead dissection is necessary. As with transtemporal approaches, this approach is also contraindicated in patients with moderate to severe medial brow ptosis.

Transforehead Limited Incision Approaches

Indications: mild lateral and central brow ptosis.
Contraindications: moderate to severe medial brow ptosis.
Ideal candidate: mild lateral and central brow ptosis; adequate frontal hair density.
Scientific basis: varies by procedure: most rely on subperiosteal elevation, superior flap advancement.

Range of Anesthesia

Limited incision approaches, by necessity, decrease to a certain degree surgical exposure and generate a "tighter" operative field. In performing these procedures, the level of anesthesia chosen should not only provide sufficient patient comfort but also ensure adequate patient cooperation. Most areas of the forehead and temple can be anesthetized with several easily applied nerve blocks. However, complete and accurate dissection with protection of important structures (especially in the temple and including the temporal crest) can be difficult in patients receiving regional nerve blockade and local infiltration only. In addition, full transpalpebral exposure and treatment of the medial brow depressors requires a degree of skin retraction patients may find uncomfortable despite adequate analgesia. The surgeon should strongly consider (at least oral) sedation in these cases. Dissection over the forehead and orbital rim is generally well tolerated after supratrochlear and supraorbital nerve blocks. Of course, patients should be provided with appropriate analgesia and anxiolysis, and general anesthesia should be considered as well, based on the patient's health and preferences.

Equipment

Limited incision forehead and temple techniques generally require a minimal number of instruments in addition to those found in a standard facial plastic surgical soft tissue tray. Transtemporal dissection is facilitated by narrow right-angle retractors and a Freer elevator, and although not necessary, a flat endoscopic periosteal elevator can aid in dissection. Transpalpebral approaches to the forehead and brow can be performed quickly with Senn, Desmarres, or narrow right-angle retractors, cautery (monopolar and bipolar), and a Freer or endoscopic elevator. If bony fixation is to be performed through either a transpalpebral or a forehead dissection, a drill is additionally required. Good overhead lights and a strong headlight or lighted retractor enable excellent visualization.

Operating Room Setup

As with all forehead procedures, complete access to the entire head of the patient should be ensured, with the patient's occiput resting at the top of the operating room table. The surgeon is seated at the head of the table, but should always have access to both sides of the patient's head. Ironically, it is with the transpalpebral approach that access to the patient's side is most important, because the surgeon needs an unobstructed visual axis to visualize the supraorbital rim, lower forehead, superomedial orbit, and glabella underneath the wound margins.

Techniques

Transpalpebral Approaches

Incision

Transpalpebral approaches use a standard upper blepharoplasty incision, which is placed at the supratarsal crease (**Figure 8-1**). When a blepharoplasty is to be performed concurrently, the planned skin excision is marked preoperatively with the patient in a seated upright position, and the supratarsal and superior incisions are marked while the brow is held manually in its desired location (**Figure 8-2**). Skin excision should be deferred until after the brow elevation is complete, at least until the surgeon has gained sufficient experience with the procedure.

Plane(s) of Dissection

All transpalpebral brow approaches utilize the relatively avascular suborbicularis/preaponeurotic plane to access the orbital rim. When a concurrent blepharoplasty is planned, it is best to defer incision of the orbital septum and resection of

pseudoherniated fat until the brow procedure has been performed, thus keeping the tissue planes unobstructed. The suborbicularis fascia is easily swept off the septum with a cotton tip applicator, and a Desmarres retractor can expose the central and lateral orbital rim. With this maneuver, the arcus marginalis is easily visualized (**Figure 8-3**). Further pre-periosteal dissection may require a minimal amount of sharp dissection.

Tissue Modifications

Glabellar Myoplasty. In patients with moderate medial brow ptosis, glabellar myotomies can provide sufficient elevation of the medial brow as well as reduce glabellar rhytids. The orbital septum is followed medial to the supratrochlear neurovascular bundle and the superomedial orbital rim is exposed. A Senn or Desmarres retractor assists in exposure (**Figure 8-4A–D**). The origin of the corrugator supercilii muscle is identified medial to the trochlea; often, the muscle can be identified by "strumming" over its surface with a blunt instrument (**see Figure 8-4E**). The muscle is then grasped and both sides of a 5-mm strip are cauterized with a bipolar cautery and the muscle strip excised (removing with it a portion of the depressor supercilii muscle) (**see Figure 8-4F, G**). Next, a 5 × 5-mm square of superiomedial orbicularis oculi muscle is excised from the undersurface of the flap at the medial head of the brow. In patients with horizontal glabellar rhytids, the

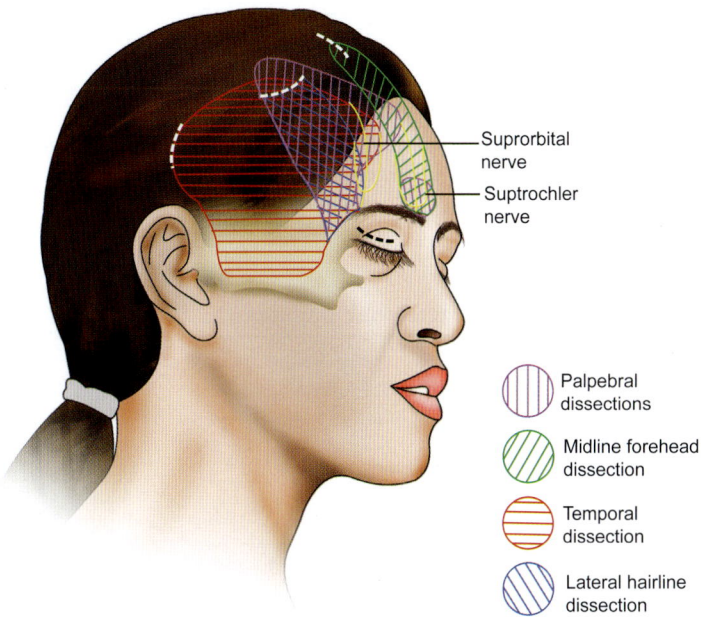

Figure 8-1. Ranges of dissection possible through various minimal incision approaches.

Suprorbital nerve

Suptrochler nerve

Palpebral dissections

Midline forehead dissection

Temporal dissection

Lateral hairline dissection

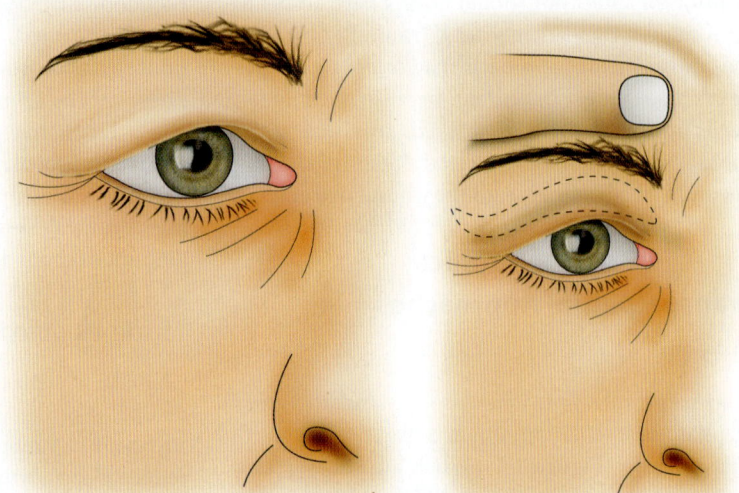

Figure 8-2. (A, B) Transpalpebral approaches to the brow and forehead use a standard upper blepharoplasty skin excision. If skin excision is not necessary, the lower, supratarsal crease, incision is used alone.

A　　　　　　**B**

procerus muscle is then incised by sliding a curved Stevens or small Metzenbaum scissors medially under the skin in a blunt fashion (**see Figure 8-4H**).

Browplasty. McCord and Doxanas[7] described a method to improve the aesthetics of the "heavy" brow. In these patients, an adequate brow *position* may be obscured by excessive brow *bulk* (**Figure 8-5A**). Anatomically, this situation has been described by Knize[2,14-16] in his extensive forehead dissection in cadavers (see Chapter 2). Knize delineated a number of fascial layers derived from the deep galea that envelop and surround the galeal fat pad. In addition, he noted that in some specimens, the two layers of deep galea that should fuse together and form a lower limit to the galeal fat pad compartment may be relatively insubstantial. Knize postulated that this weak lower boundary to the galeal fat pad would allow significant lateral brow descent, as well as inferior pseudoherniation of the galeal fat pad, which can abut and augment upper lid preseptal fat, producing unwanted volume below the brow.

In these cases, the patient would benefit from direct excision of this descended fat. Through the transpalpebral approach, the orbital rim is accessed. With proper superior retraction, the bulge of the galeal fat pad can be seen on the undersurface of the flap (**see Figure 8-5B–D**); careful dissection with a needle cautery can excise this unwanted fat (**see Figure 8-5E**). The surgeon must carefully dissect the fat, avoiding the underlying muscle and dermis, staying lateral to the supraorbital nerve. Medially, the corrugator supercilii muscle crosses into and then above the galeal fat pad as it runs laterally. The transverse head of the corrugator generally extends 1 cm lateral to the supraorbital nerve, and whereas in this location it is usually superior and superficial to the galeal fat pad, the surgeon should be aware of its proximity. If no other brow modification is necessary, the supratarsal crease incision is then closed (**see Figure 8-5F**).

Transpalpebral Limited Incision Approaches
Incisions: upper blepharoplasty supratarsal crease.
Tissue modifications: vary by procedure: subperiosteal elevation with/without fixation or brow depressor myotomies.
Fixation: varies by procedure.
Wound closure: standard upper blepharoplasty single-layer skin closure.
Complications: hematoma; temporary forehead hypesthesia (rare).

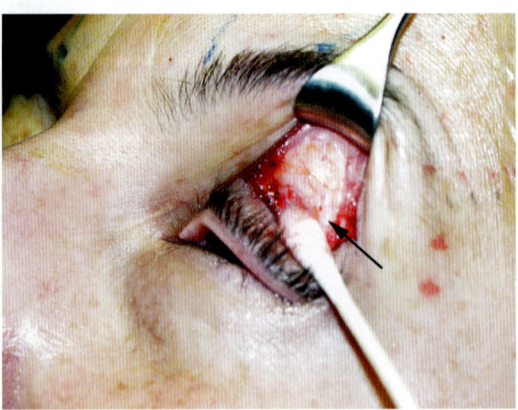

Figure 8-3. Once the orbicularis oculi muscle is incised and elevated superiorly, the septum orbitale can be followed up to the arcus marginalis, easily identified as a white condensation along the orbital rim.

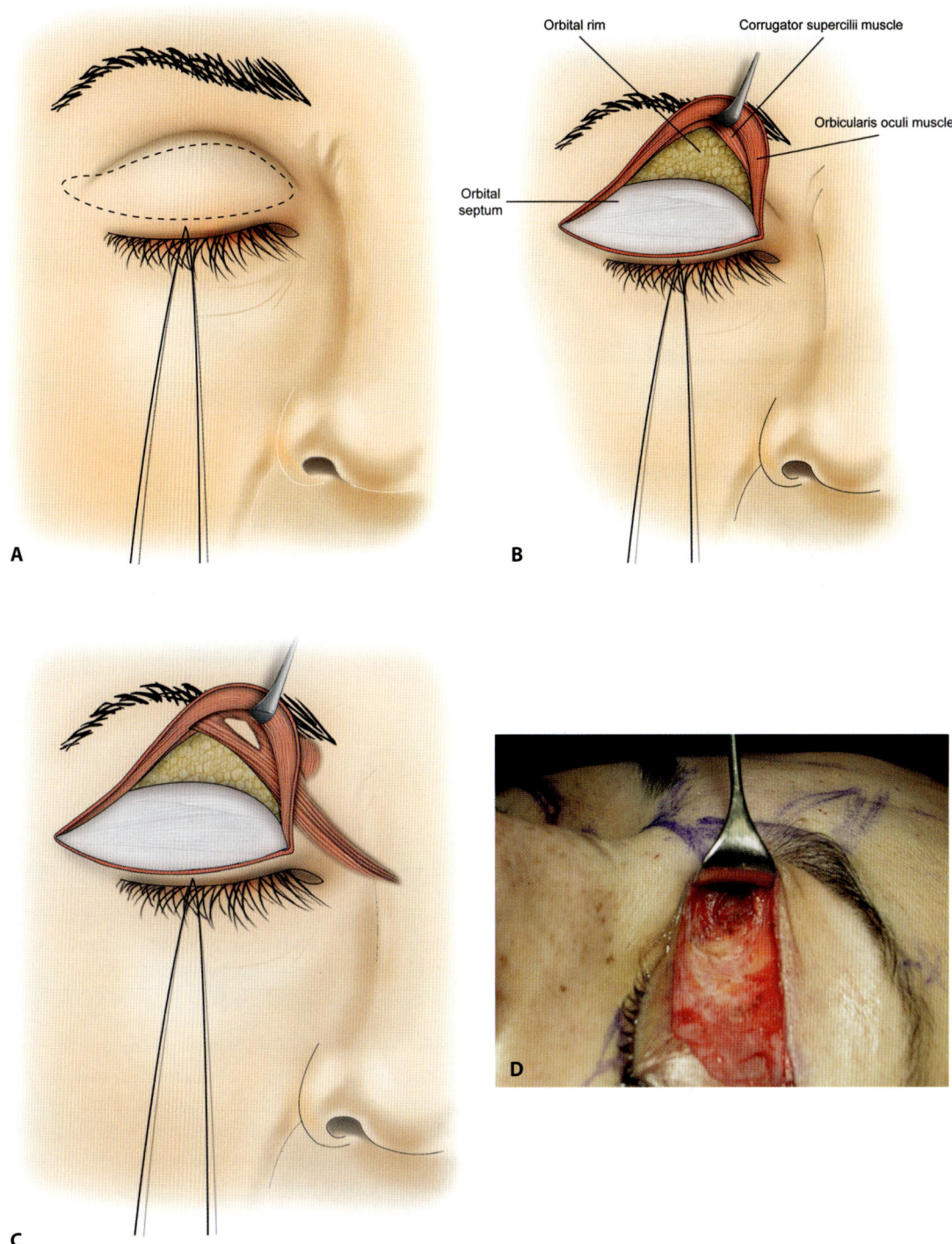

Figure 8-4. Glabellar myoplasty. (A) The upper lid is placed on traction and the upper lid skin is resected as in a standard upper blepharoplasty. (B) The orbicularis oculi muscle is incised and retracted superiorly over the orbital rim. The corrugator supercilii muscle is identified medially under the orbicularis muscle. (C) Further medial retraction gains improved corrugator exposure. (D) Close-up view of the left glabellar dissection. *(Continued)*

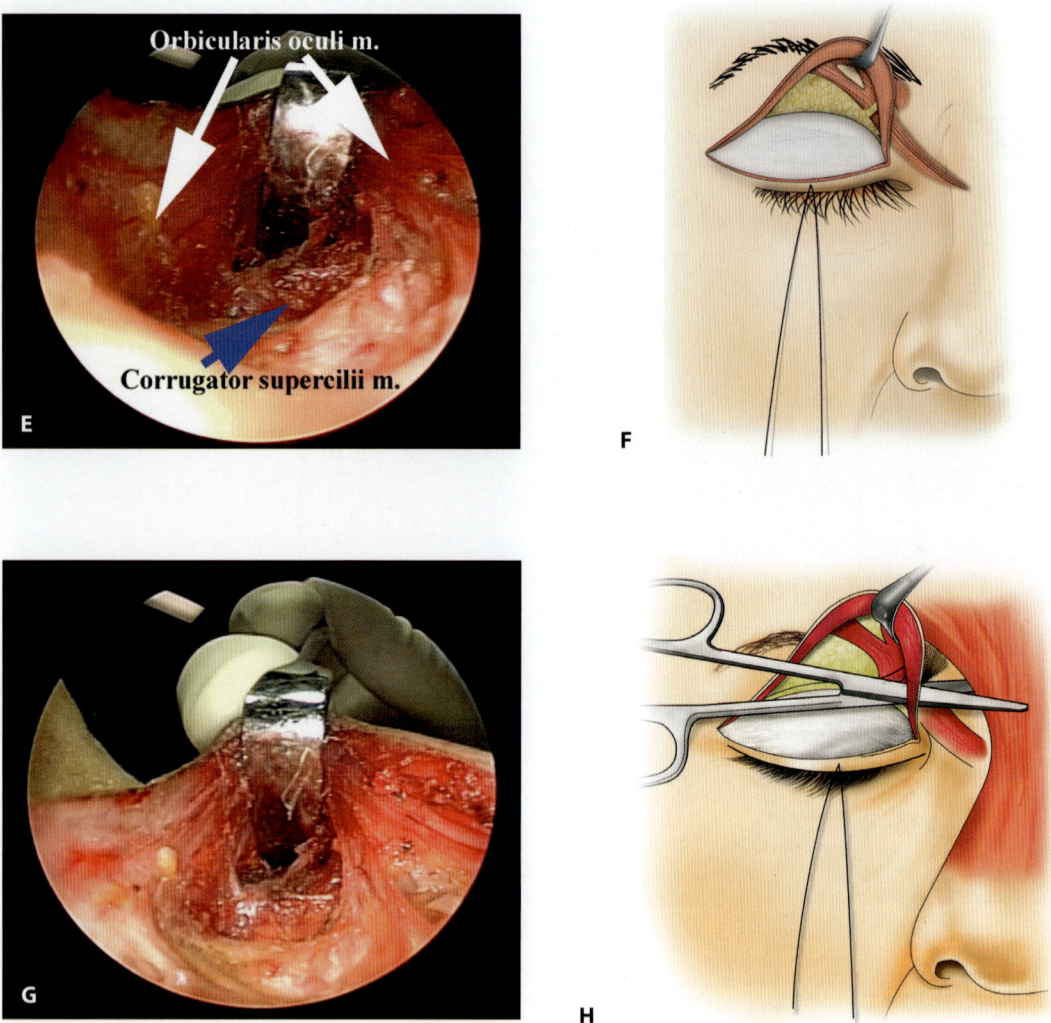

Figure 8-4. *(Continued)* (E) Left medial periorbital dissection. (F) A segment of corrugator supercilii muscle is excised and the edges cauterized. (G) Left orbital dissection demonstrates resection of a segment of corrugator muscle. (H) For horizontal glabellar rhytids, the procerus muscle can be divided blindly with scissors.

Lateral Browpexy. A number of authors have described methods to elevate the lateral brow through a transpalpebral approach. Difficulties encountered with this approach included limitations on medial forehead dissection and elevation owing to the location of the supraorbital neurovascular bundle; restraint of brow elevation by the orbital ligament; difficulty in providing adequate fixation high enough above the orbital rim through a relatively small (upper blepharoplasty) incision; and difficulty in providing sufficiently robust fixation to maintain brow elevation.

From previous discussion of brow anatomy (see Chapter 2), it should be recognized that a "pre-periosteal" plane of dissection of the forehead accessed through an upper blepharoplasty incision is in actuality performed in an "intragaleal" plane, because a leaf of the deep galea fuses tightly with the periosteum roughly 2 cm above the orbital rim. It should also be recalled that the deep branch of the supraorbital nerve generally runs in this plane as it travels superolaterally toward the temporal crest. Hence, any continued intragaleal dissection of the forehead beyond a 5- to 7-mm strip over the lateral orbital rim puts this nerve at risk for injury, which can cause postoperative crown anesthesia or neuralgia.

Before the introduction of bony fixation, stabilization of the brow elevated through a transpalpebral

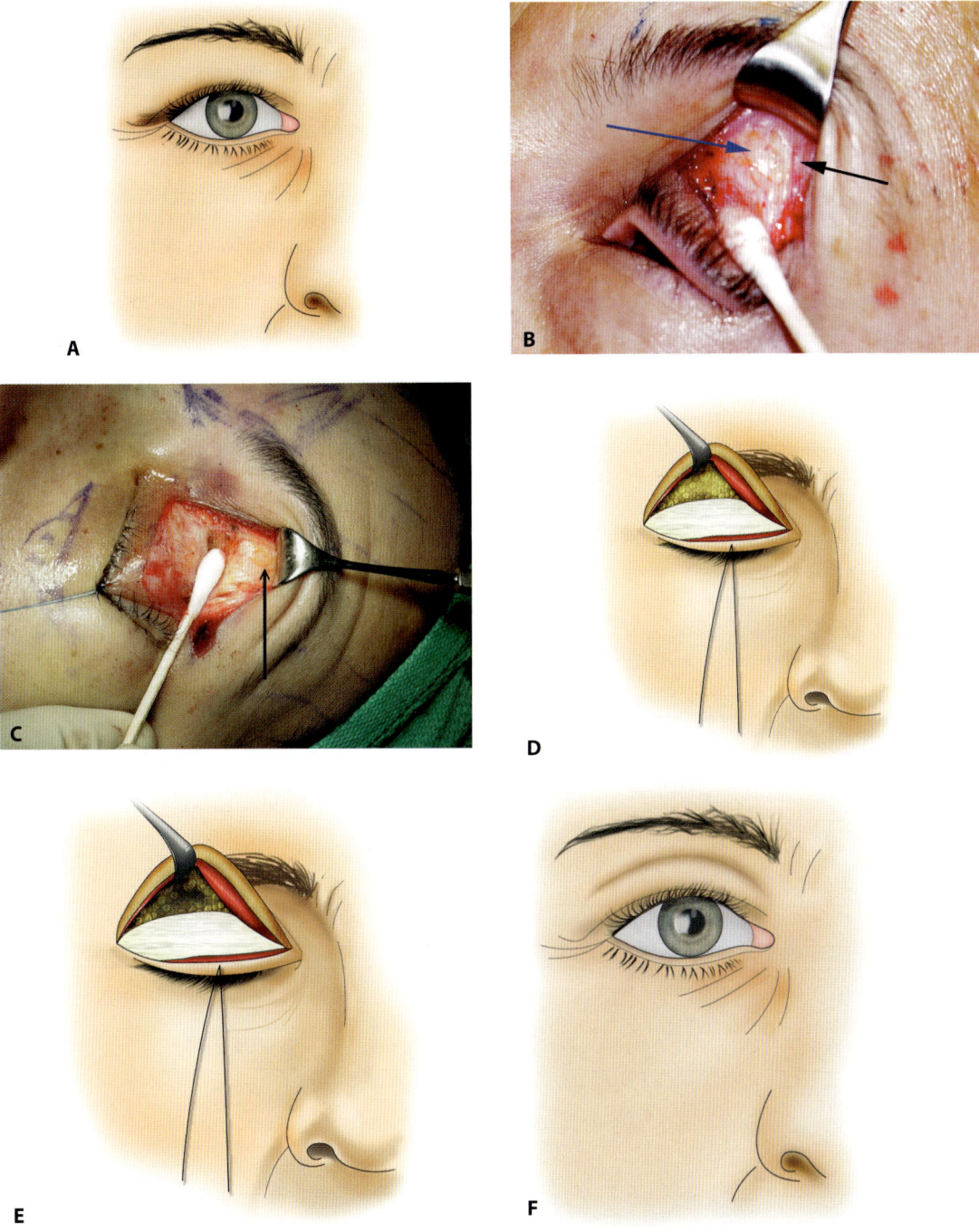

Figure 8-5. (A) Patients with excessive brow bulk will appear to have "heavy" brows, especially centrally and temporally. (B) Bulging orbital fat can be seen over the central and temporal orbital rim. (C) The brow fat can be accessed by following the septum orbitale up to the orbital rim. (D) Further retraction of the orbicularis oculi muscle allows complete access to this fat. Bulging fat is resected and cauterized (E), improving the contour of the upper eyelid (F).

incision relied on soft tissue scarring. Sokol and Sokol[8] described creation of bileaved flaps of orbicularis oculi muscle and periosteum at the lateral orbital rim. By suturing these together, they attempted to provide significant adhesion of the soft tissues *below* the brow to the orbital rim, thus elevating the lateral brow *above* the rim of the orbit. Niechajev[17] described suturing the orbicularis oculi muscle superiorly to the frontalis muscle, and Zarem and colleagues[18] noted that "modest" elevation of the lateral brow could be attained by suturing the orbicularis muscle superiorly to the arcus marginalis. McCord and Doxanas[7] placed these periosteal sutures 1 cm above the orbital rim (**Figure 8-6A**). A permanent 3-0 monofilament suture is passed transcutaneously at the lower limit of the brow (**see Figure 8-6B**); the needle is grasped and then placed through the periosteum at the desired height of the lower brow border (as measured preoperatively in millimeters above the inferior aspect of the orbital rim while manually elevating the brow). At this point, the suture tail (left in place to mark the lower brow border position on the undersurface of the flap) is removed and a mattress suture placed in the flap at this location (**see Figure 8-6C**). Multiple sutures are placed lateral to the supraorbital nerve but should not be tied until all have been placed.

Transpalpebral Endotine Browpexy. The recent introduction of slowly resorbable device for bony fixation in forehead surgery has made stabilization of the elevated brow more reliable. Currently, a crescent-shaped, slowly resorbable implant made of a copolymer of 82/18 L-lactide/glycolide (Endotine Transbleph Implant, Coapt Systems, Inc., Palo Alto, CA) is available to stabilize an elevated brow. The orbital rim is accessed through a transpalpebral approach (**Figure 8-7A, B**). The periosteum is incised with cautery about 4 mm above the inferior aspect of the orbital rim (**see Figure 8-7C**) from the frontozygomatic suture laterally and extending as far medially as the supraorbital notch (**see Figure 8-7D**). An endoscopic or Freer elevator is then used to raise the periosteum up to the hairline from the temporal crest (zone of fixation; see Chapter 2) to as far medially as possible (**see Figure 8-7E**). Care must be taken to protect the supraorbital nerve at the orbital

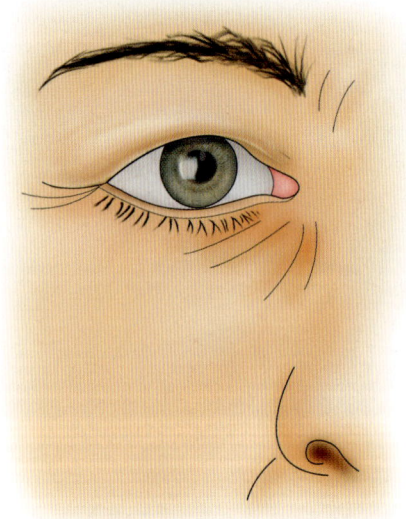

A

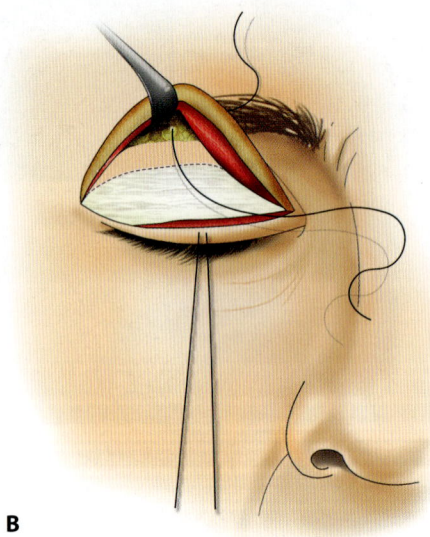

B

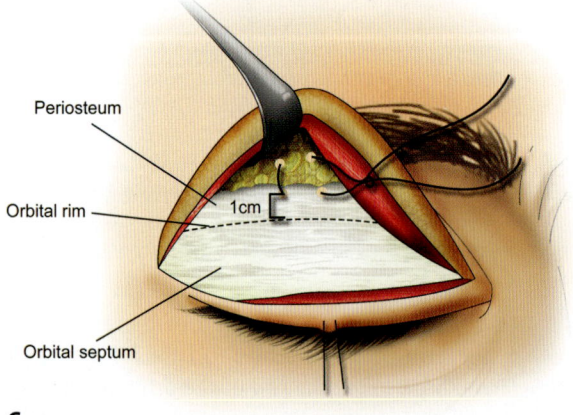

Periosteum

Orbital rim

1cm

Orbital septum

C

Figure 8-6. Transpalpebral suture browpexy. (A) Mildly ptotic brow. (B) A suture is passed transcutaneously at the lower border of the brow and the tail left in place to mark the position of the inferior brow. (C) The suture is placed through the frontal periosteum the number of millimeters above the orbital rim the surgeon desires to position the lower brow. The suture is then passed back through the brow soft tissue at the site marked by the transcutaneous suture; the suture tail is then removed and the suture tied.

rim. An instrument placed subperiosteally lateral to the nerve can be angled to elevate up to the midline forehead except the glabella (**see Figure 8-7F**). For safety, the surgeon's nondominant thumb should be placed firmly over the supraorbital notch to prevent dissection into the neurovascular bundle. After bilateral dissection, only a small triangle over the glabella remains unelevated in between the temporal crests, above the orbital rim and below the hairline.

Once the periosteum is elevated, the flap is retracted to expose at least 1 cm of calvarium superior to the orbital rim (5–6 mm above the periosteal incision) (**see Figure 8-7G**). A monocortical hole is drilled to accept the Transbleph Endotine implant (**see Figure 8-7H, I**). The hole is placed at a distance above the periosteal incision equal to the desired amount of brow elevation plus 2 mm; the hole is drilled directly above the desired high point of the brow arch (**see Figure 8-7J**). The post on the deep surface of the fixation device is then secured in the drilled hole; the superficial surface has three 3.0-mm (reserved for thin skinned patients) or 4.0-mm tines extending at a 45° angle. The upper flap is then redraped superiorly so that the tines engage the soft tissue just below the cut edge of the periosteum; the skin flap is then pushed at the same 45° angle as the tines to impale the soft tissues on the tines, essentially suspending the brow by the superior edge of the periosteum (**see Figure 8-7K**).

Wound Closure

Regardless of the specific internal modifications, the upper lid is managed similarly. If blepharoplasty is to be performed, the orbital septum is opened and pseudoherniated fat is resected as necessary. If excess upper lid skin was not excised initially, it is removed now. The skin is then closed in the same fashion as a standard upper blepharoplasty. The author's preferred method is simple sutures lateral to the lateral canthus and a running subcuticular suture medial to the canthus, both of 6-0 polypropylene. Recovery is generally quite rapid, periorbital ecchymosis is fairly limited, and patients can generally return to routine activities within a few days (**see Figure 8-7L–Q**).

Transtemporal Approaches

Whereas a transpalpebral approach can be an excellent option for correction of lateral hooding and ptosis of the brow, its effectiveness is somewhat limited by the lack of wide undermining of the lateral forehead and temple and the inability to fully release the orbital ligament and zone of fixation. Transtemporal approaches, with or without a concurrent transpalpebral procedure, can more completely mobilize the lateral segment of the brow.

Incision

Tardy and associates[19] described a "temporal lift," performed through an irregular post-trichial temporal incision. With the incision placed 2 to 3 cm posterior to the temporal hairline and designed in a sawtooth pattern, the scar was felt to be easily camouflaged. Other authors have advocated curvilinear incisions in the same location.

Plane(s) of Dissection

Most temporal brow procedures have employed dissections performed between the temporoparietal and the deep temporal fasciae. As noted earlier (see Chapter 2), the superficial temporal artery runs within the temporoparietal fascia, but no branches penetrate deep to it, and hence, this interfacial plane is fairly avascular. Also, the twigs of the temporal branch of the facial nerve run within the temporoparietal fascia. In addition, the deep division of the supraorbital nerve is still in a preperiosteal plane in the lower two thirds of the forehead medial to the zone of fixation, and skin incision and subtemporoparietal fascia dissection should not endanger this nerve. More medially, adequate mobilization of the lateral brow also requires subperiosteal elevation of the forehead, and hence, the surgeon must carefully transition to this plane after breaking through the zone of fixation medial to the temporal crest.

Tissue Modification

Tardy and associates'[20] "bitemporal lift" was, in essence, the superior continuation of the rhytidectomy incision. This was performed in a subtempo-

---

Transtemporal Limited Incision Approaches

Incisions: in/behind the temporal hair tuft.
Tissue modifications: vary by procedure.
Fixation: typically suspension of the temporoparietal fascia.
Wound closure: two-layered skin closure.
Complications: incisional alopecia (1–6%); widened scar; facial nerve injury (temporary: 5–7%; permanent: <1%); hematoma (rare).

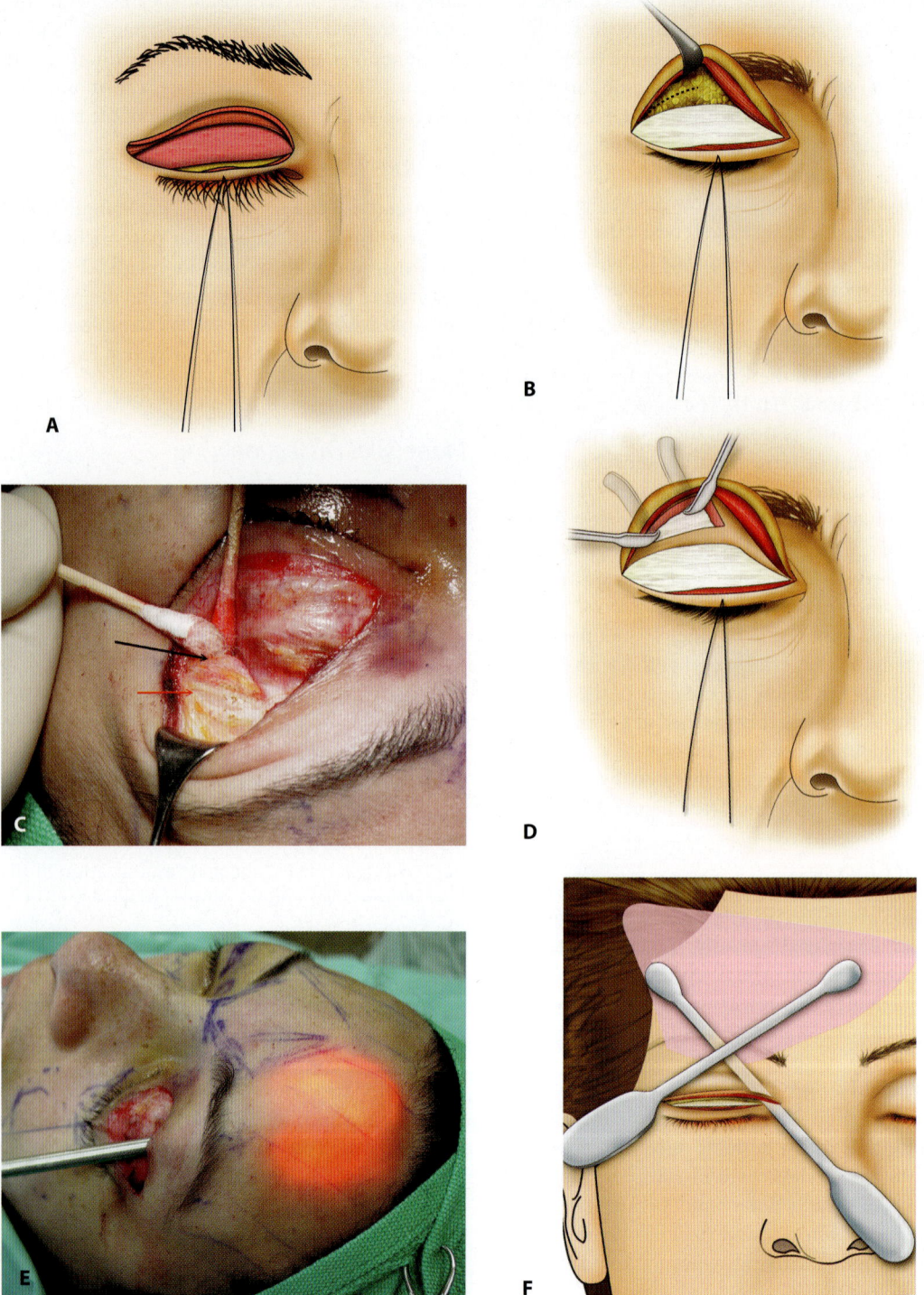

Figure 8-7. Transpalpebral Endotine browpexy. (A) Upper eyelid skin excision and exposure of the septum orbitale. (B) Soft tissue is retracted and the lateral orbital rim is identified. The periosteum is incised *(dotted line)* about 4 mm above the orbital rim. (C) Left orbital rim dissection. *Black arrow* indicates the septum orbitale; *red arrow* points to the incision in the deep fascia and periosteum. (D) Completed periosteal incision allows subperiosteal dissection. (E) Light of an endoscope shows the extent of the dissection possible through this lateral transpalpebral approach. (F) Elevators then sweep superiorly to the anterior hairline, medially to the midline, and laterally to the temporal crest. *(Continued)*

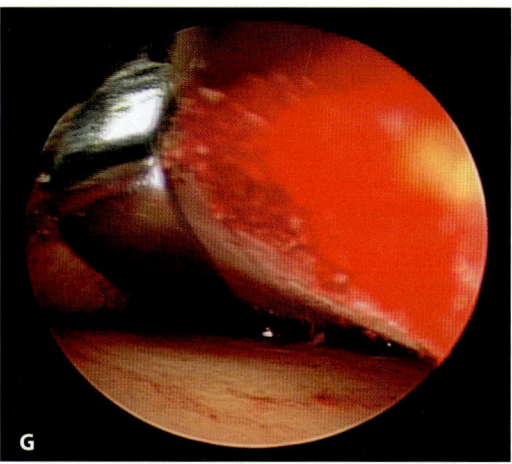

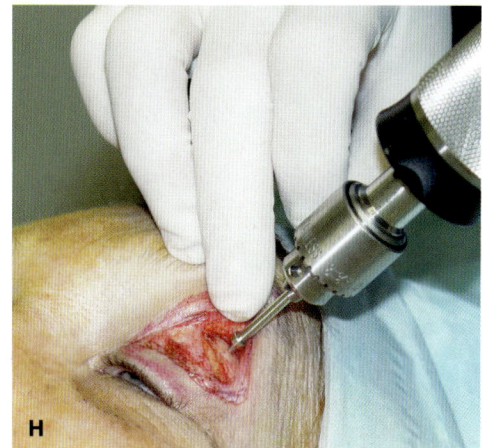

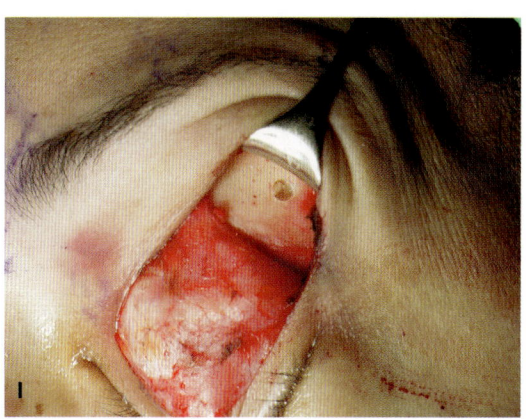

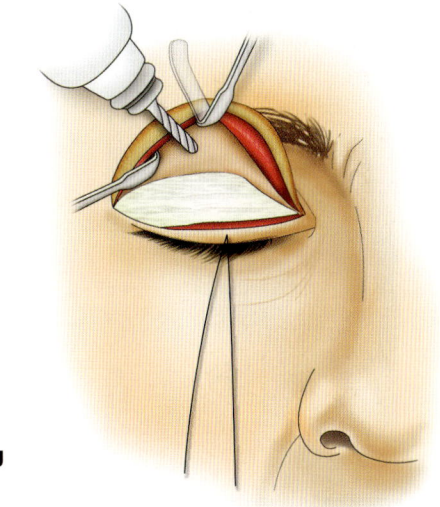

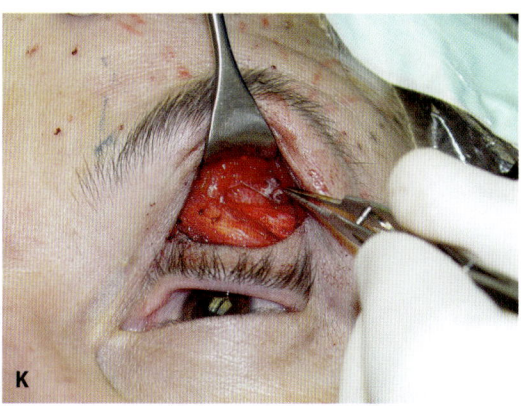

Figure 8-7. *(Continued)* (G) When the elevation is complete, view is similar to that of an endoscopic forehead lift. (H) The hole for the Endotine implant is easily drilled with a hand drill. (I) The monocortical hole is seen approximately 1 cm above the orbital rim. (J) Drill hole should be placed in line with the desired brow peak. (K) Endotine implant in place directly on bone with tines impaled into the overlying periosteum and bone. *(Continued)*

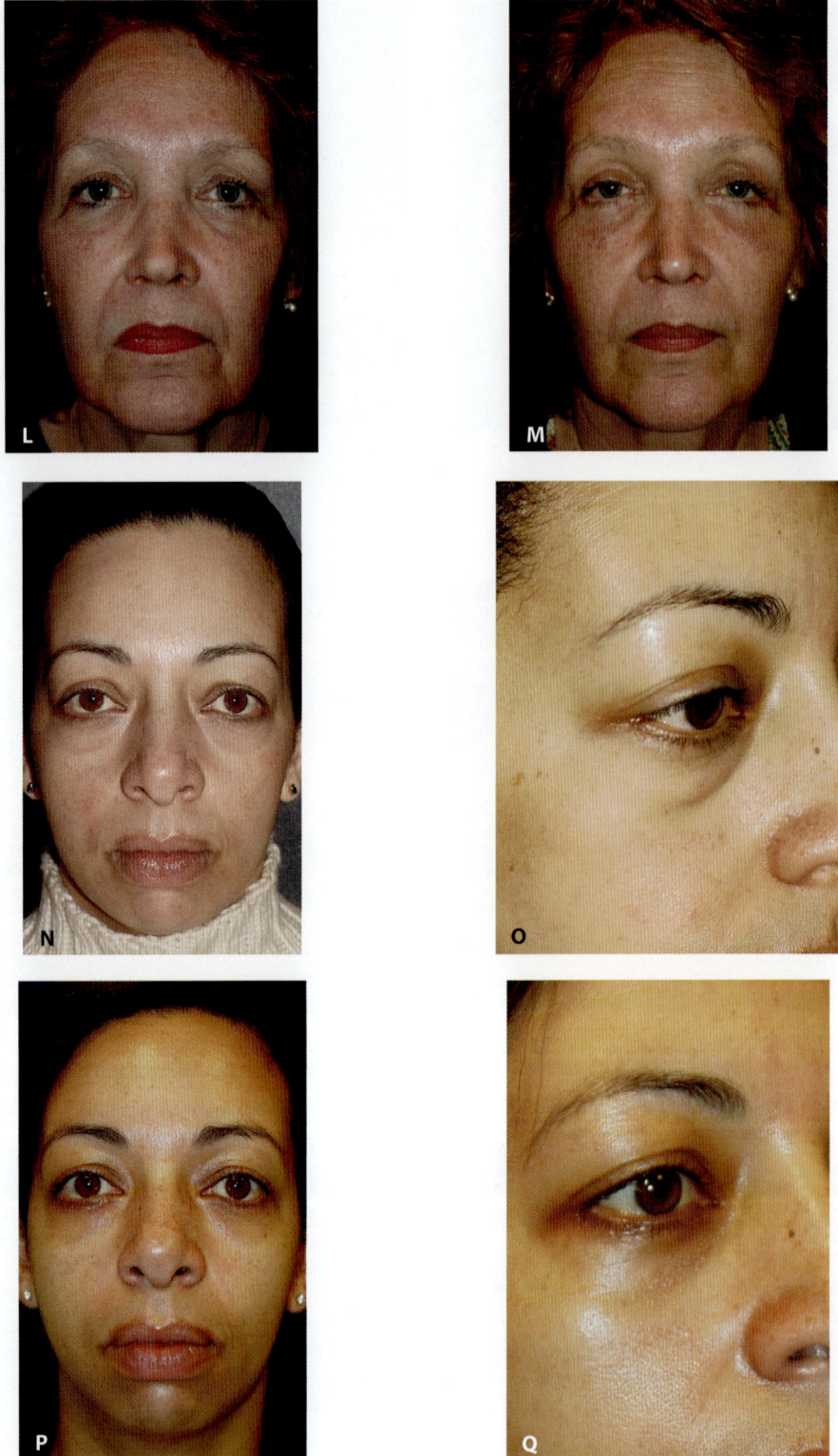

Figure 8-7. *(Continued)* Preoperative (L) and postoperative (M) views (18 mo) of a patient who underwent transpalpebral Endotine browpexy in conjunction with a midface lift. Preoperative (N, O) and postoperative (P, Q) views (1 yr) of a patient who underwent transpalpebral Endotine browpexy with corrugator resection in addition to a midface lift.

roparietal fascia plane with dissection performed to the orbital rim and zygomatic arch. No release of any specific structures was mentioned, but the orbital ligament can be divided here to improve flap mobility. After posterior mobilization of the flap and skin excision, the brow is maintained in position by reapproximation of the fasciae and skin under tension.

Fogli[20] used a temporal incision to access and undermine in a subtemporoparietal fascia plane up to and beyond the temporal crest, releasing the zone of fixation in the process. Temporally, approximately halfway from the hairline to the lateral brow, the dissection transitions to a subcutaneous plane. It is essential to carry the subfascial dissection low enough to protect the temporal branch of the facial nerve. The subcutaneous dissection then proceeds to the orbital rim. When the temporal skin is pulled posterosuperiorly, the temporoparietal fascia bears much of the strain, transferring this pull to the loose skin of the lateral brow and crow's feet, reducing redundant and ptotic skin, and smoothing this area.

Knize[2,14-16] has performed extensive anatomic dissections of the temple and brow and has embraced the temporal approach. Although he advocates concurrent use of the transpalpebral approach for glabellar myoplasty, his temporal approach can be used alone for isolated lateral brow ptosis. Again, dissection is performed in the subtemporoparietal fascia plane, inferiorly to the zygomatic arch and medially to the area of the temporal crest. The zone of fixation is elevated and the central forehead dissection is then continued inferiorly in a subperiosteal plane down to the orbital rim. The arcus marginalis can then be elevated lateral to the supraorbital nerve and continued laterally to also mobilize the orbital ligament. Once a window of deep temporal fascia is excised from the upper portion of the dissection (to provide a "bed" for postoperative fibrosis), the temporoparietal fascia is advanced posterosuperiorly and sutured down to the deep temporal fascia, and excess skin is excised. This dissection more fully releases the retaining structures of the brow and, thus, requires less skin tension for secure brow fixation.

Wound Closure

The temporal incision is easily closed with 3-0 polypropylene sutures or skin staples. It is essential to avoid skin-strangulating wound closure methods to prevent incisional alopecia. Especially in procedures relying on temporal skin tension for elevating the lateral brow, a layered closure should be performed.

Forehead Approaches

Access via the forehead to the brow is a more direct minimal incision technique and may offer enhanced protection of the supraorbital nerves (by direct vision) and the temporal branch of the facial nerve (by avoiding it entirely). However, these approaches must generate sufficient release of tissues to allow for adequate mobilization as well as provide for stable fixation. Three approaches are described below.

Lateral Subcutaneous Browlift

Miller and coworkers[10] described an approach to the lateral brow through a hairline incision in the temporal recess. Hair must be dense enough and no significant hair loss be anticipated for these incisions to be useful. The skin is undermined in a subcutaneous plane, laterally to the temporal crests and medially to the midpupillary line. Dissection is carried inferiorly no closer than 1.5 cm from the orbital rim. If significant glabellar rhytids are present, glabellar crease incisions are made and the corrugator muscles directly exposed and bluntly avulsed. No release of the zone of fixation, orbital ligament, or arcus marginalis is performed. The hairline skin is elevated and resected and brow elevation maintained by skin closure tension. The skin incisions should be closed in layers with 4-0 resorbable sutures in the dermis and 5-0 polypropylene skin sutures. Obviously, this approach leaves visible glabellar scars, is associated with a high probability of recurrent glabellar wrinkles (which may be distorted because of incomplete corrugator resection), treats primarily the lateral brows, and is unlikely to produce long-lasting results. It may, however, be useful in nonsmoking patients with heavily creased lateral forehead skin, minimal to mild brow ptosis (lateral brow only), and no significant glabellar rhytids (so that direct corrugator incisions are unnecessary).

Lateral Trichophytic Browpexy

Similarly, Chisholm and Lew[21] described a trichophytic approach to elevate the lateral brow. A hairline incision is made in the temporal recession, and a subperiosteal plane is dissected down to the orbital rim between the temporal crest (and zone of fixation) and the approximate position of the supraorbital nerve (roughly 24–27 mm from the midline). No myoplasty is performed. The lateral brow is then advanced superiorly and secured in place by skin excision. The wound is closed in layers with 4-0 polyglactin 910 braided resorbable sutures in the galea and dermis and 5-0 polypropylene skin sutures.

This technique releases the lateral brow to a greater degree, but still is somewhat limited by not addressing the zone of fixation in the temple and, similarly, does not address glabellar rhytids or central and medial brow ptosis. In addition, the hairline incision puts the deep division of the supraorbital nerve at risk for injury.

Limited Incision Nonendoscopic Browlift

Most recently, Tabatabai and Spinelli[11] have advocated a limited incision approach to the forehead lift that does elevate all segments of the brow without the use of expensive and often cumbersome endoscopic equipment.

Incisions. The limited incision nonendoscopic browlift utilizes the same paired paramedian and midline post-trichial incisions as the endoscopic browlift. These incisions are planned to give adequate exposure of the central and lateral forehead as well as allow dissection at the temporal crest. These incisions are 2 cm in length and are oriented sagittally, and they must be placed so as to remain behind the hairline even in the setting of continued hairline recession.

Plane(s) of Dissection. The access incisions are carried down through the periosteum, allowing the surgeon to perform the entire procedure in the subperiosteal plane. This plane also provides for maximal protection of the deep branch of the supraorbital nerve, which runs above the periosteum. The periosteum is elevated down to the nasal root medially, along the superior orbital rim, extending laterally to the frontozygomatic suture and then along the temporal crest. The periosteum is also elevated posteriorly to the vertex.

Tissue Modification. Once the central forehead has been elevated, the "dense adhesions of periosteum" along the temporal crest (zone of fixation)

Transforehead Limited Incision Approaches

Incisions: vary by procedure: generally trichophytic.
Tissue modifications: vary by procedure: subcutaneous or subperiosteal elevation with elevation and fixation, with/without glabellar myotomies.
Fixation: varies by procedure: galeal/periosteal reapproximation or resorbable fixation implant.
Wound closure: two-layered skin closure.
Complications: temporary forehead hypesthesia; hematoma; hair loss (rare).

---

are elevated, but the dissection does not extend into the temporal fasciae. Inferiorly, the periosteum is stripped along the orbital rim, both medial to the supratrochlear nerve and lateral to the supraorbital nerve. These locations are marked preoperatively either by palpation or based on historical averages (supratrochlear nerve 14–17 mm, supraorbital nerve 24–27 mm from the midline). No discrete myotomies are performed. The forehead is then advanced posteriorly and fixated to the calvarium at an appropriate height using a Coapt Forehead Lift device (Coapt Systems, Inc., Palo Alto, CA) deep to each paramedian incision. These are similar in nature but thicker and larger with more tines than the Endotine Transbleph device.

Wound Closure. Once the forehead flap has been elevated and placed symmetrically on the fixation devices, the brow shape and position are assessed; if suboptimal, the flap can be elevated off the tines with a Freer elevator and the entire flap repositioned and then re-impaled on the fixation devices. Once positioning is deemed acceptable, the wounds are closed in layers with 4-0 polyglactin 910 dermal sutures and skin staples.

Combined Approaches

Transtemporal/Transpalpebral Approaches

Paul[5,6] described a combination of transtemporal and transpalpebral approaches (see earlier) to browplasty (**Figure 8-8**). Wide release of the zone of fixation, orbital ligament and lateral arcus marginalis is performed through the temporal approach, and release of the brow depressors is done using a transpalpebral approach. Once the soft tissue dissection is performed, the lateral brow is elevated by excising an appropriate amount of temporal skin before wound closure; elevation of the medial brow occurs with the sectioning of the glabellar musculature.

Kikawa and colleagues[3] also advocated a combined transtemporal and transpalpebral approach, but additionally added paramedian incisions to elevate the central forehead as well as to stabilize the elevated brows with paramedian temporary transcutaneous monocortical screws.

Postoperative Management

Regardless of the approach, postoperative management of patients undergoing limited incision procedures of the brow is similar and relatively straightforward. At most, a lightly compressive dressing is placed on the forehead for up to 24 hours. Patients can return home on the day of surgery if they choose not to stay in an overnight facility for convenience. Ice compresses are applied frequently to the forehead, temple, and eyes for the first 24 to 36 hours postoperatively to reduce ecchymosis. Patients are instructed to keep their heads elevated and to avoid head-hanging or strenuous activities for 1 week. Patients are allowed to shower on postoperative day 1, but are cautioned that they should avoid hot showers, because there may be diminished sensation on the scalp for several weeks to months. Patients taking *Arnica Montana* and bromelain preoperatively are instructed to continue the use of these for 2 weeks.

Complications: Incidence, Management, and Avoidance

Hematoma

Transtemporal Approaches

If appropriate care is taken during dissection, bleeding from a temporal approach should be minimal. Any oozing should be carefully and meticulously controlled with bipolar cautery. Exceptional care should be taken in the lower portions of the dissection, because the middle zygomaticotemporal ("sentinel") vein runs in close proximity to the branches of the temporal division of the facial nerve. If it is necessary to cauterize this vessel, the bipolar tips should be applied where the vessel first pierces the deep temporal fascia and remain as far as possible from the facial nerve branches.

Forehead Approaches

The majority of the dissection in lateral and central forehead approaches to the brow is performed subperiosteally (a fairly avascular plane) and is rarely problematic. The most complete of these procedures, the limited incision nonendoscopic browlift, does incise the periosteum medial and lateral to the supratrochlear and supraorbital neurovascular bundles, respectively. Because there is no direct visualization of these vessels, the surgeon must ensure protection of these structures.

Transpalpebral Approaches

Hemostasis during the transpalpebral approach is obviously critical, because the brow portion of the wound is in continuity with the retrobulbar space once the septum orbitale is opened. Bleeding from the lateral and central brow is generally minimal and easily controllable with bipolar cautery. Central forehead subperiosteal dissection, as noted earlier, should be relatively bloodless. Glabellar dissection and myotomy/myectomy should be carefully performed, especially when treating the corrugator muscle. Supratrochlear vessels wrap over the muscle near its origin, and muscle edges should be cauterized with the bipolar to ensure meticulous hemostasis.

Hair Loss/Wide Scar

Hair loss should be minimal after a transtemporal brow procedure and is generally more likely if there is a widened scar. Although exact statistics do not exist for these transtemporal procedures, the incision is similar to the temporal incision used during an endoscopic browlift, for which a widened scar (more likely temporally) has been reported in 1% to 7% of cases. Permanent hair loss, in endoscopic brow procedures not utilizing transcutaneous fixation, has been reported in approximately 6% of cases (a number that includes both the forehead and the temporal scars). Methods to reduce the risk of visible scars due to hair loss or scar widening include appropriate preoperative evaluation and patient selection to avoid patients at high risk for genetic temporal hair thinning or hairline recession; placing the incision sufficiently posterior to the temporal hairline; beveling the incision parallel to the hair follicles to minimize follicular transaction; avoiding monopolar or extensive bipolar cautery of the wound edges; strong and reliable fixation of the elevated tissue at a fascial (not a dermal) level; and meticulous and tensionless nonstrangulating multilayer closure of the wound.

Nerve Injury

Transtemporal Approach

Temporal dissection to the orbital rim passes the temporal branch of the facial nerve, which is subject to potential injury. Knize[16] has reported a 5% to 7% incidence of temporary facial nerve injury, with a 0.4% incidence of permanent injury to the nerve. Possible mechanisms of injury include transection (unlikely if dissection is performed in the correct plane), stretching of the nerve during aggressive dissection, and thermal injury during cauterization. The surgeon should ensure that the dissection remains below the temporoparietal fascia in the temple, carefully ensure that tissue planes are gently

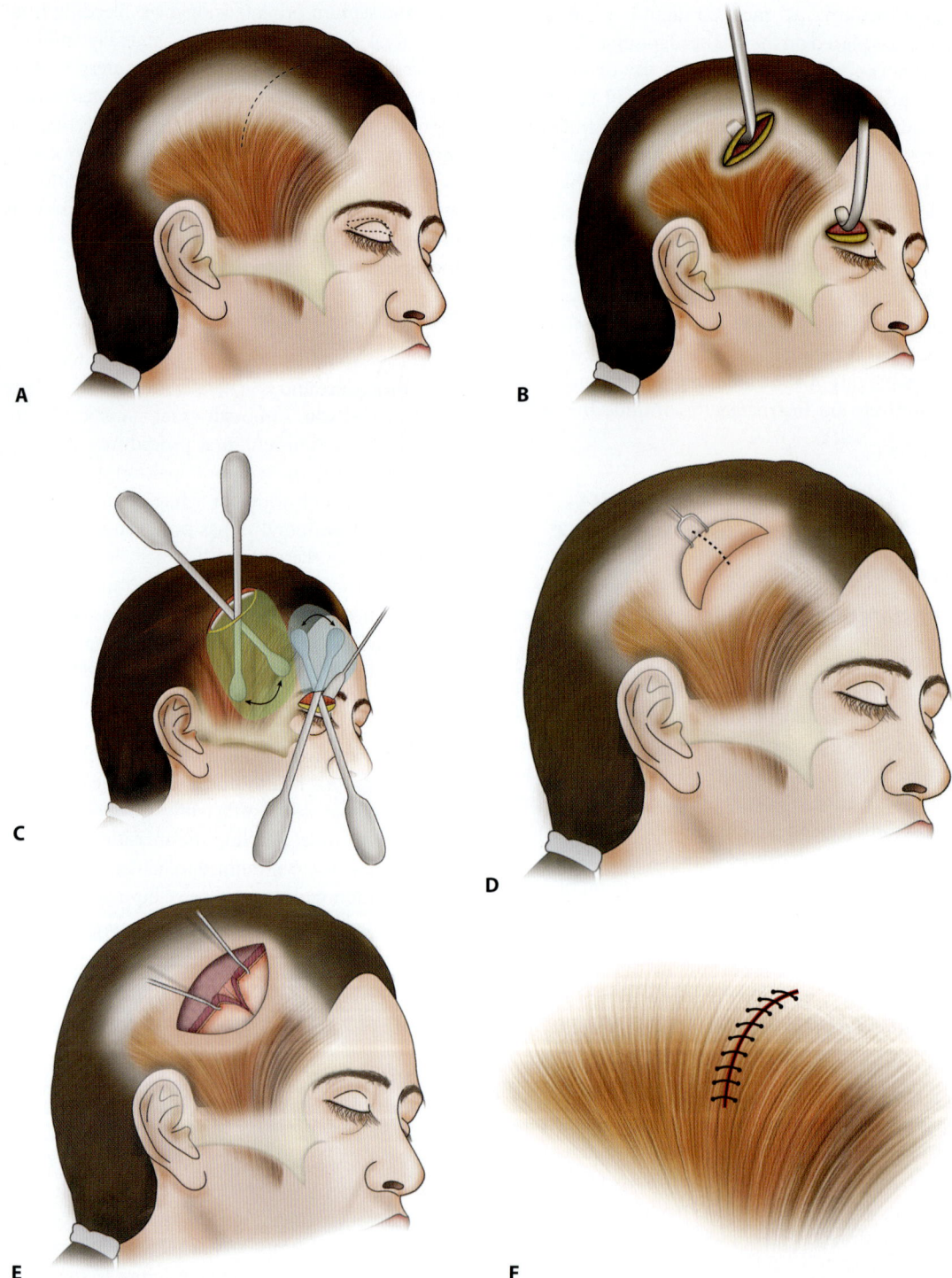

Figure 8-8. Transtemporal/transpalpebral browplasty. (A) An upper blepharoplasty skin excision, dissection down to the orbital rim, and incision of the periosteum is combined with a temporal approach. (B) Central forehead dissection (lateral to the supraorbital nerve) is combined with a subtemporoparietal fascia dissection in the temple. (C) Wide release of the zone of fixation near the temporal crest, lateral arcus marginalis, and orbital ligament allows full mobility of the central and temporal brow. The temporal skin is retracted superiorly (D), the redundant skin is split and resected (E), and the wound is closed (F).

separated (particularly in the area of the projected path of the temporal branch; see Chapter 2 for methods to project the nerve's approximate course), and limited and judicious use of cautery. When necessary, bipolar cautery should be utilized; if it is necessary to cauterize the middle zygomaticotemporal vein, the temporoparietal fascia should be appropriately elevated and cautery applied to the vein as it emerges from the deep temporal fascia.

Transpalpebral and Transforehead Approaches

Motor nerve injury should be uncommon after only a translid approach to the brow. If appropriate care is taken during dissection, permanent central forehead anesthesia should be uncommon, although temporary hypesthesia is common and occasionally persists for several months. Most likely, this is related to stretching of the nerve during flap elevation or direct injury to the supraorbital and supratrochlear nerve during glabellar myotomies. Knize[2,16] reported one of 500 limited transtemporal/transpalpebral dissections developed temporary neuralgias.

Conclusions

As surgeons search for the ideal rejuvenative brow procedure, they have attempted to correct the chronopathology of the forehead with fewer, smaller, and more easily hidden incisions and have limited dissections. As we evaluate these procedures, our understanding of the structures and forces at work in the forehead and brow becomes even more important. We have begun to understand that no surgery is ideal for every patient, but rather through careful preoperative analysis, we can choose operations that specifically target each individual patient's needs. These limited incision techniques for brow and forehead rejuvenation can focally address specific brow and forehead needs in correctly selected patients.

Human subtlety . . . will never devise an invention more beautiful, more simple or more direct than does Nature, because in her inventions nothing is lacking, and nothing is superfluous.

Leonardo da Vinci (1452–1519)

Suggested Readings

1. Parkes ML, Kamer FM, Bassilios M. Surgical treatment of the ptotic brow. Laryngoscope 1976;86:1435–1436.
2. Knize DM. Limited-incision forehead lift for eyebrow elevation to enhance upper blepharoplasty. Plast Reconstr Surg 1996;97:1334–1342.
3. Kikkawa DO, Miller SR, Batra MK, Lee AC. Small incision nonendoscopic browlift. Ophthal Plast Reconstr Surg 2000;1:28–33.
4. Knize DM. Transpalpebral approach to the corrugator supercilii and procerus muscles. Plast Reconstr Surg 1995;95:52–62.
5. Paul MD. Subperiosteal transblepharoplasty forehead lift. Aesthetic Plast Surg 1996;20:129–134.
6. Paul MD. The surgical management of upper eyelid hooding. Aesthetic Plast Surg 1989;13:183–187.
7. McCord CD, Doxanas MT. Browplasty and browpexy: an adjunct to blepharoplasty. Plast Reconstr Surg 1990;86:248–254.
8. Sokol AB, Sokol TP. Transblepharoplasty brow suspension. Plast Reconstr Surg 1982;69:940–944.
9. Sclafani AP. Comprehensive periorbital rejuvenation with resorbable Endotine implants for trans-lid brow and midface elevation. Facial Plast Surg Clin North Am 2007;15:255–264.
10. Miller TA, Rudkin G, Honig M, et al. Lateral subcutaneous brow lift and interbrow muscle resection: clinical experience and anatomic studies. Plast Reconstr Surg 2000;105:1120–1127.
11. Tabatabai N, Spinelli HM. Limited incision nonendoscopic brow lift. Plast Reconstr Surg 2007;119:1563–1570.
12. Georgescu D, Anderson RL, McCann JD. Brow ptosis correction: a comparison of five techniques. Facial Plast Surg 2010;26:186–192.
13. Walden JL, Brown CC, Klapper AJ, et al. An anatomic comparison of transpalpebral, endoscopic, and coronal approaches to demonstrate exposure and extent of brow depressor muscle resection. Plast Reconstr Surg 2005;116:1479–1487.
14. Knize DM. An anatomically based study of the mechanism of eyebrow ptosis. Plast Reconstr Surg 1996;97:1321–1333.
15. Knize DM. Anatomy of a frown: basis for a limited incision approach to treatment of eyebrow ptosis and glabellar lines. Perspect Plast Surg 1996;10:1–37.
16. Knize DM. Limited incision forehead lift for eyebrow elevation to enhance upper blepharoplasty. Plast Reconstr Surg 2001;108:564–567.
17. Niechajev I. Transpalpebral browpexy. Plast Reconstr Surg 2004;113:2172–2180.
18. Zarem HA, Resnick JI, Carr RM, Wootton DG. Browpexy: lateral orbicularis muscle fixation as an adjunct to upper blepharoplasty. Plast Reconstr Surg 1997;100:1258–1261.
19. Tardy ME, Thomas JR, Brown RJ. Temporal lift. In Facial Aesthetic Surgery. St. Louis, Mosby–Year Book, 1995, pp. 196–206.
20. Fogli AL. Temporal lift by galeapexy: a review of 270 cases. Aesthetic Plast Surg 2003;27:159–165.
21. Chisholm BB, Lew D. Modified brow lift: an adjunct to blepharoplasty. J Oral Maxillofac Surg 1996;54:281–284.

9

ENDOSCOPIC FOREHEAD LIFT

Do not remove a fly from your friend's forehead with a hatchet.

Chinese Proverb

Introduction

The endoscopic forehead lift is a "keyhole" surgical approach to the structures of the forehead and brow based predominantly upon the principles of dynamic brow positioning. The procedure provides elevation of forehead tissues, release of brow retaining structures, elimination of inferiorly directed vectors of muscle contraction, and (usually) fixation of brow position during the period required for biologic adhesion of the elevated tissues to underlying structures. Maintenance of brow position relies on these more physiologic mechanisms as opposed to soft tissue excision alone.

The endoscopic forehead lift was developed in response to dissatisfaction with the morbidity and often extended recovery associated with the coronal forehead lift, the gold standard forehead procedure at that (and, some would argue, present) time. The ongoing dispute between proponents and opponents of the endoscopic forehead lift as to which procedure is more effective may not be easily answered, because each has distinct advantages and indications as well as drawbacks.

History

The development of high-quality surgical endoscopes for genitourinary, laparoscopic, arthroscopic, and endoscopic nasal surgery in the late 1980s led the way to endoscopic facial plastic surgery. Several workers (Aiache, Isse, Ramirez, and Vasconez) presented their results in 1992, and after an initial

Endoscopic Forehead Lift

Indications: mild to moderately severe ptosis of any/all segments of the brow; glabellar furrows.
Contraindications: severe frontal/temporal scarring; high hairline (unless trichophytic modification used).
Ideal candidate: normal or low hairline with normal hair density; mild to moderately severe brow ptosis and forehead/glabellar rhytids; concurrent midfacelift planned.
Scientific basis: elimination of activity of the brow depressor muscles with preservation of brow elevator muscle activity; forehead tissues released and suspended superiorly, mechanically maintained in position until tissues heal at the elevated position.

Endoscopic Forehead Lift

Incisions: paired temporal and paramedian incision, midline incision (some authors have recommended between 3 and 6 incisions vary by procedure): post-trichial; trichophytic modification possible.
Tissue modifications: central forehead subperiosteal or subgaleal elevation; temporal subtemporoparietal fascia elevation; release at temporal crest, orbital rim, and orbital ligament; myotomies of corrugator and depressor supercilii and procerus muscles.
Fixation: long-term or permanent fixation.
Wound closure: two-layered skin closure.
Complications: temporary pruritus (20–37%); wide scar (0.1–6%), incisional hair loss (3–6%), recurrent brow ptosis (4%), hematoma/seroma (3%), neuralgias (temporary, 2%, permanent, rare), temporal branch of cranial nerve 7 (temporary, 1–2%, permanent, rare).

rush of enthusiasm, there has been an ebb and flow of interest in the procedure. At the same time, there has also been a lively debate on several technical points of the procedure.

Chajchir[1] described a subperiosteal dissection followed by release at the orbital rim and myotomies. Isse[2] dissected subperiosteally to the orbital rim but subgaleally to the crown, and included a subtemporoparietal fascia dissection as well; this was subsequently reinforced by Core and coworkers[3], and Aiache. Isse[4] attempted to better categorize the endoforehead lift, describing the standard, extended, and lateral forehead and temple endoscopic lift. In the extended endoscopic forehead lift, dissection extended along the orbital rim past the frontozygomatic suture and better elevated the lateral brow, whereas the lateral endoscopic lift eliminated the midline incision and dissected over the temporal fossa and forehead lateral to the supraorbital nerve for elevation of the brow tail and lateral canthal area only. Ramirez[5] and Oslin and colleagues,[6] responding to the criticism that forehead elevation without skin excision would cause excessive hairline elevation, described a combination of a trichophytic approach coupled with endoscopic dissection of the glabellar muscles.

Descriptions of the endoscopic forehead lift technique have included myotomies of the corrugator and depressor supercilii and procerus muscles. Whereas various authors have described many different methods of muscle modification, glabellar myotomies are relatively constant. Conversely, methods of fixation have ranged from no fixation at all to soft tissue sutures in the central forehead or temple to transcutaneous or subcutaneous bone-anchored devices.

However, it should be noted that questions about the efficacy of the endoscopic forehead lift have hindered its widespread acceptance. Chiu and Baker[7] noted that in one New York City hospital, there was a 70% decrease in endoscopic forehead lifts from 1997 to 2001. This decline, which undoubtedly is evidence of a certain level of dissatisfaction with the procedure, does not necessarily impugn the utility of the endoscopic forehead lift nor does it prove the superiority of open forehead procedures. The decline in number of endoscopic forehead lift procedures performed may have been a result of several patient and surgeon factors, such as (1) the depletion of a large pool of patients who were candidates for a forehead lift but had refused a coronal forehead lift; (2) the introduction and popularization of minimally inva-sive procedures for forehead and brow rejuvenation, including botulinum toxin injections; (3) unrealistic expectations of both patients and surgeons of the results possible with this procedure; (4) a better definition and understanding of the ideal candidate for the endoscopic forehead lift; (5) an evolving understanding of the critical steps in the endoscopic forehead lift and methods of fixation during that time period; and (6) a steep learning curve that may have frustrated some surgeons. Most surgeons who currently perform the endoscopic forehead lift are quite confident they are providing their patients with appropriate and durable aesthetic results.

Rationale and Scientific Basis

Of all brow procedures, the endoscopic forehead lift is the one most reliant on an understanding of the active, tonic, and passive forces that act on the forehead and brow. The endoscopic forehead lift is grounded on the suppositions that the general position of the forehead and brow tissues is restrained and maintained by the soft tissue–to–bone attachments—the periosteum, including the arcus marginalis, and the orbital ligament—and that the specific position and shape of the brow are determined by the interaction between and relative activity of the brow depressor (corrugator and depressor supercilii, procerus, and orbicularis oculi) and elevator (frontalis) muscles.

Knize[8,9] has illustrated the various structures and planes that allow the inferior descent of the brow. Noting that the majority of vertical movement of the brow occurs in the lower half of the brow, he points out the importance of the glide plane space. This plane allows the superficial tissues to glide over the deep layer in response to brow muscle contraction. General positioning at this level is mediated by tonic contraction of the brow muscles and specific movement by overt active contraction of the corrugator and depressor supercilii, orbicularis oculi, and procerus muscles.

Manipulating any of these muscles affects the balance of forces acting on brow position. Any change to the brow elevator or depressor muscles will directly affect the brow. Significantly, this tonic muscle contraction may not be readily apparent; for example, brow position may drop up to 3 mm after an upper blepharoplasty, as the subtle tonic contraction of the frontalis muscle (which preoperatively had been involuntarily used to subtly raise the brow and improve the superior visual field) relaxes and allows the brow depressor forces to predominate and lower the brow. By preserving the integrity of the frontalis muscle (brow elevator) and significantly weakening or totally sectioning the brow depressors, the forehead can relax and the brow rise. Superior mobilization of the forehead flap is facilitated by this reduction in depressor forces.

In theory, frontalis contraction should facilitate maintenance of an elevated brow position, but with time, it is expected that this tonic contraction should relax, and if the brow position has not been stabilized in some manner by this time, relapse of brow ptosis may occur. As the elevated forehead tissues re-adhere at either a periosteal or a galeal level (depending upon the plane of elevation used), brow position is stabilized; therefore, the brow must be maintained in position long enough for this healing to occur. A number of factors will affect how long this period of critical brow stabilization will be: the preoperative tonic activity of the frontalis muscle; the time course of frontalis muscle relaxation; the preoperative depressor muscle activity; the thoroughness of depressor myotomy; the thoroughness of forehead tissue release; and the soft tissues themselves and the natural course of re-adherence strong enough to resist displacement. Experimentally, periosteal re-adherence to bone has been reported to reach control strength by as little as 8 days[10,11] to as long as 4 to 6 weeks. However, two separate groups noted that periosteal healing was histologically similar to soft tissue healing, and it is reasonable to expect a similar time course.[12,13,14] In choosing methods of and devices for fixation, it is essential to fully evaluate long-term maintenance of the intraoperative brow position in the context of periosteal or galeal wound healing. The use of any extrinsic stabilization of the forehead tissues that is not applied for a sufficiently long time will lead to "failure" of the procedure or "recurrence" of brow ptosis. Preoperative administration of botulinum toxin A to the brow depressor muscles will help to reduce inferiorly directed pull on the brow. Also, newer methods of fixation are simpler and easier to apply and provide a more predictable level of support; an enhanced understanding of these processes now allows the surgeon to utilize them to her or his advantage.

Advantages, Disadvantages, and Alternatives

The most obvious advantage of the endoscopic forehead lift is the small incisions, and from that, many of the other potential benefits follow. Three to six 15- to 20-mm sagittal incisions behind the hairline are more easily camouflaged than a long coronal incision. Similarly, these incisions, when appropriately oriented, are less likely to lead to significant postoperative alopecia. There is significantly less edema associated with the endoscopic forehead lift when compared with the coronal forehead lift, and patients have a significantly more rapid recovery. If proper precautions are taken and the appropriate tissue planes respected, there should be a very low risk of injury to the temporal branch of the facial nerve as well as forehead paresthesias from injury to branches of the supratrochlear and supraorbital nerves.

Conversely, the endoscopic forehead lift requires specialized and expensive equipment that limits direct access to the tissues of interest. There is a steep learning curve, because the surgeon must learn to visualize the two-dimensional images on the monitor as a three-dimensional space. The efficacy of the endoscopic forehead lift may be limited in patients with severe brow ptosis, and if fixation and/or release is inadequate, relapse of brow ptosis may occur. Dissection must be carefully performed, because even minor hemorrhage will obscure visualization and may require cautery; thermal injury may be a prime mechanism of nerve injury. As with all other brow procedures, the endoscopic forehead lift can be used to address brow ptosis and forehead and glabellar rhytids. In cases of severe brow ptosis with or without glabellar furrows, a coronal forehead lift may be an acceptable alternative to the endoscopic forehead lift, assuming there is adequate hair density and distribution to camouflage the scar. More mild cases of brow ptosis can often be treated with minimal incision approaches based on the pattern of brow ptosis (see Chapter 8). Significant forehead and glabellar rhytids can alternatively be treated with skin resurfacing techniques (CO_2 or erbium:yttrium-aluminum-garnet [Er:YAG] laser, phenol or trichloroacetic acid peel), botulinum toxin chemodenervation, or soft tissue filler injections.

Indications and Contraindications

The endoscopic forehead lift is indicated for cases of mild to moderately severe brow ptosis, glabellar furrows, and forehead rhytids. Unilateral forehead paralysis and significant asymmetries of the brow can be addressed by the endoscopic forehead lift. The endoscopic forehead lift should be considered especially when a concurrent lateral midface lift is contemplated, because the endoscopic dissection leads readily to the midface dissection. However, adequate hair density is required to make the incisions cosmetically acceptable. Severe frontal or temporal scarring is a relative contraindication to the endoscopic forehead lift, because elevation in the correct planes may be impossible. Because there is no skin excision in the standard endoscopic forehead lift, patients with elevated foreheads should not undergo an endoscopic forehead lift without a trichophytic modification, because the hairline will otherwise shift unacceptably posteriorly.

Range of Anesthesia

The endoscopic forehead lift is a relatively straightforward procedure, easily completed in 2 hours or less. Incisions are small, and areas of dissection are easily anesthetized with blockade of the supratrochlear, supraorbital, and zygomaticotemporal nerves, supplemented by local infiltration. However, patients generally benefit from intravenous sedation and anxiolysis. Because patient participation is not needed to ensure appropriate positioning of the brow, preoperative patient assessment and management is performed and the patient screened for contraindications to any sedatives or potential respiratory depression; unless medically contraindicated, patients may be given general anesthesia. If combined with other procedures, a greater degree of sedation may be needed to ensure patient comfort during the longer operative period.

Equipment

One of the more significant drawbacks to the endoscopic forehead lift is the need for somewhat expensive and highly specialized instruments. The additional endoscopic equipment necessary is required because of the distance tissue modifications are performed from the small access incisions. This equipment consists of a 25° to 35° rigid endoscope coupled to a digital video camera and video monitor, long-handled endoscopic elevators, and long-shafted tissue dissectors (scissors, forceps, knives, and hooks). After flap elevation and tissue modifications, some form of fixation is generally desirable (methods and materials to be discussed later).

The rigid surgical telescopes used typically have viewing angles turned downward 25° to 35°, are illuminated with a xenon light source, and are inserted into dissection sheaths with distal flanges of various shapes (**Figure 9-1A**). These flanges assist in supporting the overlying tissues and provide an optical cavity designed to maximize the surgeon's view of the underlying soft tissue and bone. The angle of the lens also compensates for the convexity of the calvarium. Because the skin flap can be elevated only a short distance from the bone, the pertinent forehead and brow structures curve away from the endoscope tip as the dissection proceeds inferiorly; the flange supports the overlying tissue while the downward angle of the endoscope maintains visualization to the orbital rim. Although it is theoretically possible for the surgeon to operate visualizing tissues directly through the endoscope eyepiece, this positioning makes accessing and handling instruments in other ports awkward and cumbersome. A small video camera (single or triple chip with acceptable resolution) should be mounted on the eyepiece and the image displayed on a color monitor placed near the foot of the operating table, in line with the surgeon's axis of vision.

Tissue elevators come in various shaft lengths and curvatures, and the tips are designed for specific uses. At a minimum, an adequate set of endoscopic elevators should have straight, curved, and highly curved, flat, spatula-tipped elevators (**see Figure 9-1B**). Additional elevators, such as the highly curved, spatulated elevator for elevating the arcus marginalis, are helpful but not absolutely necessary. Other instruments, such as endoscopic scissors or knives (to incise the periosteum) and nerve hooks, are useful for specific functions during glabellar dissection. Finally, insulated forceps are helpful to control hemorrhage from muscle edges and small vessels during corrugator myotomy (**see Figure 9-1C**). In addition, a small plastic surgery tray with right-angle and Senn retractors and a Freer elevator as well as a bipolar cautery should also be available.

Operating Room Setup

Proper positioning of the patient and arrangement of equipment and personnel are critical in facilitating and efficiently performing the endoscopic forehead lift (**Figure 9-2**). The patient should be positioned with the patient's occiput in a round head pillow at the end of the operating table; access to the sides of the patient's head should be unencumbered. This provides access to all incisions and allows the use of long-handled instruments without hindrance. The surgeon is positioned at the head of

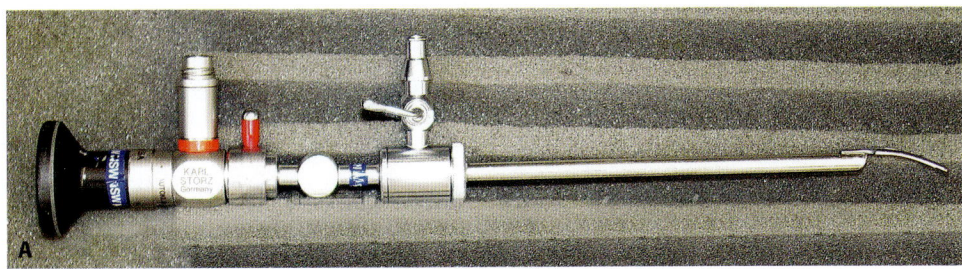

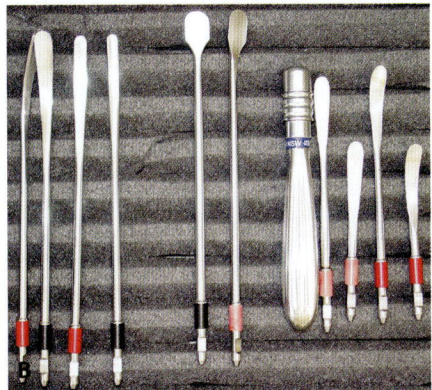

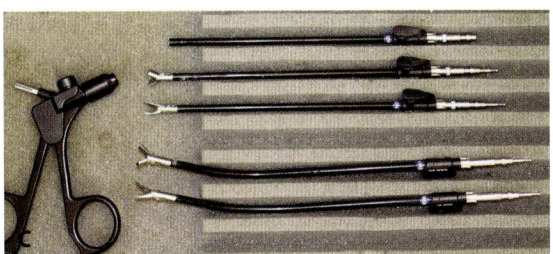

Figure 9-1. (A) A Hopkins II 30° down-turned endoscope with dissector sheath. The distal tip of the sheath is designed to keep forehead tissues elevated and help maintain an optical cavity. (B) Elevators with universal handle for an endoscopic forehead lift. Note the varying handle and blade lengths and curvatures and shapes of elevator tips. (C) Insulated forceps, scissors, and suction cautery with universal handle. (A–C Advanced Endobrow Facelift Set, Karl Storz Endoscopy-America, Inc., Culver City, CA.)

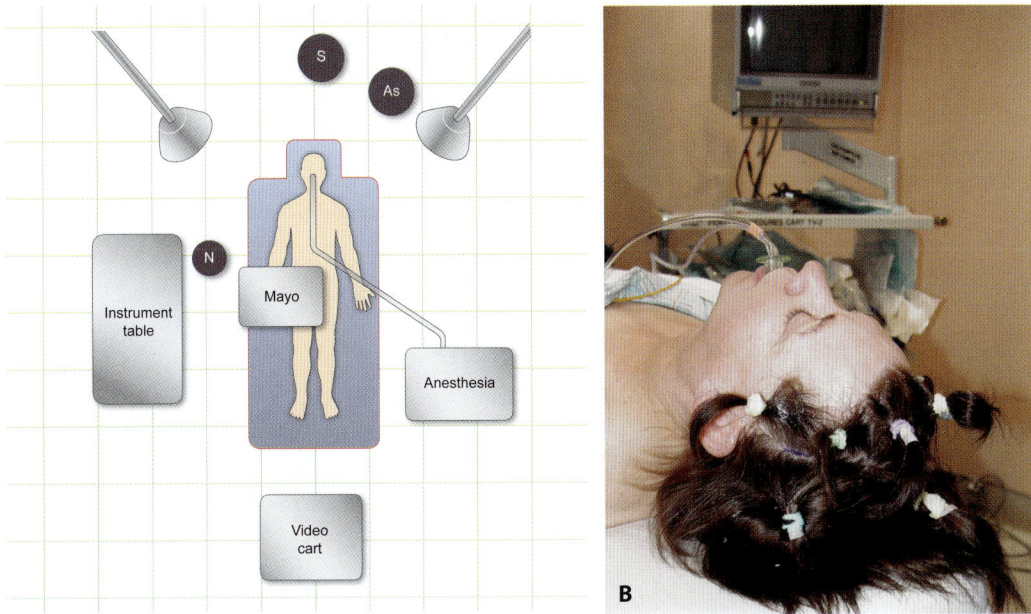

Figure 9-2. Operating room setup. (A) Video cart and monitor are located near the patient's feet to allow visualization of the screen in the same axis as that of the surgical field. The remainder of the operating room personnel and equipment is positioned to provide the surgeon with maximal access to the patient's forehead, temples and scalp. As = assistant; N = scrub nurse; S = surgeon. (B) Locating the monitor near the patient's feet allows a direct line of sight as the surgeon faces the patient.

the table, and the video monitor is positioned near the foot of the table, allowing the surgeon to sit facing the head and view the video monitor in the same visual axis. The scrub nurse is positioned at the side of the patient, with a small Mayo stand with a few frequently used instruments positioned over the patient's chest. Overhead lights should be positioned symmetrically angled over the patient's head in order to reduce camera glare.

Incisions

The standard endoscopic forehead lift elevates a flap continuously from one temple to the other across the forehead (**Figure 9-3A**). Whereas some authors have advocated as few as three or as many as six incisions, most surgeons use two temporal, two paramedian, and one midline incision 15 to 20 mm behind the hairline. The endoscope and camera are inserted into one port, while instruments are placed through another port. This angled approach helps the surgeon convert the two dimensions of the video image into a spatial map of the surgical cavity.

The temporal incision is generally 3 to 4 cm in length and is made about 2 cm posterior to the temporal hairline. This incision is a gently curved arc bisecting a line running from the ipsilateral alar crease through the lateral canthus. The temporal incision is taken down through skin until the temporoparietal fascia is identified; this is then incised and the deep temporal fascia is visualized. Before dissection proceeds inferiorly between these two fascial layers, a registration mark is incised in the deep temporal fascia, exposing the underlying temporalis muscle,

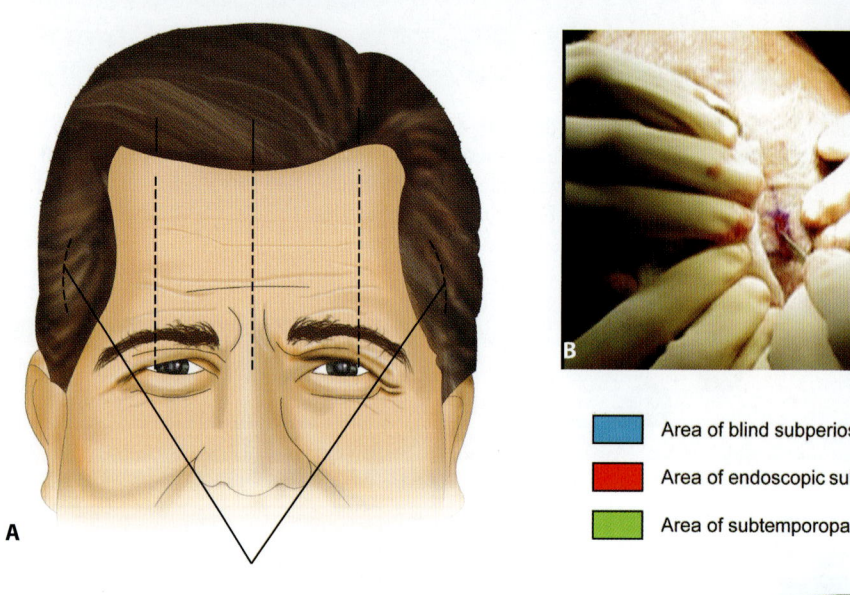

Area of blind subperiosteal dissection

Area of endoscopic subperiosteal dissection

Area of subtemporoparietal fascia dissection

Figure 9-3. (A) Typically, five incisions are used in the endoscopic forehead lift: two temporal, two paramedian, and one midline incision. (B) Incisions are made at least 1 cm behind the hairline and should take into account anticipated hair loss and hairline recession. (C) Central and paramedian incisions allow access for subperiosteal dissection over the central forehead. Temporal incisions are used for subtemporoparietal fascia dissection.

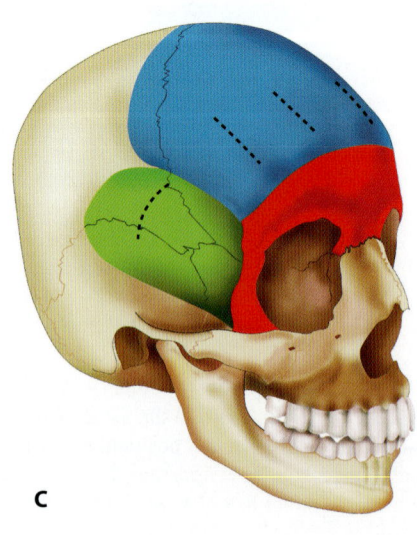

directly below the incision in the temporoparietal fascia. This deeper incision marks the position of the temporoparietal fascia incision. After flap elevation, the temporoparietal fascia is retracted and elevated a predetermined distance superolaterally above this mark.

The midline and paramedian incisions are oriented sagittally and are also placed about 2 cm posterior to the hairline (**see Figure 9-3B**). These incisions are typically 15 mm in length and can be easily made to minimize damage to the hair follicles by carefully parting the hair. The position of the paramedian incisions can be located anywhere between the midpupillary line and the lateral canthus but, in general, is placed above the location of the desired peak of the brow arch. These incisions are carried directly through all soft tissue with a #15 blade, incising the periosteum as well (**see Figure 9-3C**). The periosteum is then swept sideways with a Freer elevator to expose the bone; while the soft tissues are retracted laterally with Senn retractors, a registration mark is drilled at the anterior edge of the skin and periosteal incisions (**Figure 9-4**). Flap elevation is then performed as described later.

Plane(s) of Dissection

Two schools of thought exist as to the optimal central forehead plane of dissection during the endoscopic forehead lift. Advocates of the subgaleal plane suggest that this approach makes muscle identification and resection simpler and more direct, allows more focal contouring of the medial brow, and in general, is an easier plane to elevate (**Figure 9-5A**). Nassif and associates[15] found little difference in flap elevation tension between subgaleal elevation and subperiosteal elevation with release, and more recently, Thomas and coworkers[16] reported faster wound healing of elevated galea compared with elevated periosteum.

Conversely, proponents of the subperiosteal plane argue that this plane provides a better optical cavity (because calvarial bone reflects source light more effectively than soft tissue) (**see Figure 9-5B, C**), is associated with less bleeding (because this plane is relatively avascular), develops a highly vascularized flap (spares the vascular connections between the deep galea and the periosteum), and provides access to the midface in a subperiosteal plane. Also, the subperiosteal dissection avoids the glide plane space, which is necessarily violated and entered during a subgaleal dissection, and scarring here could profoundly limit postoperative brow mobility. Moreover, in comparison with the subgaleal plane, the subperiosteal plane better protects the deep branch of the supraorbital nerve (which runs above the periosteum as it ascends in the lateral forehead). Periosteum is thought to densely re-adhere to the underlying bone within 6 weeks, although a few authors have claimed that this may occur within 2 weeks in animal models.

In a national survey of 570 plastic surgeons, six-sevenths performed their forehead dissection subperiosteally. Both dissection planes have been proven to be effective in procedures to lift and contour the brow, and both have been advocated by

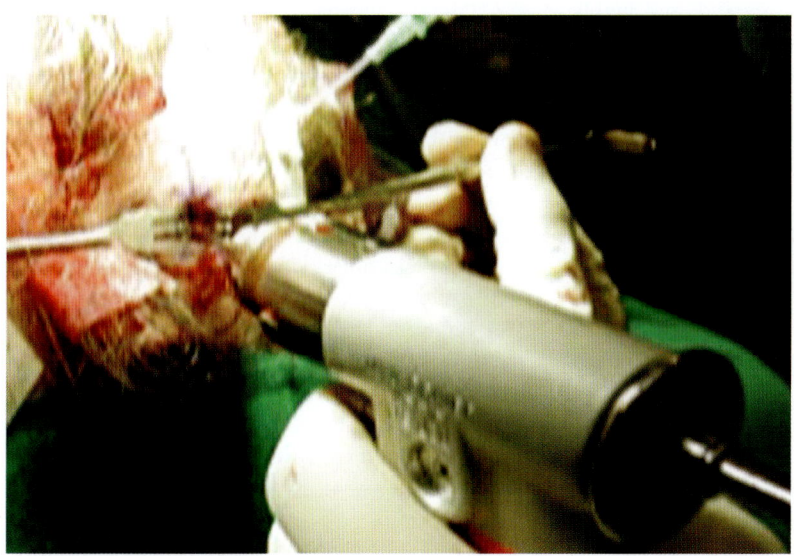

Figure 9-4. A registration mark is made on the outer table of the calvarium at the anterior extent of the skin incision before the forehead soft tissues have been elevated.

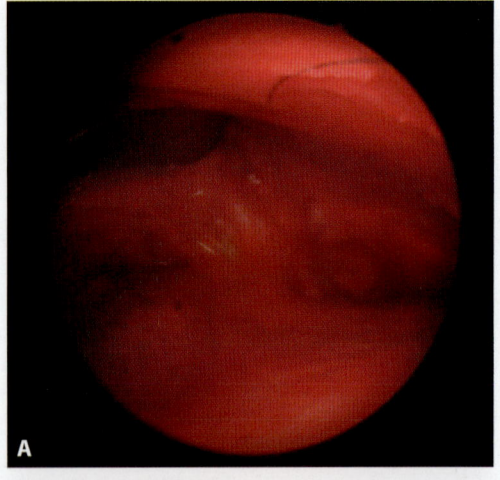

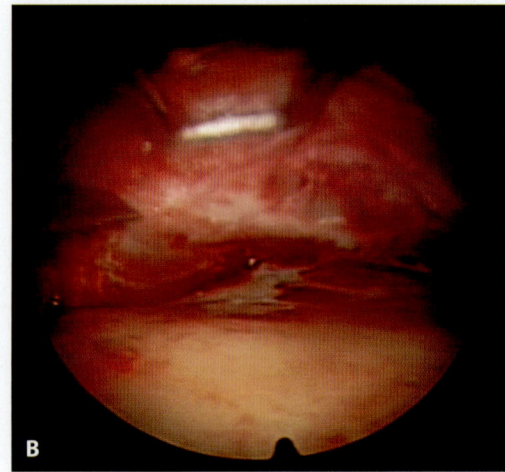

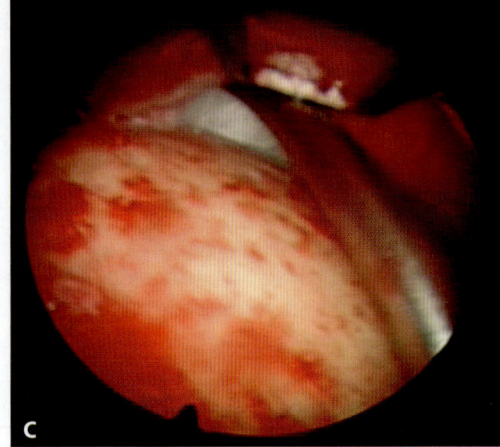

Figure 9-5. (A) Subgaleal dissection is fairly avascular and allows the surgeon to directly approach the glabellar muscles. (B) Subperiosteal dissection is performed in a less vascular plane and is "brighter," because the light from the endoscope reflects better off the white calvarium than off soft tissue. (C) The orbital rim is more easily skeletonized in the subperiosteal dissection.

well-respected surgeons. The actual plane chosen is a surgeon's personal preference. Freer elevators are used to begin this dissection over the central forehead, followed by straight, curved, and highly curved endoscopic elevators. This can be done blindly up to the vertex and down to within 2 cm of the orbital rim (**Figure 9-6A**). Subsequent inferior dissection is performed with endoscopic visualization, because at this point, the final leaf of deep galea fuses to periosteum and the periosteum becomes tightly adherent to the calvarium (**see Figure 9-6B**). The dissection proceeds to the level of the orbital rim, at which point, the corrugator and procerus muscles come easily into view (subgaleal approach), or just over the orbital rim, where often the arcus marginalis (seen as a white condensation of the periosteum) can be elevated (subperiosteal approach) (**see Figure 9-6C**).

Regardless of the central forehead dissection plane chosen, the temporal dissection is performed in a subtemporoparietal fascia plane. This plane is loose, avascular, and easily developed. Careful elevation in this plane protects the temporal branch of the facial nerve (within the elevated temporoparietal fascia); conversely, elevation below the deep temporal fascia is more vascular, makes inferior release more difficult, and risks trauma to the temporal fat pads, potentially leading to postoperative temporal hollowing. Again, once the correct plane is defined (**Figure 9-7A**) as being just below the temporoparietal fascia (above the deep temporal fascia), a registration mark is made at the level of the skin incision (which by extension is at the level of the incision through the temporoparietal fascia) (**see Figure 9-7B**). A Freer elevator is used to dissect this plane toward the zygoma inferiorly and toward the temporal crest medially (**see Figure 9-7C**). If a right-angle retractor is used for exposure and a strong headlight used for illumination, much of this dissection can be done under direct vision. When the temporal crest and area above the zygoma are neared, the endoscope is used for better visualization

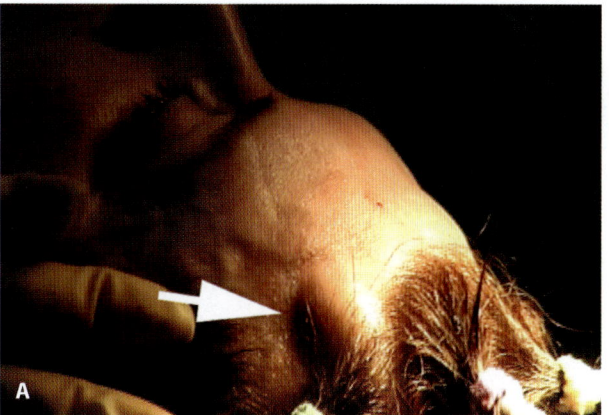

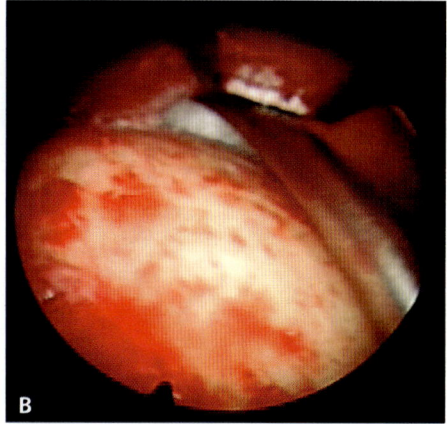

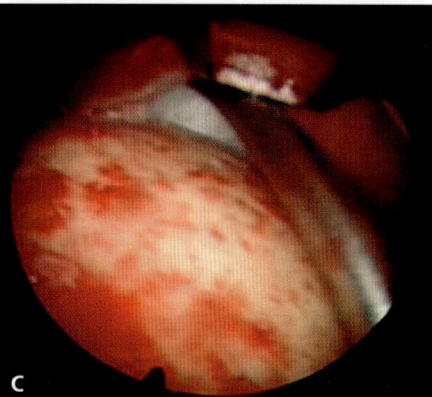

Figure 9-6. (A) Subperiosteal posterior scalp elevation and central forehead dissection can be performed blindly down to a point 2 cm above the orbital rim. Note the outline of the elevator below the skin *(arrow)*. (B, C) Further inferior dissection is done with endoscopic visualization as the orbital rim is approached; more curved elevator tips are generally used more inferiorly.

(**see Figure 9-7D**). In the area superolateral to the tail of the brow (**see Figure 9-7E**), the area of the temporal branches of the facial nerve is heralded by the middle zygomaticotemporal vein ("sentinel vein"; see Chapter 2 for topographic methods to plot the anticipated course of the nerve; see **Figure 9-7F–H**). Careful dissection around this vessel should be performed; if the vein limits adequate dissection, it can be cauterized near its entry into the deep temporal fascia with an insulated forceps and then transected. Cautery use should be limited and should never near the temporoparietal side of the vessel, because thermal injury to the facial nerve branches can occur. The temporoparietal fascia is elevated until the zone of fixation (see Chapter 2) is reached (**Figure 9-8A**); the endoscope is then moved into the central forehead pocket (**see Figure 9-8B**) while a gently curved spatulated elevator is place through the temporal incision under the temporoparietal fascia up to the zone of fixation. The elevator is then directed down against the bone and advanced into the central pocket under endoscopic visualization (**see Figure 9-8C**). Once the tip of the

elevator is seen in the central subperiosteal/subgaleal pocket, the spatula end is angled downward against the bone and swept up and down along the temporal crest (**see Figure 9-8D**) to completely elevate the zone of fixation. Once this is done bilaterally, the remainder of the lower brow is elevated: the endoscope is placed through one incision and the dissecting instruments through another. A gentle pushing motion is used to elevate the soft tissues; as the dissection progresses closer to the orbital rim, a more curved elevator is needed to adequately dissect in this area (**Figure 9-9**). The dissection proceeds inferiorly until the soft tissue has been elevated off of the entire supraorbital rim from one lateral canthus to the other. Having an assistant hold the endoscope allows the surgeon to place the thumb and forefinger of his or her nondominant hand over the orbital rim for external reference while dissecting with the other hand (**Figure 9-10**). Alternatively, external traction sutures can be placed through the skin at the upper border of the brow and the assistant can pull on these for soft tissue countertraction during dissection. Complete dissection along the lateral

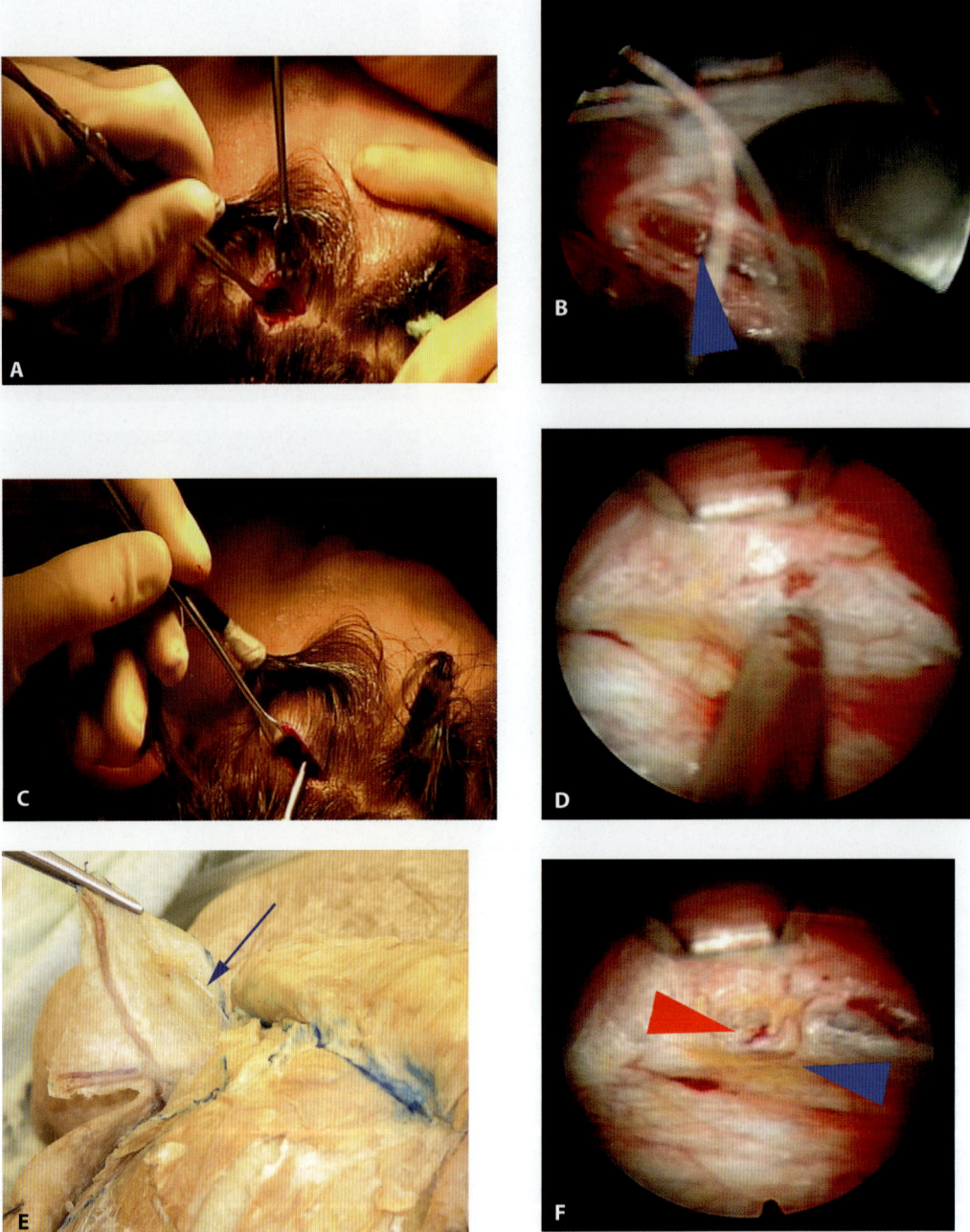

Figure 9-7. (A) Temporal dissection is begun by identifying the temporoparietal fascia, incising it, and then identifying the deep temporal fascia. (B) An incision in the deep temporal fascia confirms the identity of this fascia (temporalis muscle seen below this fascia) and is made directly below the skin incision to serve as a registration mark. (C) A Freer elevator can then be placed below the temporoparietal fascia and this fascia elevated from the deep temporal fascia under direct vision. (D) As dissection proceeds more medially and inferiorly, an endoscope is used for better visualization. The yellow glint of the superficial temporal fat (seen below the superficial layer of the deep temporal fascia) serves as a marker for the approximate position of the zygomaticotemporal ("sentinel") vein, which, in turn, can be used to locate the temporal branches of the facial nerve. (E) In this cadaver dissection, the temporal branches of the facial nerve are seen running within the temporoparietal fascia. (F) The zygomaticotemporal vein *(red arrowhead)* can be seen running from the temporoparietal fascia into the deep temporal fascia and superficial temporal fat pad *(blue arrowhead)* *(Continued)*

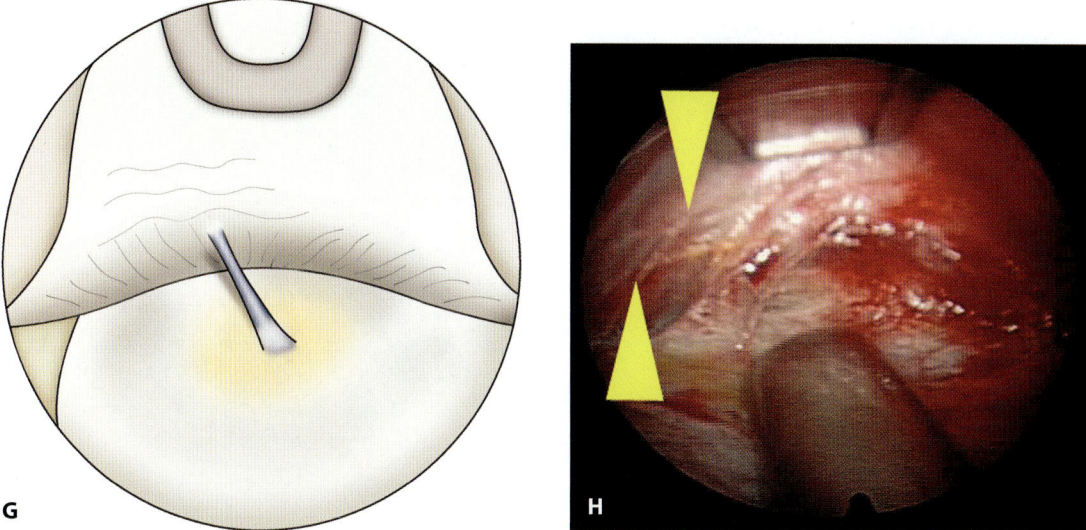

Figure 9-7 *(Continued)* (G) The zygomaticotemporal vein *(red arrowhead)* can be seen running from the temporoparietal fascia into the deep temporal fascia and superficial temporal fat pad *(blue arrowhead)*. (H) Temporal branches of the facial nerve *(yellow arrowheads)* in close proximity to the zygomaticotemporal vein.

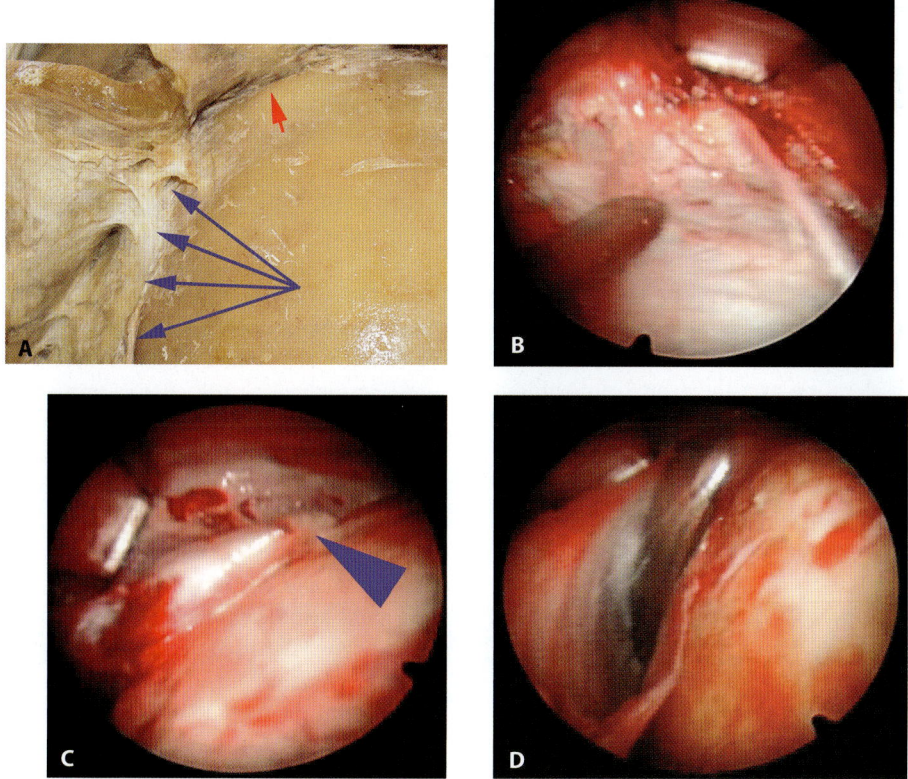

Figure 9-8. (A) Zone of fixation *(blue arrows)* is a dense condensation of deep and superficial temporal fascia layers just medial to the superior temporal line *(red arrow* marks the superior orbital rim). (B) Left zone of fixation as seen from the endoscopic central pocket. (C) Elevator is placed directly above the deep temporal fascia through the temporal incision, and the outline of the elevator tip *(blue arrowhead)* can be seen. (D) The elevator tip is pushed through the last fascial fibers, connecting the dissection pockets, and then the elevator is swept up and down along the temporal crest to complete the elevation of the zone of fixation.

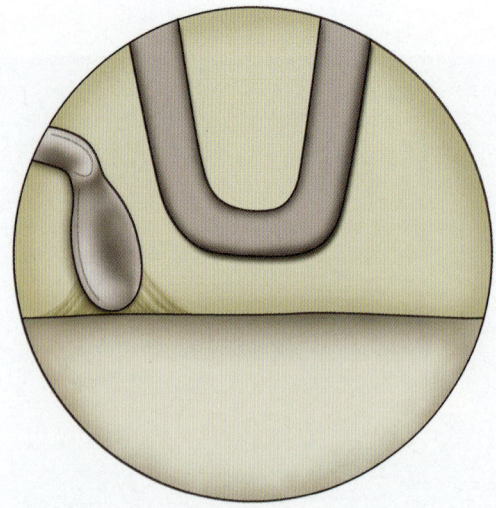

Figure 9-9. More highly curved instruments are used to dissect along the orbital rim.

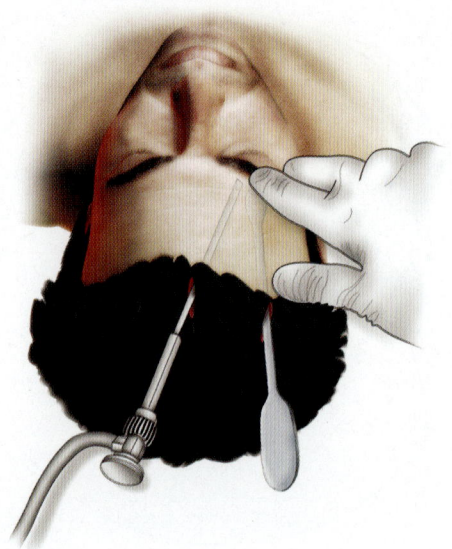

Figure 9-10. Significant feedback useful for orientation can be gained by external palpation.

orbital rim to the lateral canthus ensures release of the orbital ligament, necessary for adequate mobilization of the lateral brow.

If the subgaleal plane is chosen, this dissection will allow direct visualization of the glabellar muscles. In subperiosteal central forehead dissections, it is critical that the periosteum be elevated inferiorly to include exposure and mobilization of the arcus marginalis at the orbital rim. This can be both felt during dissection as an area of dense attachments as well as visualized as a thickening or condensation of the elevated periosteum at the orbital rim **(Figure 9-11)**. This dissection can be facilitated by an orbital rim dissector, which has a highly curved, downward-oriented distal tip of the elevator and is useful for elevating over the orbital rim without penetrating into orbital fat. Once the periosteum is adequately elevated, it is incised with an endoscopic knife or scissors along the full length of elevation. An endoscopic forceps, scissors, or nerve hook is then used to spread the edges of the cut periosteum apart.

Tissue Modifications

Whereas some early authors argued that elevation, mobilization, and fixation of forehead tissues is sufficient, most workers agree that some form of glabellar myoplasty is necessary to fully elevate the brow and maintain its elevated position as well as smooth glabellar furrows. This may take the form of myotomy, myectomy, or muscle disinsertion to reduce the activity of that particular muscle. Early

in the development of the procedure, Core and coworkers[3] additionally advocated frontalis weakening by transverse cuts below deep transverse rhytids; however, frontalis muscle incision would weaken the sole elevator of the brow and most surgeons would agree that skin resurfacing with or without soft tissue augmentation is a more appropriate treatment for any postoperative residual forehead rhytids.

Glabellar myoplasty generally includes treatment of the corrugator and depressor supercilii and procerus muscles and may also include myotomy of the superolateral orbicularis oculi muscle. After the dissection reaches the area just above the supraorbital rim (subgaleal dissection) or after incision of the periosteum 3 to 5 mm above the arcus marginalis (subperiosteal dissection), myoplasties of the corrugator and depressor supercilii are performed. Care must be taken in this dissection to avoid violation of the periorbita, which will lead to increased ecchymosis and edema postoperatively. As the endoscope is advanced inferiorly, the brow depressor muscles are visualized near the orbital rim. The appropriate treatment of these muscles must take into account the method of fixation to be used, the postoperative result desired, and the risk of postoperative deformity. Aggressive treatment of the procerus muscle may leave a postoperative depression; if this muscle is completely sectioned, a small amount of fat can be harvested and placed into the defect to prevent both muscle re-adhesion and a postoperative deformity.

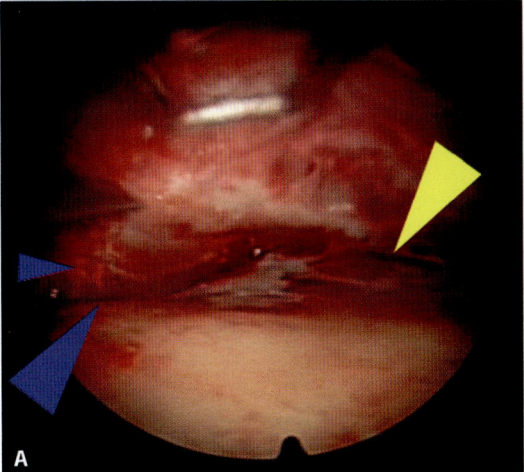

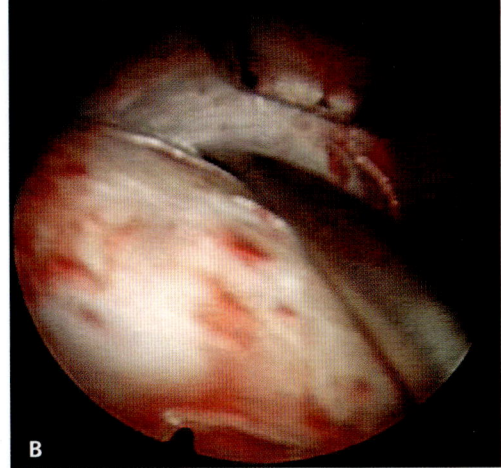

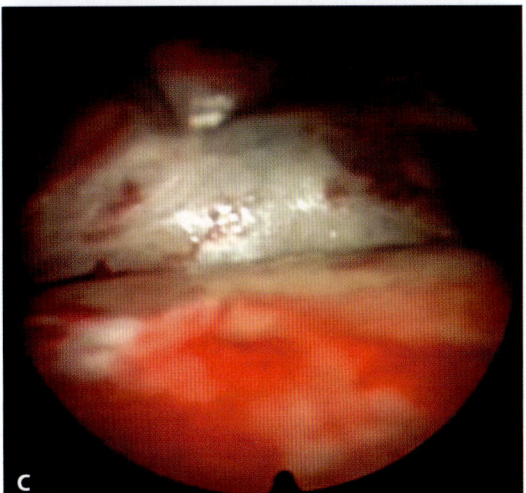

Figure 9-11. (A) Dissection near the orbital rim. *Yellow arrowhead = nasal root; blue arrowhead = arcus marginalis.* (B) An inferior/anterior pushing/stretching motion is useful to fully elevate the arcus marginalis. (C) Full elevation of the arcus marginalis is confirmed by the solid and uniform white condensation as well as by palpation.

Aggressive treatment (overly-through myotomy or distinct myectomy) of the corrugator supercilii muscle releases the medial brow attachment[17] and can lead to excessive separation and overlatereralization of the medial brow. Using endoscopic scissors, forceps, or a nerve hook, the muscle fibers of the corrugator supercilii and procerus muscles can be stripped parallel to the direction of the fibers of each muscle as well as the supraorbital and supratrochlear nerves and vessels (**Figure 9-12**). If performed carefully, bleeding is generally minimal and can usually be controlled with external pressure but may occasionally require cauterization. The dissection proceeds until fat is easily visible, tranversed by twigs of the glabellar nerves and vessels (**Figure 9-13**). More laterally, the edges of the periosteum are spread radially away from the orbital rim to release the lateral orbicularis oculi muscle. The dissection

hugs the orbital rim laterally past the frontozygomatic suture up to the area of the lateral canthus.

Once the tissues of the forehead and temple have been elevated, retaining structures (including periosteum) have been released and the depressor forces that act on the brow have been weakened or eliminated. The brow can be elevated to the desired height but must be maintained in this position long enough for the elevated tissues to re-adhere sufficiently. The method and length of time required for tissue fixation remains one of the more hotly debated technical issues in performing the endoscopic forehead lift.

Based on the dynamic theory of brow positioning, after soft tissue elevation and the release of the brow and depressor myotomies, the preoperative tonic contraction of the frontalis muscle (brow elevator) alone will support the brow in a new,

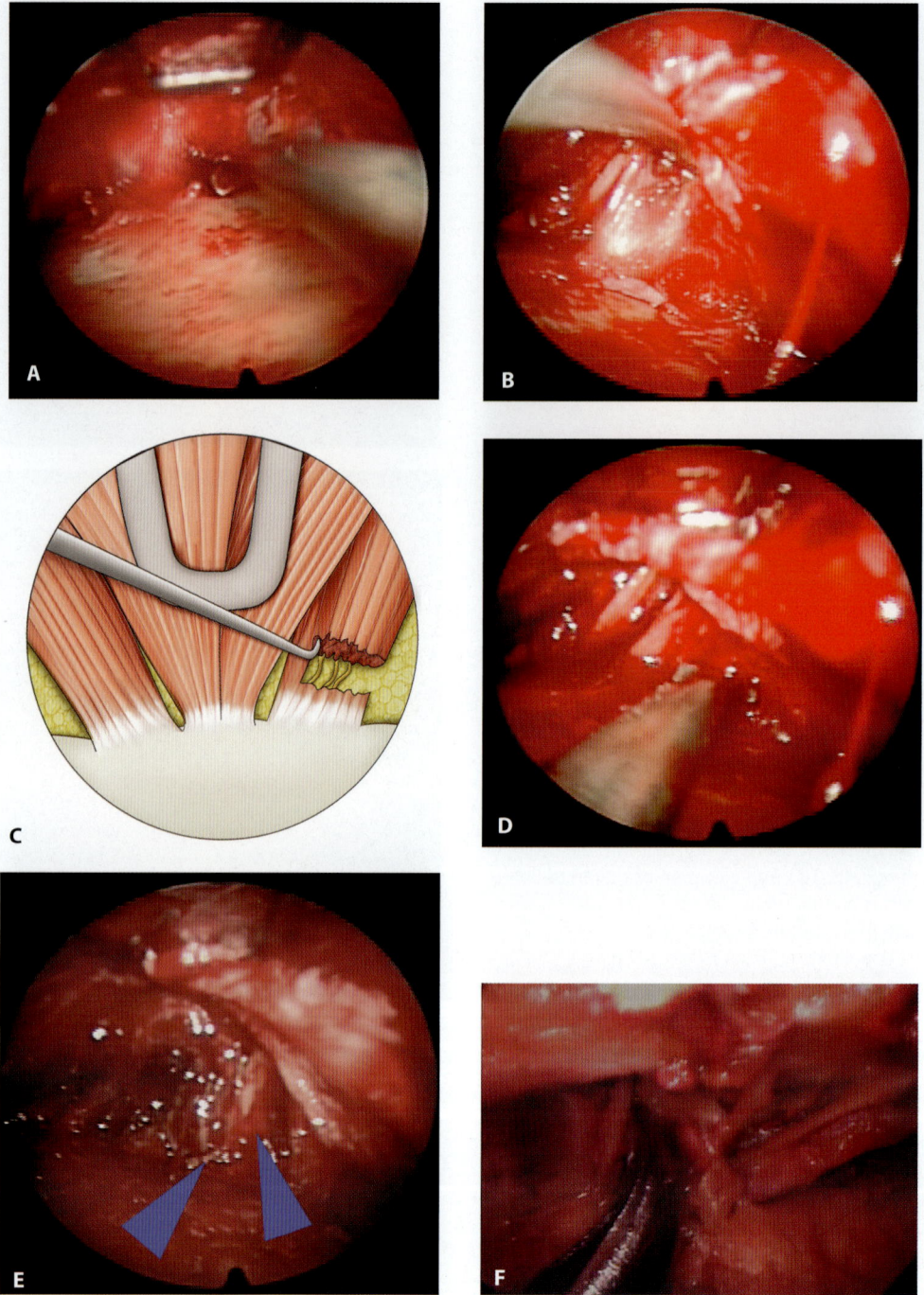

Figure 9-12. Glabellar myoplasty. (A) Dissection is begun (if subperiosteal plane used) by piercing the periosteum with a sharp instrument such as scissors, chisel, or nerve hook. (B) By stripping the periosteum radially away from the orbital rim, the edges of the periosteal cut are separated and the corrugator supercilii muscle is teased away from the supratrochlear and supraorbital nerves. (C) Careful dissection skeletonizes the branches of the supratrochlear and supraorbital nerves. (D) Dissection should progress in between nerve fibers, and dissection is always parallel to these fibers. (E) Branches of the supraorbital and supratrochlear arteries will also be seen and should be preserved and carefully cauterized only if necessary. (F) Spreading dissection with endoscopic forceps or scissors can help skeletonize the glabellar neurovascular structures.

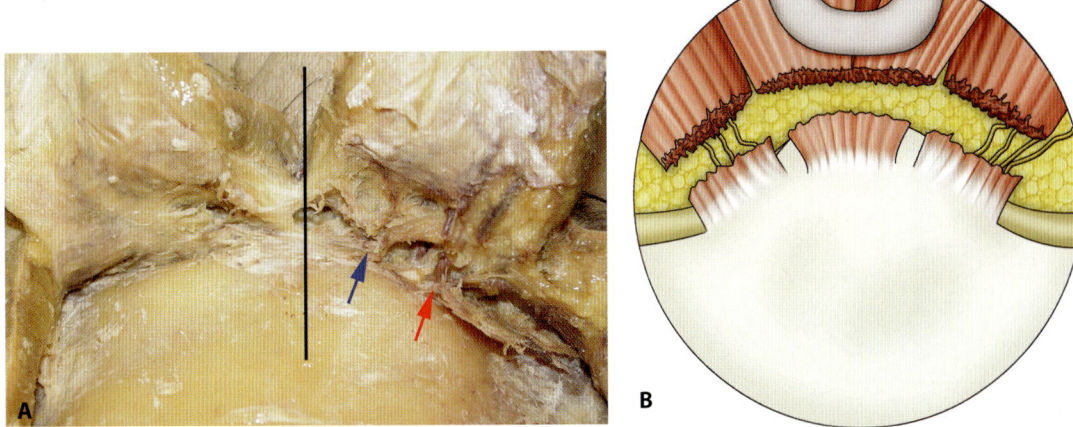

Figure 9-13. A Cadaver dissection of the orbital rim, as seen from above (same view as the endoscopic forehead lift shown in Figure 9-3). Supratrochlear *(blue arrow)* and supraorbital *(red arrow)* nerves with vessels shown. *Black line* marks the midline. B At the completion of the endoscopic glabellar dissection, brow fat should be seen behind the fibers of the supraorbital and supratrochlear nerves and arteries.

elevated position (**Figure 9-14**). Over time, the frontalis muscle does relax, as evidenced by the reduction/elimination of transverse forehead rhytids. Theoretically, if the frontalis muscle maintains its tonic contraction longer than the time necessary for secure re-adherence of the elevated tissue (galea or periosteum) down to the deeper layer (galea-periosteum or bone), no additional measures are required to stabilize the brow position. Some early authors advocated no fixation or short-term

methods, such as skin staples placed posterior to temporary transcutaneous screws (**Figure 9-15**), skin or galeal mattress sutures, or fibrin glue. However, signs of the inadequacy of short-term fixation are evident in early reports of the need for "overcorrection" or "early failure"/ "early recurrence of brow ptosis." The fact that not all patients suffered early recurrence of brow ptosis is a testament to the fact that in some patients, the thoroughness of depressor myotomies, the persistence of elevated

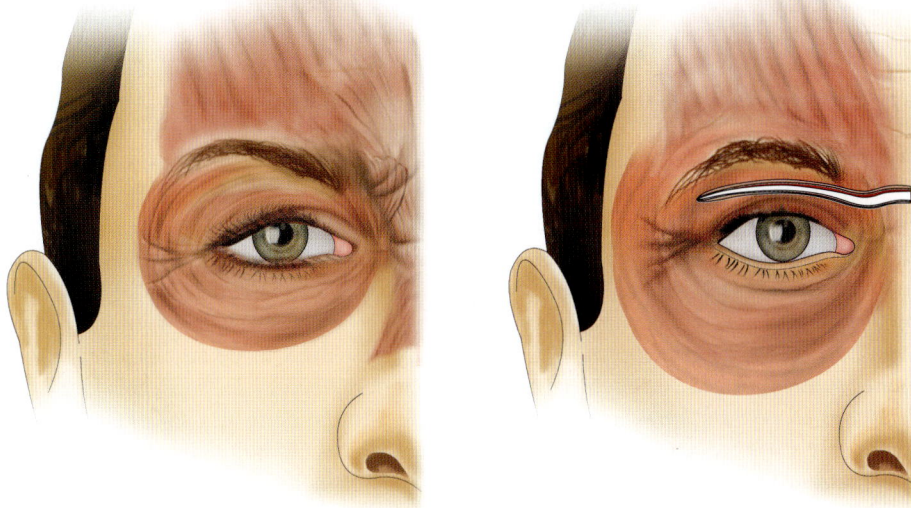

Figure 9-14. In the absence of effective brow depressor muscle activity, brow position will rise to a more neutral height.

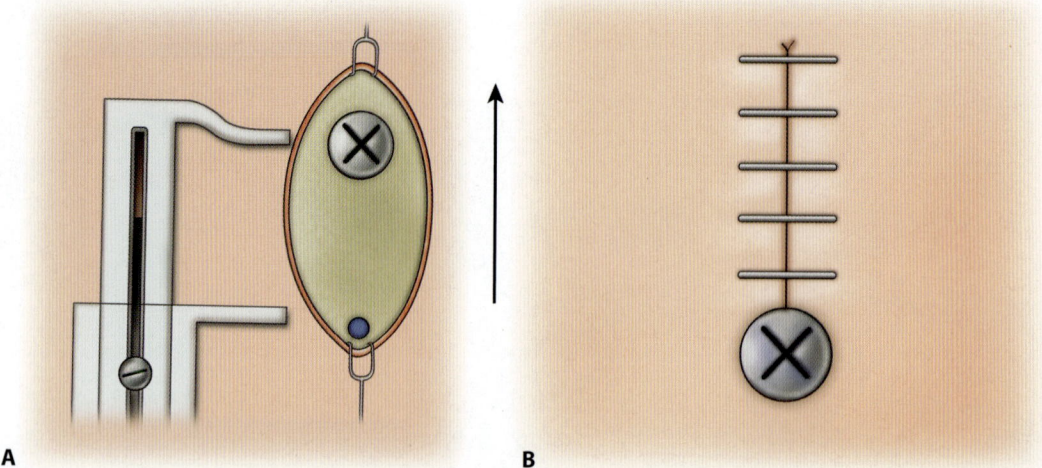

A   **B**

Figure 9-15. (A) Temporary transcutaneous screw fixation of brow position. Transcutaneous screw is placed a measured distance superior to the registration mark made at the anterior end of the skin incision. The skin flap is then mobilized superiorly so that the anterior end of the skin incision rests against the screw post. (B) Surgical staples are then used to close the wound. The scalp is maintained in its elevated position because the staples are held up by the screw head.

frontalis tone, and the rapidity of tissue re-adherence is sufficient to allow the brow to heal in its desired position. In a study of endoscopic forehead lifts for unilateral brow ptosis due to facial paralysis, Ducic and Adelson[18] fixed the forehead in its desired position with temporary transcutaneous screws. These patients had no depressor function from the ipsilateral orbicularis oculi, corrugator and depressor supercilii, and procerus muscles, yet the authors described a 1.3-mm loss of elevation at 12 months postoperatively. In these cases, even the limited effect of the *contralateral* brow depressors, coupled with the effect of gravity on the brow, led to descent of brows that were inadequately healed to deep tissues by 2 weeks.

However, in a review of 220 patients undergoing an endoscopic forehead lift with subperiosteal dissection and muscle "debulking,"[19] fixated postoperatively with either cortical tunnels or fibrin glue, overall patients averaged 6 mm of elevation at the midpupil. However, patients whose brows were fixated with fibrin glue averaged 2-mm loss of elevation between 1 and 6 months after surgery, compared with no change in brow position when polydiaxanone sutures placed through cortical tunnels were used to provide long-term fixation. McKinney and Sweis[20] noted that in 93 patients undergoing endobrow lift, fixation with Vicryl sutures in the temple and around central forehead cortical tunnels was inadequate, because the average of 6 to 7 mm of intraoperative brow elevation

decreased to 4.1 mm postoperatively. This also supports the concept that fixation should be maintained for somewhat longer than 3 weeks to allow for periosteal re-adherence.

The variability of results led many surgeons to abandon the endoscopic forehead lift as inadequate; however, others persisted to improve the reliability of this procedure. Some surgeons advocated simply overcorrecting by a factor of two or more (while still using short-term fixation methods), but again, the unpredictability of the specific brow position left patients as likely to be overcorrected as undercorrected. Alternatively, some surgeons changed to methods of permanent fixation using surgical hardware such as bone microplates as suture anchors or buried titanium tacks. As a compromise, methods of long-term (but ultimately temporary) fixation (with or without hardware) have been developed. These methods suspend the (mobile) elevated forehead tissues to the (stable) calvarium. Cortical tunnels and calvarial bone hooks take advantage of the dual cortex of the calvarium to define bone upon which a (semi-) permanent suture from the galea or periosteum can be suspended. A cortical tunnel is developed by drilling a hole in the outer table of the frontal bone at a 45° angle, stopping when the diploic space is entered. A complementary hole is drilled at a 90° angle to the first hole, meeting it in the diploic space (**Figure 9-16**). This defines an overlying 3- to 4-mm bone bridge; a needle is then passed through one hole and out the other and then

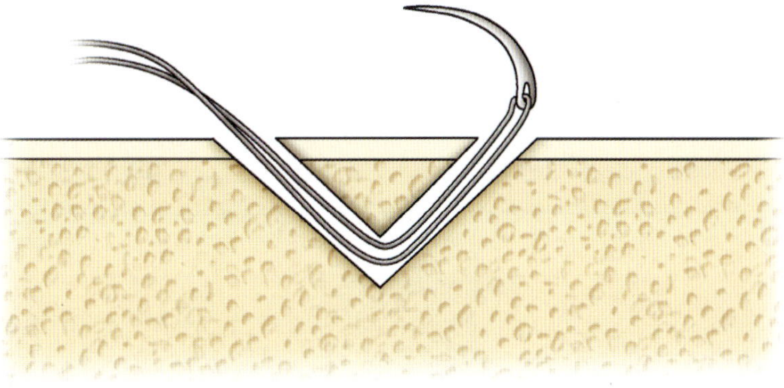

Figure 9-16. Cortical tunnels are created by drilling two holes through the outer cortex of the calvarium at complementary 45° angles, meeting within the diploic space. A suture is then passed through this tunnel and then sutured to the forehead skin flap.

passed through the elevated flap tissue. The brow is thus suspended by sutures from this bone bridge. The bone hook technique similarly utilizes the outer cortex for suture stability. An inverted "U" shaped trough is drilled through the outer cortex, leaving a vertically oriented extension of cortical bone to serve as a "hook" for suture placement. Both of these techniques are simple and rapidly performed, although they may be complicated by diploic space oozing, which can be controlled with bone wax.

A number of resorbable (made of polylactic acid derivatives) fixation devices are available and are essentially countersunk screws through or around which forehead fixation sutures can be placed. Finally, a "rake" implant is also available that is fixed to calvarium by a post on its deep surface inserted into a monocortical hole and suspends the soft tissue of the forehead with externally oriented, angled tines that impale the periosteum and galea. All of these devices are designed to provide significant tensile strength for at least 12 weeks but are fully hydrolyzed and resorbed within a year of placement.

The author's personal preference is Lactosorb 2.0 × 5.0-mm forehead fixation screws. Preoperatively, with the patient seated in an upright position, specific points along the brow (above the medial canthus, in the midpupillary line, and at the desired brow peak) are first marked and then individually elevated to the desired height. The distance to be elevated is measured and recorded. After the forehead tissues have been elevated and myotomies performed, a distance posterior to the registration bone mark in the central incision equal to the length of elevation desired for the medial brow is measured, and a 5.0-mm deep hole drilled to accommodate a 2.0-mm-diameter resorbable screw. The same is then done for each of the paramedian incisions, using the distance desired for elevation of the midpu-

pillary brow. A Lactosorb screw placed in each hole. A 3-0 polydiaxanone suture is then passed through the periosteum and galea at the most anterior aspect of the skin incision (corresponding to the site of the registration mark prior to elevation), the suture tail is passed through a hole in the screw head in each of these three incisions, and the suture is tied. This elevates the anterior edge of the scalp incision exactly the same distance as the desired brow elevation for each of these points (**Figure 9-17**). Ultimately, the method of fixation used by a given surgeon should be chosen based on the safety and efficacy of the method, the amount of permanent hardware left in place, and the perceived length of time for which extrinsic fixation is necessary.

Whereas most authors do acknowledge the need for some form of central forehead fixation, others have argued that temporal fixation only is necessary. Because the frontalis muscle does not extend beyond the temporal line (thus elevating the tail of the brow by secondary movement of forehead skin only), the frontalis tone should not be expected to significantly elevate the brow tail, based on the dynamic theory of brow position. Rather, a suture is placed to suspend the elevated temporoparietal fascia up to the posterosuperior deep temporal fascia. Because the suture is directed at an angle, rather than completely vertically, there needs to be greater advancement of the temporoparietal fascia than that desired for brow elevation. Mathematically (**Figure 9-18**), the amount of superolateral movement needed increases as the desired high point of the brow moves more medially. In theory, this factor can be calculated; however, 2 to 3 mm of additional movement (beyond the number of millimeters desired for brow peak elevation) is generally sufficient. Before placing suture, a square of proximal deep temporal fascia is removed to provide a highly vascular bed for fibrosis to

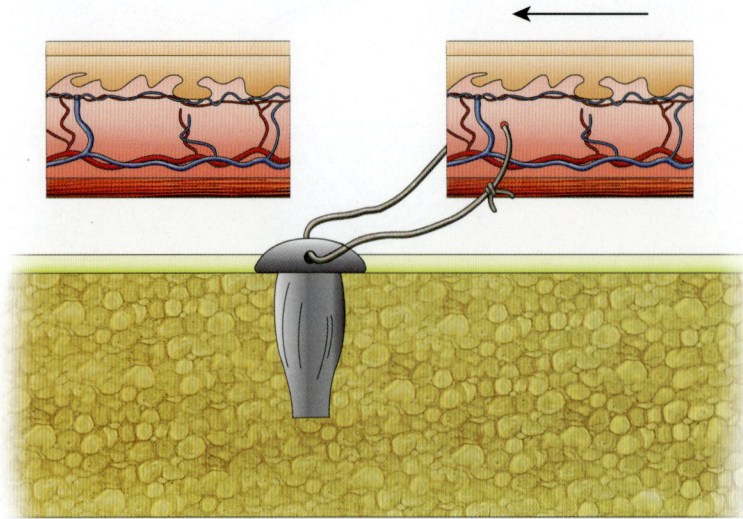

Figure 9-17. Resorbable bone screws can also be used to maintain fixation. These screws have a hole in their heads to accept sutures after placement in the outer cortex of the calvarium.

occur between the mobilized temporoparietal fascia and the temporalis muscle for increased adhesion. Once the temporoparietal fascia–deep temporal fascia suture has been placed, lateral brow positioning is assessed as *the point beyond which the lateral brow cannot be manually depressed easily.* Indeed, some authors have advocated using the temporal fossa sutures alone as a means of fixation. However, even if central forehead fixation is employed, temporal fixation is essential to adequately control the lateral brow position and overall brow shape.

Wound Closure

Before wound closure, a fluted suction drain is draped under the flap over the upper forehead and both temples and brought out through a separate stab incision laterally. The temporal elevation may produce some skin redundancy, which is conservatively resected. All incisions are then closed in layers with 4-0 absorbable dermal sutures and skin staples.

Dressings

A lightly compressive dressing of cotton or fluffed gauze covered by an elastic bandage is placed over the forehead and around the drain site. The lower edge of the dressing is taped to the suprabrow area to prevent its displacement, and a stockinette over the dressing may be helpful to maintain the dressing in place.

Technique Modifications

When properly performed and the brow position stabilized for a sufficient period of time, the endoscopic forehead lift can be a highly accurate technique for moderate brow repositioning without the need for overcorrection. As such, it is rarely necessary to elevate the brows more than 7 to 8 mm. Hence, the frontal hairline is rarely overelevated except in cases of a preexisting high hairline. In these cases, a trichophytic incision is necessary; this can be incorporated into the endoscopic forehead lift. Originally described by both Ramirez[5] and Oslin and colleagues[6] in 1995, a trichophytic central incision allows a subcutaneous dissection of the upper 2 to 4 cm of the central forehead between the temporal crests. This incision then continues into the hair-bearing temple or along the temporal hairline (determined by the distance between the temporal hairline and the lateral brow). The degree of central subcutaneous dissection is increased by the need for forehead reduction, deep transverse forehead rhytids, and brow asymmetry and balanced by a patient history of tobacco use or vascular insufficiency. The frontalis muscle is plicated between the supraorbital nerve branches. Sagittal slits are then made in the frontalis muscle to allow endoscopic modification (subperiosteal or subgaleal) of the brow depressor muscles (**Figure 9-19A**). Once the myoplasties are performed, the skin is redraped, redundant skin along the hairline is excised (**see Figure 9-19B**), and the skin is closed in layers.

Postoperative Management

Patients undergoing endoscopic forehead lifting may be discharged home on the day of surgery, unless they also undergo multiple concurrent

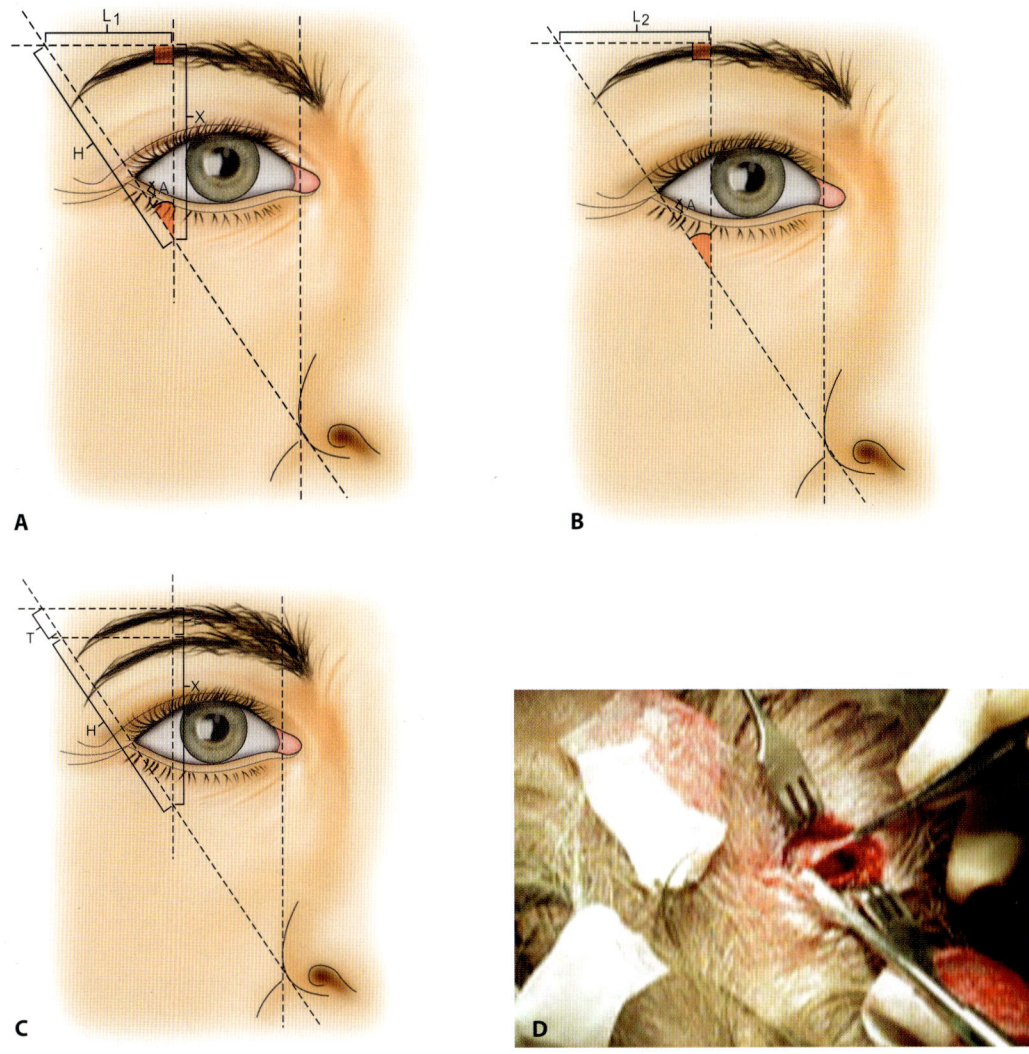

Figure 9-18. (A–C) Mathematical expression of the amount of temporal elevation (T) needed to achieve desired elevation of the brow peak (E). It can be seen that the amount of oblique temporal elevation necessary increases as the distance from the brow peak to the temporal incision (L) increases. (D) Temporoparietal fascia is the carrier structure, allowing elevation of the brow. Temporal suspension is performed by suturing the temporoparietal fascia superiorly to the deep temporal fascia.

procedures or wish to stay in an overnight facility for convenience. In patients without contraindications, a preoperative stress dose of an intravenous corticosteroid is followed by a rapid taper over the first 3 days postoperatively. Prophylactic antibiotics are given for 5 days, and a prescription for a narcotic analgesic is provided to the patient as well. Although patients frequently describe the sensation of a severe "tension headache" on the night of surgery, discomfort rarely requires narcotics use for more than 24 to 48 hours postoperatively. Patients are instructed to keep their heads elevated for the first 48 hours,

and ice compresses are applied to the forehead and periorbital area for the first 24 hours. Patients taking *Arnica Montana* and bromelain are instructed to continue their use for 10 to 14 days postoperatively.

Patients are seen on postoperative day 1, at which time, drain removal is generally appropriate. The dressing is removed at this time, and patients are instructed to apply antibiotic ointment to the skin staples three times daily. They are allowed to shower after drain removal, but are cautioned to avoid hot showers, because the scalp is generally numb from the brows to the vertex for some time after

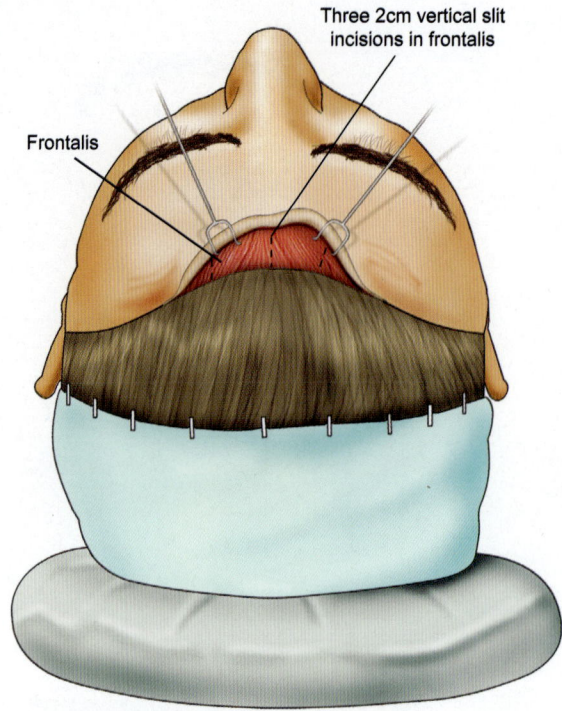

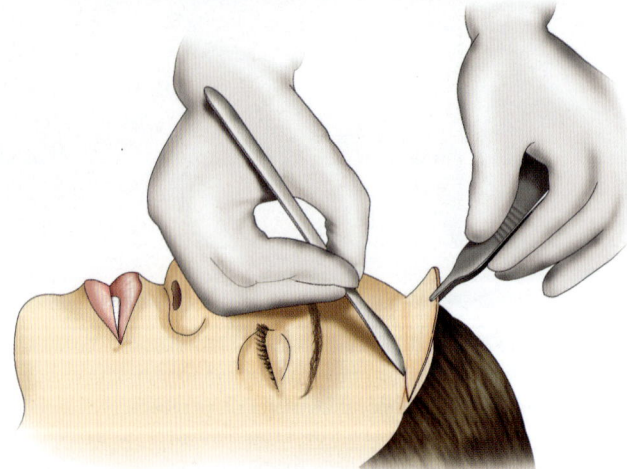

Figure 9-19. Trichophytic endoscopic forehead lift. (A) An incision along the anterior hairline continues along the temporal hairline or reflects back into the temporal hair. After a skin flap is developed, three sagittal incisions are made for glabellar myoplasty. (B) After glabellar myoplasty is performed (similar to standard endoscopic forehead lift), redundant skin is excised and the incision is closed.

surgery. Staples are removed 5 to 7 days after surgery, at which time there is little to no discoloration or edema of the forehead and only minimal periorbital ecchymosis and edema. Patients typically can return to work within 4 to 5 days and can resume normal activities by 14 days after surgery.

Complications: Incidence, Management, and Avoidance

When properly performed, the endoscopic forehead lift is a highly successful procedure with mild temporary morbidity and few potential permanent complications.

Hair Loss/Wide Scar

Permanent hair loss after an endoscopic forehead lift is generally considered uncommon. In a national survey, Elkwood and colleagues[21] noted only 2.9% of cases had reported hair loss, which compares favorably with the 4% reported for the coronal forehead lift. Withey and associates,[22] interestingly, noted a 29% incidence of incisional alopecia when fixation was provided with skin staples suspended upon a temporary transcutaneous bone screw and contrasted that with a 6% incidence when any other technique of fixation was used. Postoperatively, areas of incisional alopecia can be excised and resutured or the area grafted with single-unit hair transplants. Clearly, edge-to-edge tensionless two-layer wound closure should be performed to minimize these complications, and if cautery is necessary to control bleeding from skin edges, only bipolar cautery should be used.

Widened Scar

Roberts and Ellis[23] noted that the coronal forehead lift was significantly more likely (15.3%) to leave a widened scar than the endoscopic forehead lift (6.6%). Conversely, Elkwood and colleagues[21] revealed in their survey that surgeons reported a 0.8% incidence of widened scar in open procedures compared with less than 0.1% in the endoscopic forehead lift. Again, transcutaneous screw fixation accounts for a majority of widened central forehead scars; however, widening of the temporal scar may be related to its use as a drain exit site or if inadequate lateral brow release has been performed and a tension wound closure used to elevate the lateral brow. As with incisional alopecia, widened scars can be excised or the area transplanted with single-unit hair grafts. Using buried fixation devices, exiting drains separately, performing a two-layered wound closure, and avoiding wound tension should reduce scar widening to an acceptable level.

Hematoma/Seroma

Although it might be expected that hematomas or seromas develop more commonly after subgaleal than subperiosteal dissections because of the vascular anatomy of the scalp, neither approach is particularly associated with this complication. Isse[2] reported a seroma rate of 6.6%, whereas multiple workers[1,16] have reported a hematoma rate of about 3%, similar to the coronal forehead lift. These are rarely problematic if wounds are drained and can either be expressed or simply aspirated. Careful dissection near the orbital rim should protect the supraorbital and supratrochlear vessels, and any oozing can be controlled with cautery.

Pruritus

Pruritus can be quite disturbing to patients, even if temporary, and generally lasts 3 to 9 months.

Adamson and Johnson[24] reported temporary pruritus in up to 18% of patients undergoing a coronal forehead lift, whereas Roberts and Ellis[23] noted this complaint in almost 60% of coronal forehead lift patients. These workers contrasted this with a 20% incidence in patients undergoing endoscopic forehead lifting and carbon dioxide laser resurfacing and 21% incidence in those patients undergoing laser resurfacing only. Withey and associates[22] also reported that 37% of patients noted pruritus after endoscopic forehead lift. Patients should be counseled that, although this may persist for several months, it is rarely permanent.

Nerve Injury

Sensory

Forehead hypesthesia/aesthesia is almost universal in the first 7 to 10 days after an endoscopic forehead lift. Permanent anesthesia is unusual; Elkwood and colleagues[21] noted surgeons self-reported problematic forehead numbness in less than 0.1% in either endoscopic or open forehead lifts. Guillot et al., in a group of patients evaluated prospectively, found that numbness was greater in open browlift procedures than in endoscopic browlifts up to 14 weeks after surgery, but this difference was not significant by 6 months post-operatively. In a separate retrospective cohort, subjective sensitivity of both the forehead and scalp was more diminished in open forehead patients, while scalp mechano- and thermosensitivity was less after open browlifts than endoscopic browlifts up to 18 months after surgery; these differences were not observed after 18 months. However, if the forehead is carefully examined 8 to 12 weeks after surgery, small areas (often no larger than a fingertip in size) of diminished sensation may be identified, and even patients who note this are rarely bothered by this finding. These areas, when in the lower forehead, are generally quite small and most likely related to injury to small branches of either the supratrochlear or the supraorbital nerve during corrugator supercilii myoplasty. Areas of hypesthesia near the crown may be larger and are thought to be related to injury to the deep branch of the supraorbital nerve. Care should be taken when dissecting near the branches of the supratrochlear and supraorbital nerves. This is certainly no more (and likely less) common in endoscopic cases than in the coronal forehead lift.

Temporary neuralgias are much less common in the endoscopic forehead lift (~2%) when compared

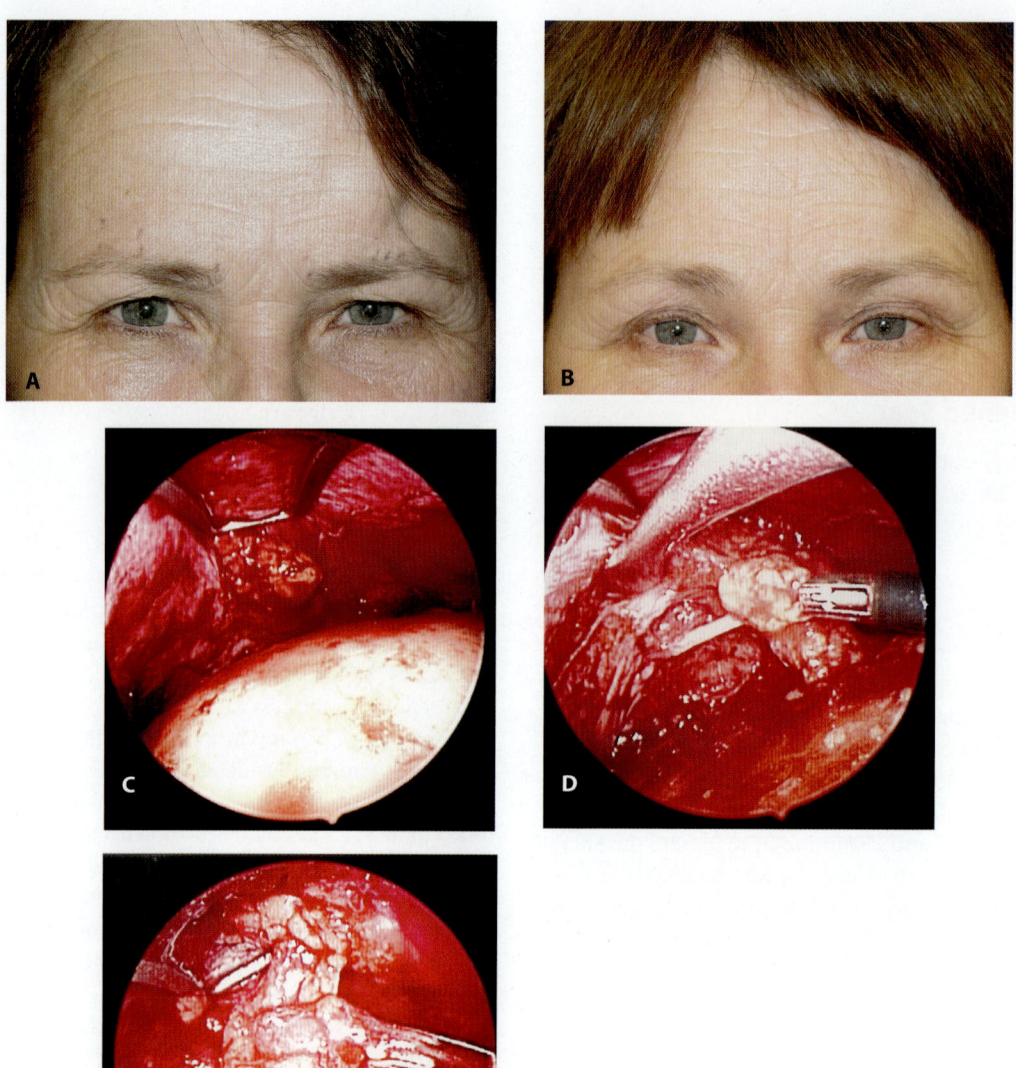

Figure 9-20. Preoperative (A) and postoperative (B; 1 yr) left views after endoscopic forehead lift and removal of a left subcutaneous lipoma. Brow position is relaxed and symmetrical, and the glabellar and forehead are smooth. (C–E) Intraoperative view of lipoma removal after periosteum, galea, and frontalis muscle are split.

with the coronal forehead lift (10–20%). Although long-term or permanent neuralgia is generally thought of as rare after the endoscopic forehead lift, Roberts and Ellis[23] reported this to occur in almost 20% of coronal forehead lift patients.

Motor

Permanent injury to the temporal branch of the facial nerve would clearly be catastrophic, and fortunately, it can usually be avoided. This nerve runs distinctly within the temporoparietal fascia, so it is essential to respect this fascia in the lower temple.

Care should be taken to establish a subtemporoparietal fascia plane immediately, identified by the loose avascular plane between the temporoparietal fascia above and the glistening deep temporal fascia below. Even if this plane is defined and maintained, excessive traction with either a right-angle retractor or the endoscope tip can cause a neuropraxia of the nerve and manifest as a temporary paresis or paralysis. Whereas surgeons self-reported a less than 0.1% incidence of temporary temporal branch paralysis (after either endoscopic or open forehead lift), most authors acknowledge a 1% to 2% incidence of

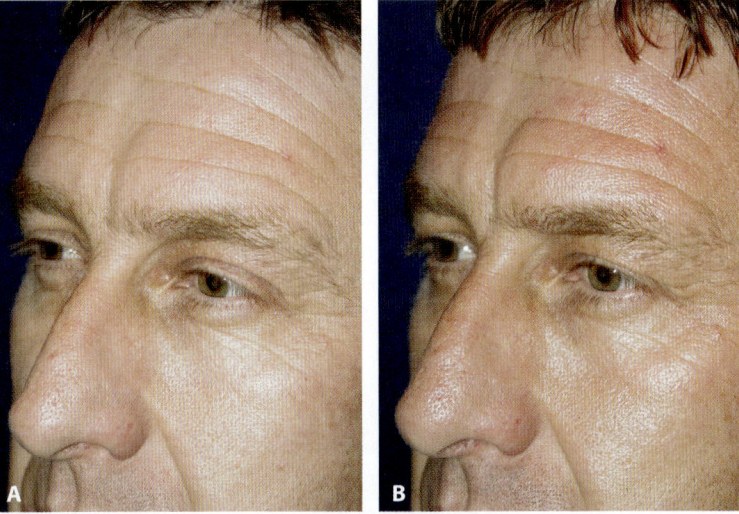

Figure 9-21. Preoperative (A) and postoperative (B; 1 yr) views after endoscopic forehead lift. The brow is now maintained in a slightly more elevated (but appropriate in this male patient) level, and glabellar and forehead rhytids are improved.

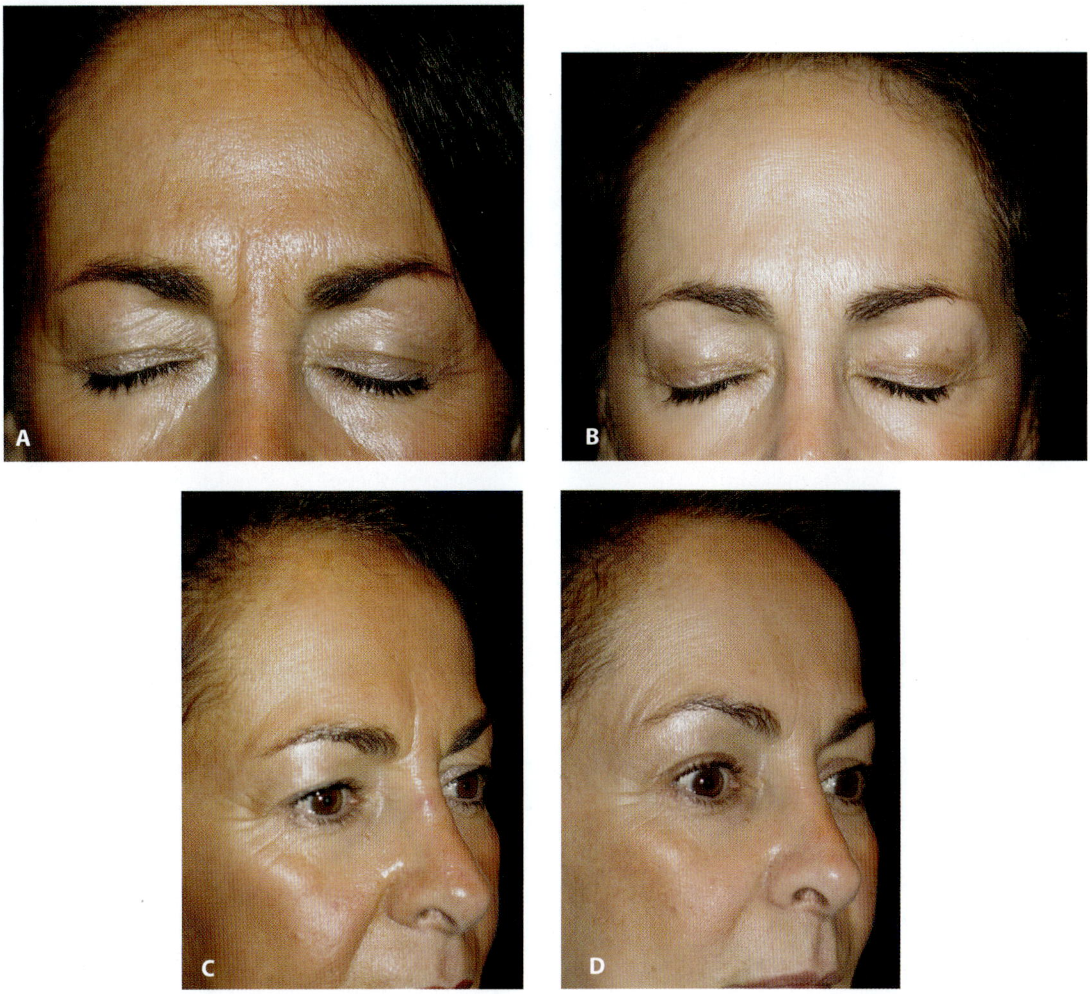

Figure 9-22. Preoperative (A, C) and postoperative (B, D; 10 mo) views after endoscopic forehead lift and upper blepharoplasty. The brows are maintained in an elevated position with improved contour and a more feminine arch. The glabella is notably smoother postoperatively.

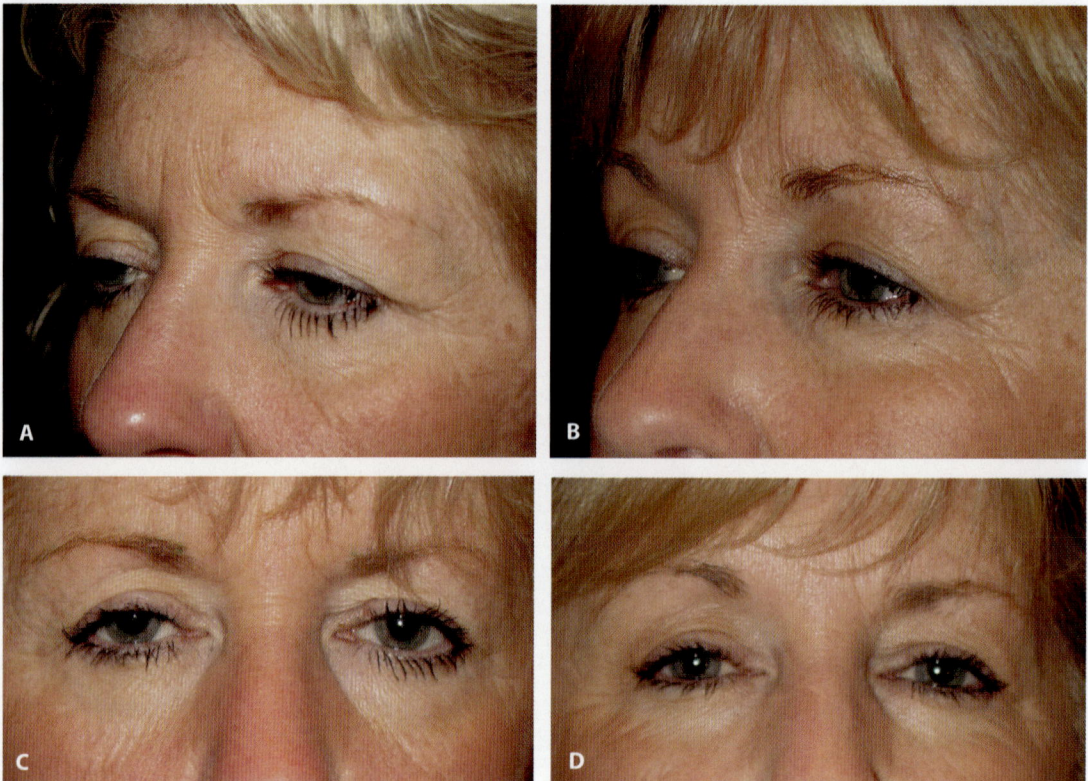

Figure 9-23. Preoperative (A, C) and postoperative (B, D; 9 mo) views after endoscopic forehead lift only. Some mild lateral upper lid skin redundancy persists, but the brow is now in a more appropriate position and the periorbital area appears refreshed.

temporary paralysis of the temporal branch. This is slightly higher than the 0.4% to 0.6% incidence reported with the coronal forehead lift.

Recurrent Brow Ptosis

If all aspects of the endoscopic forehead lift are properly performed (elevation, release, depressor myoplasties, adequate fixation), recurrent brow ptosis should be unlikely. Withey and associates[22] reported only a 4% incidence of significant loss of brow elevation after endoscopic forehead lifting with an average follow-up of 17 months. This compares favorably with a 20% brow ptosis recurrence rate in coronal browlifts (unspecified follow-up) as reported by Connell and coworkers in 1989[25] after bicoronal browlift.

Conclusions

The endoscopic forehead lift was introduced in the mid-1990s with great fanfare, because it was touted as a method to address global forehead and brow issues that could avoid the extensive dissection and morbidity of the coronal forehead lift. Early enthusiasm (before a complete understanding of the particular wound events occurring in the early postoperative period was gained) soon gave way to disillusionment and abandonment of the procedure by many. However, with a much more fundamental understanding of brow physiology and wound healing, coupled with improved techniques and materials for stabilizing the elevated brow, excellent results (**Figures 9-20 to 9-23**) can be obtained with the endoscopic forehead lift in the majority of patients. As always, careful analysis of the preoperative position of the brow, activity of the brow muscles, and associated aesthetic needs of the patient are essential for selecting appropriate candidates for the endoscopic forehead lift.

New opinions are always suspected, and usually opposed, without any other reason but because they are not already common.

John Locke (1632–1704)

Acknowledgments

The author would like to thank Karl Storz Endoscopy-America, Inc. (KSE-A), for the loan of instruments. Video images were recorded with an AIDA DVD (KSE-A, Culver City, CA) and an Endogo handheld endoscopic video camera (Envisionier Medical Technologies, LLC, Rockville, MD).

Suggested Readings

1. Chajchir A. Endoscopic subperiosteal forehead lift. Aesthetic Plast Surg 1994;18:269–274.
2. Isse NG. Endoscopic facial rejuvenation: endoforehead, the functional lift. Aesthetic Plast Surg 1994;18:21–29.
3. Core GB, Vasconez LO, Graham HD. Endoscopic browlift. Clin Plast Surg 1995;22:619–631.
4. Isse NG. Endoscopic forehead lift. Evolution and update. Clin Plast Surg 1995;22:661–673.
5. Ramirez OM. Endoscopically assisted biplanar forehead lift. Plast Reconstr Surg 1995;96:323–333.
6. Oslin B, Core GB, Vasconez LO. The biplanar endoscopically assisted forehead lift. Clin Plast Surg 1995; 22:633–638.
7. Chiu ES, Baker DC. Endoscopic brow lift: a retrospective review of 628 consecutive cases over 5 years. Plast Reconstr Surg 2003;112:628–633.
8. Knize DM. An anatomically based study of the mechanism of eyebrow ptosis. Plast Reconstr Surg 1996;97:1321–1333.
9. Knize DM. Limited incision forehead lift for eyebrow elevation to enhance upper blepharoplasty. Plast Reconstr Surg 2001;108:564–567.
10. Guillot JM, Rousso DE, Replogle W. Forehead and scalp sensation after brow-lift. A comparison between open and endoscopic techniques. Arch Facial Plast Surg 2011;13:109–116.
11. Troilus C. A comparison between subaleal and subperiosteal browlifts. Plast Reconstr Surg 1999; 104:1079–1090.
12. Romo T, Sclafani AP, Yung R, et al. Endoscopic foreheadplasty: a histologic comparison of periosteal refixation after endoscopic versus bicoronal lift. Plast Reconstr Surg 2000;105:1111–1117.
13. Sclafani AP, Fozo MS, Romo T, McCormick SA. Strength and histological characteristics of periosteal fixation to bone after elevation. Arch Facial Plast Surg 2003;5:63–66.
14. Boutros S, Bernard RW, Galiano RD, et al. The temporal sequence of periosteal attachment after elevation. Plast Reconstr Surg 2003;111:1942–1947.
15. Nassif PS, Kokoska MS, Homan S, et al. Comparison of subperiosteal vs subgaleal elevation techniques used in forehead lifts. Arch Otolaryngol Head Neck Surg 1998;124:1209–1215.
16. Thomas JR, Lee AS, Patel AB. Brow-lift: subgaleal vs subperiosteal flap adherence in the rabbit model. Arch Facial Plast Surg 2007;9:101–105.
17. DeCordier BC, de la Torre JI, Al-Hakeem MS, et al. Endoscopic forehead lift: review of technique, cases, and complications. Plast Reconstr Surg 2002;110:1558–1568.
18. Ducic Y, Adelson R. Use of the endoscopic forehead-lift to improve brow position in persistent facial paralysis. Arch Facial Plast Surg 2005;7:51–54.
19. Jones BM, Grover R. Endoscopic brow lift: a personal review of 538 patients and comparison of fixation techniques. Plast Reconstr Surg 2004;113: 1242–1250.
20. McKinney P, Sweis I. An accurate technique for fixation in endoscopic brow lift: a 5-year follow-up. Plast Reconstr Surg 2001;108:1808–1810.
21. Elkwood A, Matarasso A, Rankin M, et al. National plastic surgery survey: brow lifting techniques and complications. Plast Reconstr Surg 2001;108:2143–2150.
22. Withey S, Witherow H, Waterhouse N. One hundred cases of endoscopic brow lift. Br J Plast Surg 2002;55:20–24.
23. Roberts TL, Ellis LB. In pursuit of optimal rejuvenation of the forehead: endoscopic brow lift with simultaneous carbon dioxide laser resurfacing. Plast Reconstr Surg 1998;101:1075–1084.
24. Aiache AE. Endoscopic facelift. Aesthetic Plast Surg 1994;18:275–278.
25. Connell BF, Lambros VS, Neurohr GH. The forehead lift: techniques to avoid complications and produce optimal results. Aesthetic Plast Surg 1989;13:217–237.

10

Nonsurgical Management of the Aging Forehead and Brow

The surgeon should have a perceptive eye, ideas that are always lucid, of the nature that will still enable him always to act with promptness and assurance.

Jean Yperman (1260–1310)

Introduction

As our understanding of brow anatomy and the function has improved and the demographics of facial plastic surgery patients has shifted towards the younger patients since the 1990,s, the demand has increased for rejuvenative procedures with fewer (or no) incisions, short (or no) recovery periods, and more focused and specific results. Patients no longer wish to wait until retirement from the workforce or to take extended periods of time off work to recover from surgery. Patients are less likely to seek "dramatic" or "radical" changes, especially in the upper third of the face, because these types of results often impart an unnatural, surgical, or surprised appearance. These facial plastic surgery population changes have driven the quest for both minimal incision procedures and, as an extension, nonsurgical treatments. As experience with botulinum toxin A has increased and as soft tissue fillers have improved (in terms of better tissue blending and increased longevity of effect), these techniques increasingly have been employed. Interestingly, when properly counseled, many patients will opt for short-term (3–9 mo) results from nonsurgical techniques over surgical approaches. Although in

the long term, this approach will ultimately cost the patient more than a permanent surgical treatment, many (particularly younger) patients will use these nonsurgical modalities as means to delay ultimate surgical correction until they are emotionally and financially "ready." Nonsurgical treatments are an essential part of the facial plastic surgeon's armamentarium, both for the temporary benefits they

Brow Suture Suspension

Indications: mild brow ptosis.
Contraindications: moderate to severe brow ptosis; active infection.
Ideal candidate: young; female; minimal ptosis; minimal rhytids.
Scientific basis: mechanical suspension of the brow.

Brow Volume Augmentation

Indications: mild lateral brow ptosis.
Contraindications: moderate to severe brow ptosis; active infection.
Ideal candidate: young; female; minimal ptosis.
Scientific basis: increase lateral brow volume, causing upward angulation of the lateral brow hairs.

provide to the patients and for the opportunity they provide to develop trusting, long-term relationships with patients who will ultimately desire surgical correction of the aging forehead and brow.

History

Whereas most surgeons today would date the beginnings of nonsurgical forehead and brow rejuvenation to the early to mid 1990s, some of these treatments have been described and available for decades. Moderate (sometimes dramatic) improvement of forehead rhytids can be obtained with the use of medium to deep chemical peels. Dyschromias, some fine lines, and rough texture of the forehead skin can be improved with a medium depth peel such as a 35% trichloroacetic acid, whereas effacement of deeper lines and moderate skin tightening can be obtained with a deep peel such as a Baker-Gordon formula peel. In the mid to late 1990s, the development of carbon dioxide and erbium:yttrium-aluminum-garnet (Er:YAG) lasers added to the options for skin rejuvenation, and since the beginning of the 21st century, nonablative laser, monopolar, or bipolar radiofrequency, plasma, and fractionated laser skin resurfacing have been introduced to expand the range of treatments of the skin. Treatment of the forehead with these techniques is very similar to other areas of the face and are covered elsewhere in this series.

While using small incisions, suture suspension of the brow is an easily performed office procedure with little to no significant postoperative recovery period for patients. Although this has recently been popularized with the introduction of barbed, permanent sutures, it is important to note that this procedure was not only described by Costantino and coworkers in 2003[1] for the treatment of paralytic brow ptosis, but that the procedure itself dates back at least to 1976, when Parkes and colleagues[2] described the basic technique.

Botulinum Toxin A Brow Modification

Indications: mild brow ptosis; glabellar and/or forehead rhytids.
Contraindications: moderate to severe brow ptosis; active infection.
Ideal candidate: young; female; minimal ptosis.
Scientific basis: adjustment of balance between depressor and elevator muscle tone in specific locations to affect brow position.

Botulinum toxin A, originally used to treat essential blepharospasm and spasmodic neurolaryngeal disorders, was expanded into cosmetic use in the early 1990s. Beginning with improvement of the appearance of the crows' feet by treating the underlying lateral orbicularis oculi muscle (pars orbitalis), its use was expanded to affect the position and shape of the brow. The concept of the dynamic position of the brow could be used to predict the effect on brow position based on which specific areas of the forehead and brow musculature were treated. Concurrently, this knowledge also enhanced our ability to perform more functional forehead surgery, such as the endoscopic forehead lift and some limited incision techniques.

Intradermal volume augmentation for treatment of rhytids has been quite popular since the introduction of bovine collagen fillers in the early 1980s. Widespread use of the bovine collagens in the forehead was limited by the risk of skin necrosis in the glabella (with glutaraldehyde cross-linked bovine collagen, although possible with *any* dermal filler) and the short duration (6–8 wk) of effect of non–cross-linked bovine collagen. Since the introduction of the hyaluronic acid–derivative fillers in 2003 with their greater longevity of effect (5–7 mo or longer), there has been an increased interest in soft tissue fillers in the forehead and brow. Also, the cohesiveness of some hyaluronic acid–derived products allows placement of these fillers subdermally or even deeper with good maintenance of effect. Alternatively, autologous fat can be micrografted to augment senescent brow soft tissue. Surgeons now comprehend the five-dimensional nature of brow aesthetics (vertical and horizontal positioning, thickness [depth], muscular effects, and chronoaging), and the need to ensure an appropriate brow volume is being recognized.

Rationale and Scientific Basis

Most nonsurgical treatments of brow aging are camouflage techniques, designed to provide a modest and/or temporary improvement in the appearance of the brow. Suture suspension simply mechanically changes the lowest point to which the brow can descend. This procedure essentially supplants the galea, periosteum, orbital ligament, and skin's elasticity as the primary static restrictor of inferior brow descent, while leaving intact the forces that both depress and elevate the brow.

Botulinum toxin A can be used to selectively alter the depressor and elevator tonic forces that affect brow position and shape. If these forces are considered globally, there exists a balanced tone maintaining the brow in a specific position, whether ptotic or not. Targeting specific areas of muscles and treating with botulinum toxin decreases the activity of these specific muscle fibers and alters the balance of muscle tone.[2] If one understands the anatomy of the brow muscles and the vector of pull generated by each, individual and groups of muscles can be targeted to change the position of the brow. Paralyzing segments of certain depressor muscles allows the opposing elevator forces to predominate and raise the brow. Care should be taken to fully anticipate the effect on each segment of the brow (medial, central, and tail of the brow) when any given muscle segment is treated with botulinum toxin.

Finally, soft tissue fillers can be injected intra- or subdermally to improve brow aesthetics. In recent years, there has been an increasing recognition that not only does the brow descend differentially along its length but also patients may undergo significant atrophy of the brow soft tissues, most likely representing atrophy of the inferior galeal fat pad. By augmenting soft tissue bulk deep to and just below the brow, an infrabrow ledge is created that angles the brow upward and increases the distance between the lashes and the brow.[3]

Advantages, Disadvantages, and Alternatives

These minimally or nonsurgical treatments of the brow and forehead are easily performed office procedures with little to no significant recovery time. Effects are seen immediately or within a few days, and there is little disruption of the patient's daily routine. Compared with surgical procedures, these procedures are considerably less expensive in the short term.

Conversely, botulinum toxin A neuromodulation typically provides moderate alteration of brow position that lasts only 3 to 4 months before retreatment is required. The effect of soft tissue augmentation with hyaluronic acid derivatives (typically) persists for 5 to 7 months and, ironically, is less useful in patients with severe brow soft tissue atrophy, because the volume required for replacement can be excessive and impractical. Finally, the longevity of effect of brow suture suspension is still hotly debated and somewhat questionable. Surgical procedures can provide more significant and more permanent improvement in brow appearance than nonsurgical treatments.

Indications and Contraindications

In general, nonsurgical procedures for treatment of brow ptosis and the aging forehead are indicated for mild brow ptosis, particularly in younger patients. These procedures, either separately or combined, can treat ptosis of any or all segments of the brow. Paralytic brow ptosis cannot be treated with botulinum toxin, because in this case, brow position is due to the effects of gravity (not muscular contraction), and adding bulk with soft tissue fillers will only increase the "heaviness" of the brow appearance. Suture suspension in these cases, conversely, can be quite efficacious in correcting resting brow position.

These modalities should usually not be used in cases that require more than 4 to 5 mm of brow elevation, nor should they be used in cases in which the patient has known hypersensitivity to any material or drug used, any active inflammatory condition at the injection/incision site, or unrealistic expectations. In addition, patients with neuromuscular disorders or who are using aminoglycosides or other agent that interferes with neuromuscular transmission should not be treated with botulinum toxin.

Range of Anesthesia

These procedures are simply and easily administered in an office setting. Botulinum toxin does not require any specific anesthetic techniques, although topical anesthetic cream can be applied for 20 to 30 minutes before the procedure. The same holds true for soft tissue fillers, especially when subdermal fillers are used. In addition, an ice compress can be applied for approximately 60 seconds before treatment to lessen the discomfort of the needlestick. The patient should be in a calm and relaxed state during injection, because any furrowing of the brow will make treatment more difficult and more painful. Suture suspension techniques require small incisions that should be anesthetized with local infiltration; passage of the suture through subdermal tissue is rarely more than slightly uncomfortable and minimal (if any) local anesthetic needs to be infiltrated along the proposed suture path.

Equipment

Suture suspension of the brow can be performed with monofilament smooth or proprietary barbed sutures. A needle holder, single-toothed forceps, #11 and #15 scalpels, and a 4-inch straight needle are required.

Botulinum toxin requires a 3- to 5-mL syringe and a 25-gauge needle for reconstitution with preservative-free normal saline; a 1-mL syringe and a 30-gauge needle are needed for treatment. Currently, botulinum toxin A is commercially available in the United States as Botox Cosmetic (Allergan, Palo Alto, CA) and Dysport (Medicis Aesthetics, Scottsdale, AZ). While these two represent the same active molecule, units are not interchangeable between these two preparations. For clarity, botulinum toxin doses mentioned in this chapter will refer to Botox units (BU).

A complete discussion of soft tissue fillers is beyond the scope of this chapter, but some general observations can be made. Non–cross-linked collagen (Zyderm/Cosmoderm, Allergan, Palo Alto, CA) or mid-dermal hyaluronic acid derivatives (Restylane, Medicis Aesthetics, Scottsdale, AZ; Juviderm, Allergan, Palo Alto, CA) can be used to fill glabellar rhytids. These same fillers can be used to augment the subcutaneous tissues of the brow, although larger-particle hyaluronic acid derivatives (Perlane, Medicis Aesthetics, Scottsdale, AZ) can be used in this location.

Incisions

Incisions are used only for suture suspension of the brow. Small trichophytic incisions are made and carried down to the dermal level. If suture loops are used, stab incisions are made with a #11 blade just below the lowest brow hairs and are used to reverse the direction of the suture and return it toward the brow.

Procedures

Brow Suture Suspension

Plane of Dissection

Whereas Parkes and colleagues[2] used a subcutaneous suture loop placed above the lateral limbus, and Costantino and coworkers[1] described passing multiple suture loops subperiosteally, most authors have described passing these suture loops in a subgaleal plane (**Figure 10-1**). This allows the brow to slide superiorly over the periosteum.

Tissue Modification and Wound Closure

Suture suspension of the brow can be performed with a permanent monofilament suture passed on a 4-inch Keith needle from a stab incision located just

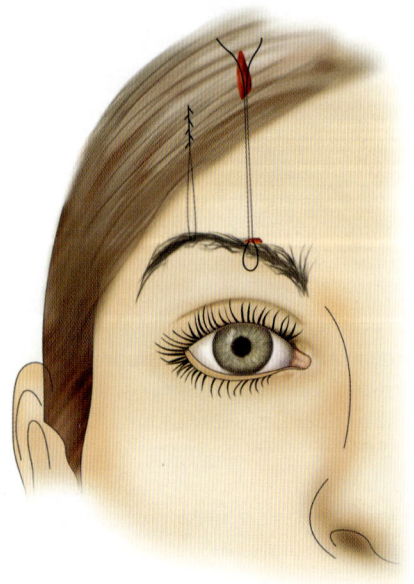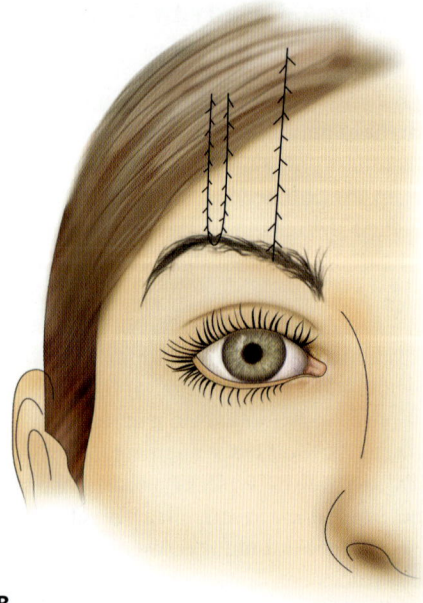

A   **B**

Figure 10-1. (A) Suture loops can be placed from the post-trichial scalp through small incisions and out through the infrabrow skin via a small stab incision, the reverse using a different path but exiting the same scalp incision. Whereas these are most effective laterally, they must be placed carefully when medial to the supraorbital nerve. (B) Uni- or bidirectional barbed sutures may obviate the need for a scalp incision, but fixation relies solely on the barbed ends of the suture engaging surrounding tissues.

Brow Suture Suspension

Incisions: trichophytic incision; infrabrow stab incision.
Tissue modifications: none.
Fixation: subcutaneous loop sutured to periosteum or dermis.
Wound closure: two-layered skin closure.
Complications: incomplete elimination; broken suture.

below the lowest brow hairs. The needle is directed down to just above the periosteum and then turned superiorly in this plane. Each end of the suture is passed superiorly just above the periosteum in separate, serpentine paths separated by approximately 1 cm and brought out the hairline incisions. The suture ends are then either tied together or sutured down to periosteum on tension, elevating the brow position. The scalp wounds are then closed with 4-0 absorbable dermal sutures and a 5-0 polypropylene suture; the brow incision is closed with a 4-0 or 5-0 chromic suture.

Postoperative Management

Ice compresses are applied to the forehead and scalp, and antibiotic ointment is applied to the skin sutures three times daily until sutures are removed 5 to 7 days after surgery. Mild brow edema is expected, but generally resolves in 48 to 72 hours.

Forehead and Brow Treatment with Botulinum Toxin A

Tissue Modification

A more thorough description of the cosmetic uses of botulinum toxin A is presented elsewhere in this series and this discussion is limited to its use in the forehead and brow. Botulinum toxin is best reconstituted freshly in preservative-free normal saline. Dilution volumes can vary from 2 to 5 mL or more, but the author's preference is 2.0 mL. As mentioned earlier, care should be taken to fully anticipate the effects on the brow and forehead of injections at

Botulinum Toxin A Brow Modification

Incisions: none.
Tissue modifications: neuromodulation/temporary paralysis of brow and forehead muscles.
Fixation: none.
Wound closure: N/A.
Complications: upper lid ptosis; altered muscle tone causing poor aesthetic result.

particular sites in the glabellar and forehead muscles, because treatment of any muscle will affect the dynamics of other brow muscles.

Transverse forehead rhytids can be treated with botulinum toxin injected just below the dermis. The entire forehead can be adequately treated with 20 to 30 Botox units (BU) distributed evenly over the midsuperior and centrolateral forehead in 2.5-BU (0.05-mL) doses (**Figure 10-2**). The surgeon should remember that the paired bellies of the frontalis muscle split in the midline; hence, any botulinum toxin injected into the midline mid or upper forehead will work only if there is sufficient diffusion laterally. It should also be remembered (see Chapter 2) that movement of the forehead occurs primarily in the lowest 2 cm, facilitated by the glide plane space. Muscular contraction of the upper two thirds of the forehead where gross movement and sliding of the forehead tissues are much more restricted will predominantly cause wrinkling and furrowing, and it is this area that is targeted for botulinum toxin treatment. The lowest 2 cm is typically *not* treated, because paralysis of the lower frontalis muscle and elimination of its tonic contraction will allow this lower portion of the brow to slide downward under the unaltered influence of the brow depressor (corrugator and depressor supercilii, procerus) muscles and worsen brow ptosis. However, by injecting the frontalis muscle no lower than fingerbreadth above the brow, this can be avoided. In addition, because lateral brow elevation is important in facial expression, injection of the lateral forehead extends slightly less inferiorly than the medial forehead.

Elevation of the lateral segment of the brow with botulinum toxin requires preservation of the function of the lower frontalis muscle (for elevator function) and treatment of the superolateral orbicularis oculi muscle below the brow (to reduce the depressor forces). For women with early brow ptosis, especially in the lateral segment, who desire minimal changes to the brow except for a more accentuated lateral brow arch, treatment with 3 to 5 BU of botulinum toxin can yield 2- to 3-mm elevation of the brow (**Figure 10-3**). It is important to center the injection directly below the desired brow arch peak.[4]

Patents with ptotic central and nasal brow segments, with or without glabellar concerns, can be treated with botulinum toxin to reposition the medial two thirds of the brow. Treating the corrugator and depressor supercilii muscles will soften the medial brow and smooth the glabella as well as raise the medial brow. Again, the lowest 2 cm of frontalis muscle should remain untreated to provide medial

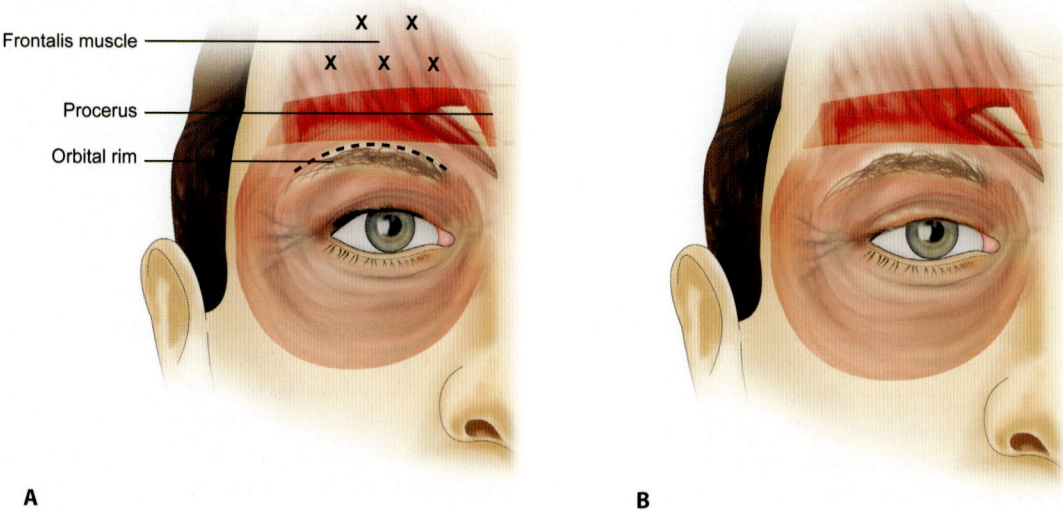

A　　　　　　　　　　　　　　　**B**

Figure 10-2. Botulinum toxin A treatment of horizontal forehead rhytids. (A) Reduction or elimination of transverse forehead rhytids can easily be achieved without eliminating expressivity. Injection sites (X) should be limited to the frontalis muscle no less than 2 cm above the orbital rim *(shaded area)*. (B) If the lowest 2 cm of the forehead remains untreated, there is generally sufficient frontalis muscle to maintain brow position and some motion without causing ptosis.

brow elevation. Typically, the corrugator/depressor supercilii complex is treated with 7.5 to 15 BU per side. Before injection, the surgeon rests the non-dominant thumb and forefinger above and below the medial half of the brow and the patient is asked to frown as the surgeon assesses the brow for maximal muscle contraction. The patient then relaxes the brow while the surgeon grasps the brow in the area of maximal muscle bulk. The finger grasping

the lower side of the brow is placed over the edge of the orbital rim (ensuring that the toxin remains above the rim) and the muscle injected, typically in three sites. An additional 5 BU can be injected into the procerus muscle to provide additional medial brow elevation (**Figure 10-4**). For particularly deep glabellar rhytids, combining botulinum toxin treatment with an intradermal soft tissue filler can provide excellent and long-lasting results (**Figure 10-5**).

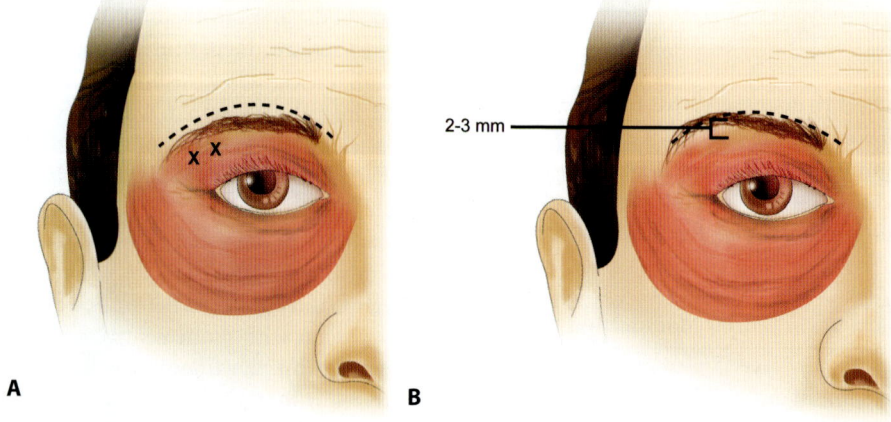

A　　　　　　　　　　　　　　　**B**

Figure 10-3. (A, B) By treating the lateral brow depressors (superior lateral orbicularis oculi muscle) just below the brow at the desired place of the brow peak with botulinum toxin, the lateral brow can be raised subtly. This can be performed in isolation or together with other facial areas.

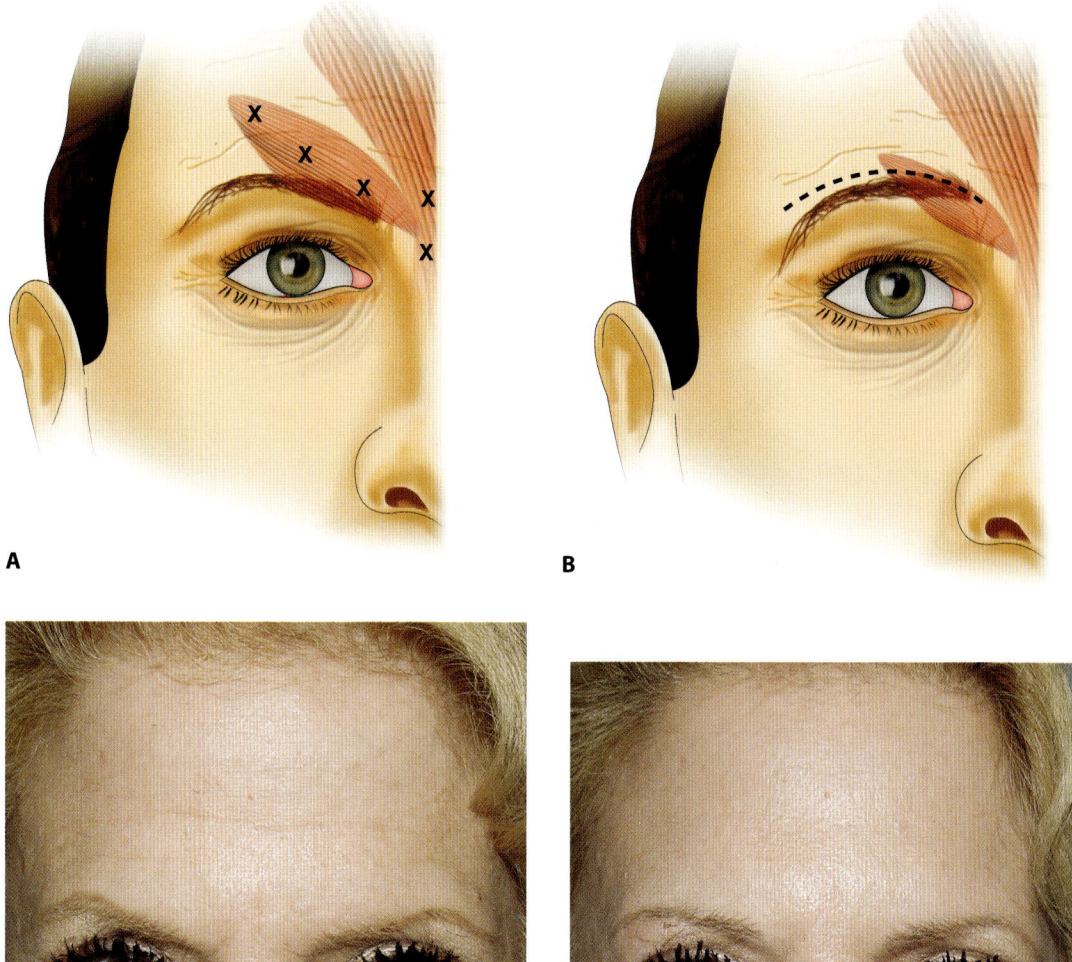

Figure 10-4. (A, B) Ptotic medial and central brows can be repositioned with botulinum toxin A treatment of the brow depressors. Glabellar rhytid effacement as well as correction of brow ptosis is achieved with relative ease. (C) The patient's pretreatment appearance suggested a "scowl" because of excessive medial brow depressor tone. (D) Two weeks after treatment of the corrugator supercilii and procerus muscles with botulinum toxin A. Note the smoothing of the glabellar, "opening" of the periorbital area, and a better balance of the brow segments.

By first carefully analyzing the patient's aesthetic needs, a combined treatment of individual brow segments can be performed to modify the brow as a whole, both eliminating hyperfunction and appropriately altering the position of the brow (**Figure 10-6**).

Postoperative Management

Patients are counseled that the early effects of botulinum toxin treatment will not be evident for at least 24 to 48 hours after treatment, and it may take up to 14 days to see the full effect. Patients are asked to apply ice compresses to the treated areas for 20 to 30 minutes to limit bruising and to avoid head hanging or recumbent position, massage of the treated areas, and vigorous activity for 6 hours after treatment. Patients are allowed to apply cosmetics 1 hour after treatment.

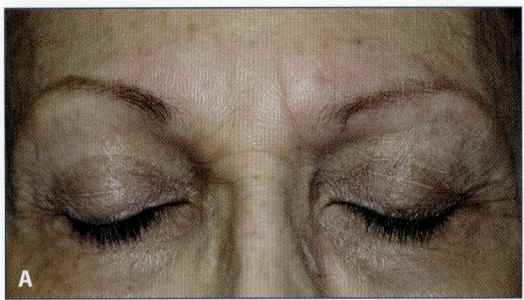

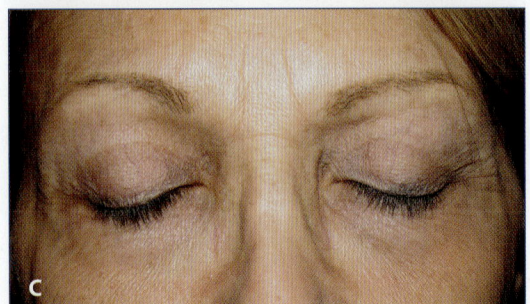

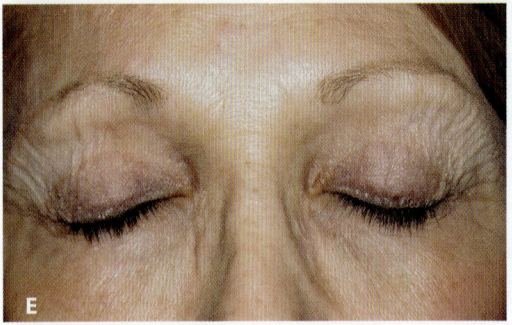

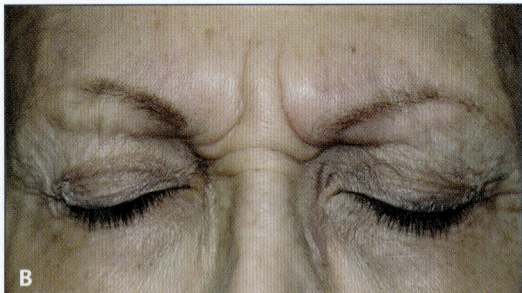

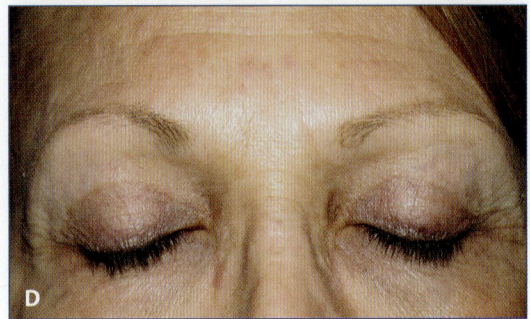

Figure 10-5. Patient with deep glabellar rhytids in repose (A) or during a frown (B). C One week after botulinum toxin A treatment of the procerus and corrugator supercilii muscles. In repose, rhytids are somewhat improved but still present. Note the slight elevation of the medial brows. One week after treatment with nonanimal stabilized hyaluronic acid (NASHA) derivative in repose (D) and during frowning (E). Note the smooth appearance of the glabella and inability to generate active rhytids.

Soft Tissue Filler Management of the Forehead and Brow

Tissue Modification

It is essential to be familiar with the physical properties of each filler material whose use is contemplated in order to avoid/minimize the risk of complications. Use of cross-linked human or bovine collagen is expressly contraindicated for the treatment of glabellar lines because of the risk of skin necrosis, although the possibility of vascular embolization and/or occlusion from extravascular compression is theoretically possible with any filler. Typically, glabellar lines are related to both muscular contraction (treatable with botulinum toxin) and focal dermal thinning (amenable to dermal augmentation). Combining these treatments judiciously can provide the most complete correction of glabellar lines and can enhance the longevity of effect of the filler. The specific techniques of dermal injections are covered elsewhere in this series.

Brow soft tissue atrophy, however, can be treated with soft tissue replacement with injectable fillers. Rather than inject intradermally or even at the dermal-subdermal border, restoration of brow volume is best performed at the preperiosteal level, which augments the galeal fat pad (**Figure 10-7**). A small wheal is raised with 0.1 mL of 1% xylocaine HCl lateral to the brow to anesthetize the needle entry site. The brow is grasped between the thumb and the forefinger and lifted away from the orbital rim. The needle is inserted parallel to the brow and the surgeon places linear strands of filler material deeply (just above the periosteum) and just below the lowest brow hairs. This is done along the lateral two thirds to three quarters of the brow and may require a second needlestick. Typical volumes used range between 0.1 mL and 0.5 mL per side (**Figure 10-8**). After the material has been injected, the brow is grasped with the thumb and forefinger of both hands and firmly massaged medially and laterally in a horizontal direction to smooth the deposited fillers and to ensure

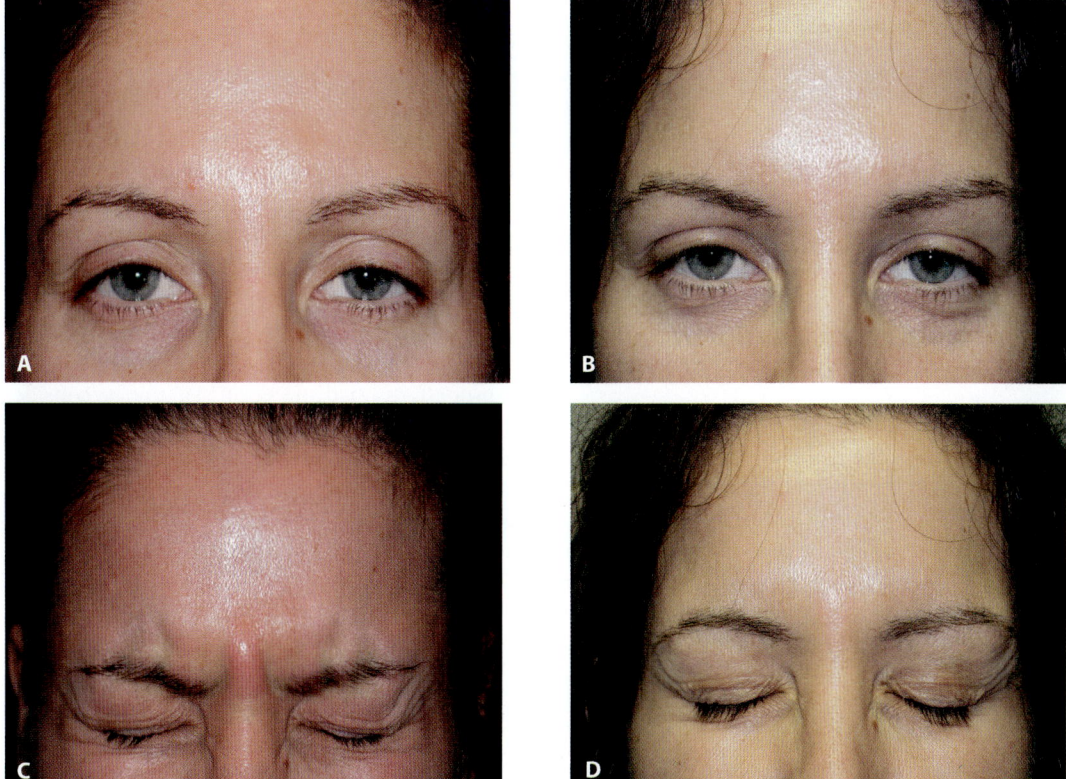

Figure 10-6. This young, athletic patient requested an improved contour to her brows and a smoother forehead. Pretreatment, in repose (A) and with maximal animation (C). Note the mild brow asymmetry and relatively flat brow arch, as well as significant contour deformity of the glabella during frowning. (B, D) One week after treatment with botulinum toxin A. The forehead is smoother and there is less "bulk" (contracted brow depressors) in the glabellar area and a more feminine arch. This required treatment of the corrugator supercilii and procerus muscles (to smooth the glabella), the upper frontalis muscle (to avoid overelevating the medial brow), and the superolateral orbicularis oculi muscle (to lift the tail of the brow slightly and to create a more arched brow).

proper placement just above the orbital rim. Injection either too superficially or too superiorly will visually increase brow "bulk" and give the brow a "heavy" appearance, rather than provide the natural brow soft tissues a platform upon which to rest. Currently, the author's filler of choice for this area is a nonanimal stabilized hyaluronic acid filler such as Restylane or Perlane (Medicis Aesthetics, Scottsdale, AZ) because of it elasticity, cohesiveness, and malleability.

This technique works best to rejuvenate the lateral two thirds of the brow. Although it may only *raise* the brow 1 to 2 mm, this technique gives the illusion of greater movement. By providing an enhanced "shelf" upon which the lateral brow rests, the brow hairs are angled less inferiorly, increasing the apparent distance between the lateral brow and the eyelashes. Combined with other nonsurgical techniques for rejuvenation of other parts of the face, soft tissue filler augmentation of the brow can

provide the patient with a dramatic degree of cosmetic improvement in a relatively simple office session (**Figures 10–9 and 10–10**).

Postoperative Management

If the patient remains in the office and applies ice compresses to the brows for 20 to 30 minutes after treatment, there is generally minimal or no bruising and scant swelling. The patient is instructed to avoid manipulation of the treated area for the following 4 hours and can apply cosmetics the following morning. The patient is advised that there may be a sensation of a "heavy" brow for 12 to 24 hours after treatment; if this treatment is applied only to patients with reasonable skin elasticity, there is little chance of accentuating brow ptosis. Pain is generally minimal, requiring (at most) over-the-counter analgesics for the first 12 hours.

Brow Volume Augmentation

Incisions: none.
Tissue modification: increase volume of lateral brow subdermis, galeal fat pad.
Fixation: none.
Wound closure: N/A.
Complications: "heavy" brow with little elevation; skin necrosis.

Complications: Incidence, Management, and Avoidance

If proper precautions are taken, complications of these nonsurgical treatments of the forehead and brow skin should be minimal. The small incisions used in the suture brow lift generally heal without sequelae, but care should be taken to avoid superficial passage of the sutures, because dermal dimpling may occur. If this is noted, the suture should be removed and replaced in a deeper plane. Under-, over-, or asymmetrical elevation can be corrected by adjusting tension on the sutures. Forehead anesthesia may occur, but should be transient. Neuralgia also may occur if the suture compresses a branch of the supraorbital or supratrochlear nerve; if this does

not resolve quickly, removal of the suture should be considered.

Complications from botulinum toxin should be rare, unless injected inappropriately. Care should be taken to properly dilute U.S. Food and Drug Administration (FDA)–approved botulinum toxin and to use properly defined amounts of active toxin. Anecdotal reports of severe complications of botulinum toxin (including respiratory failure and long-term ventilator dependence) were related to the improper dilution and use of non–FDA-approved (research grade only) botulinum toxin by an unlicensed and improperly trained physician. Failure to consider brow aesthetic needs and target the correct muscles will lead to an undesirable appearance of the brow, giving the patient a "severe," quizzical," or "sad" appearance. Alternatively, brow ptosis may worsen if insufficient function of the frontalis muscle remains owing to excessive lower frontalis treatment (**Figure 10-11**). Eyelid ptosis has been reported in up to 5% of patients; this has been postulated to be due to diffusion of the neurotoxin from corrugator treatment inferiorly into the lid and deeply through the septum orbitale to affect the levator palpebrae superioris muscle. Alternatively, it has been suggested that many, if not all, patients who devel-

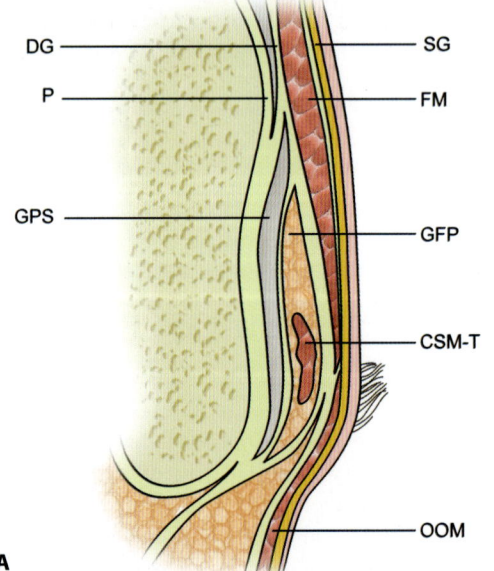
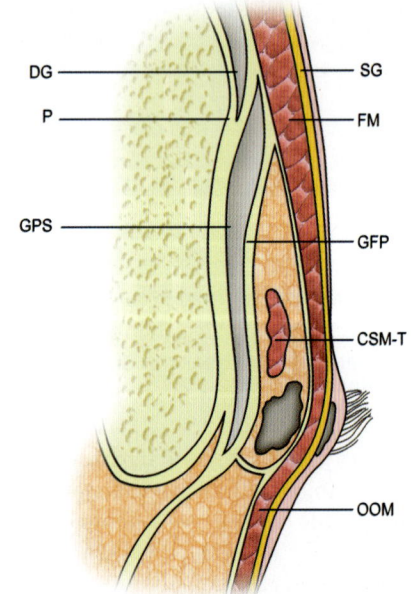

Figure 10-7. Soft tissue filler brow modification. (A) With flattening of volume loss of the galeal fat pad (GFP), the brow hairs are allowed to descend and are angled more inferiorly. (B) By adding bulk to the sub-brow soft tissues, the forehead and brow skin is redraped in such a way as to subtly elevate the position of the brow and angulation of the brow hairs. CSM-T = transverse head of corrugator supercilii muscle; DG = deep galea; FM = frontalis muscle; GPS = glide plane space; OOM = orbicularis oculi muscle; P = periosteum; SG = superficial galea.

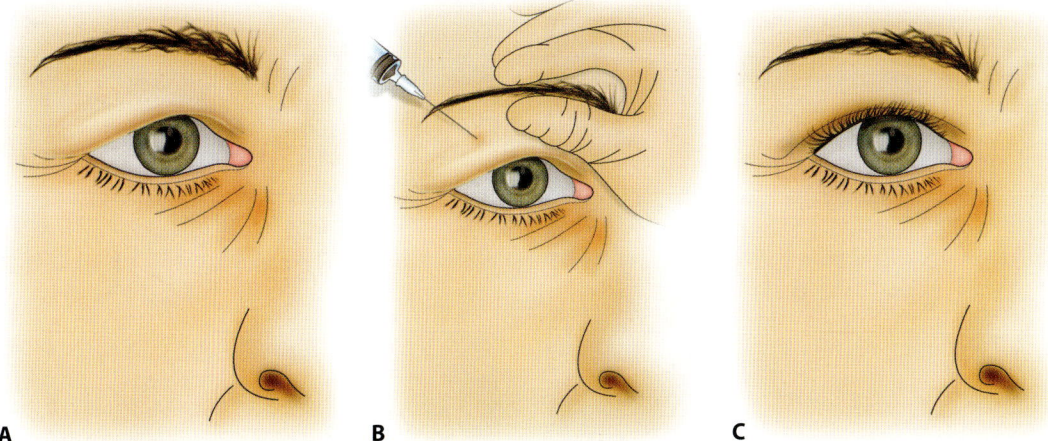

A   **B**   **C**

Figure 10-8. (A) Management of the flattened and ptotic lateral and central brow segments. (B) The brow is grasped and the filler is injected into the subdermal fat and galeal fat pad under the brow. This is then manually molded for smoothness. (C) The central and lateral thirds of the brow are subtly repositioned and rejuvenated.

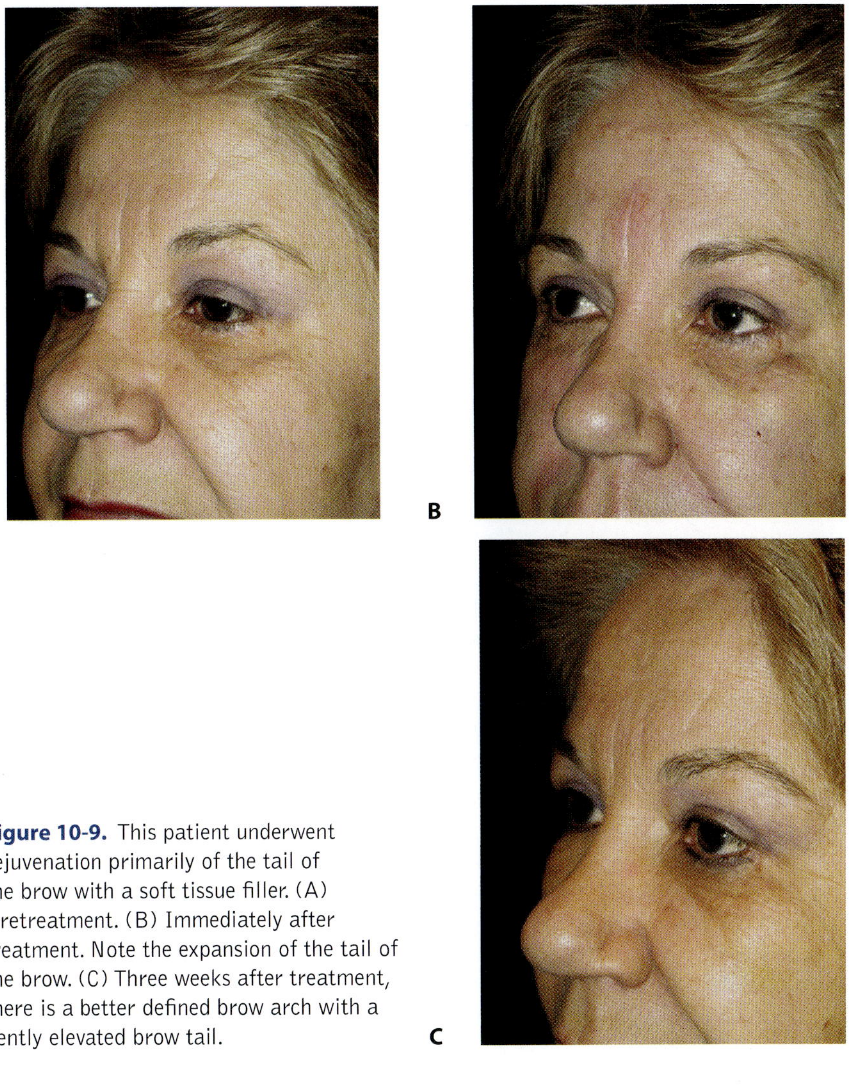

Figure 10-9. This patient underwent rejuvenation primarily of the tail of the brow with a soft tissue filler. (A) Pretreatment. (B) Immediately after treatment. Note the expansion of the tail of the brow. (C) Three weeks after treatment, there is a better defined brow arch with a gently elevated brow tail.

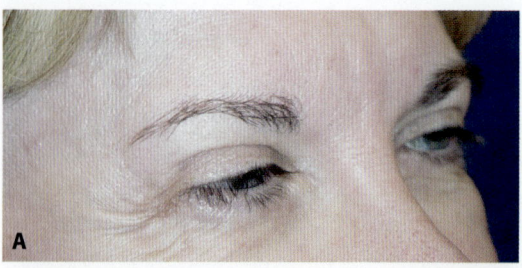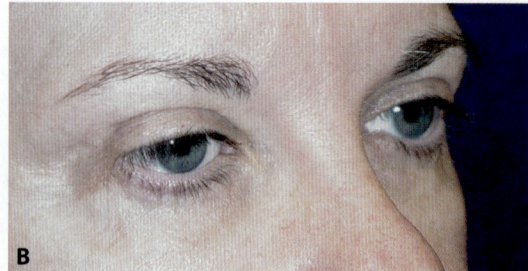

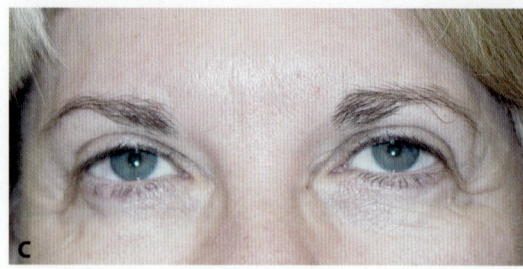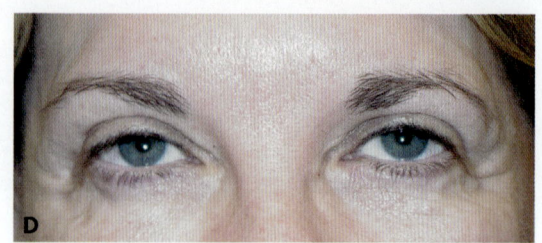

Figure 10-10. Before (A, C) and after (B, D) soft tissue augmentation of the brow. The "foundation" provided by the additional soft tissue bulk contours the brow and subtly highlights the brow arch.

op post–botulinum toxin treatment ptosis had preexisting ptosis compensated by frontalis muscle hypertonicity before treatment and that aggressive treatment of the frontalis muscle "unmasks" this condition. Generally, post–botulinum toxin ptosis is a self-limited condition, usually lasting no more than 2 to 4 weeks before resolving (far sooner than the cosmetic effects of treatment), but can be quite distressing to the patient. By increasing contraction of Müller's muscle, topical eyedrops can be used to correct up to 1 to 3 mm of ptosis. Pseudoephedrine HCl 2.5% is an over-the-counter a-agonist that can be used in patients who do not have narrow-angle glaucoma or a history of aneurysm; alternatively, 0.5% apraclonidine is an α_2-agonist and can be given three times daily until spontaneous resolution of the ptosis occurs. However, avoiding this complication is best accomplished by injecting above the orbital rim, using concentrated solutions (no less than 2.5 U/0.1 mL) and ensuring that the patient avoids rubbing, massaging, or otherwise manipulating the area for 4 to 6 hours after treatment. Bruising is not uncommon in this area but is rarely significant. Gentle application of cold compresses immediately before and after injection helps limit ecchymosis and minimize discomfort during injection.

Complications of soft tissue fillers will be highly dependent upon the properties of the material used. For hyaluronic acid derivatives, nodularity and lumpiness are uncommon after judicious intradermal injection; however, if this is noted to occur during treatment, the area can be massaged gently to smooth out any irregularities. Bruising is more likely to occur after intradermal injections, but typically is limited to the sites treated and can easily be camouflaged with cosmetics. Deeper injections to replace or augment brow soft tissue bulk are usually quite well tolerated, as long as the surgeon "molds" the deposits of filler into a smooth and uniform bulk at the time of treatment.

Milia may occur owing to general congestion of the dermis and should be treated conservatively. Herpetic outbreaks can be stimulated by injection treatment of the glabella and are clinically preceded by pain and accompanied by vesicular eruptions leading to a superficial excoriation. In the rare case of glabellar skin necrosis, significant pain and blanching of the skin that does not quickly reverse after injection may signal vascular compromise. Light massage or topical nitroglycerin can be used in an attempt to limit the extent of tissue injury, and a solution of hyaluronidase (Amphadase, Amphastar Pharmaceuticals, Rancho Cucamunga, CA or Hydase, Keystone Pharmaceuticals, Inc., Laguna Hills, CA) should be injected into the hyaluronic acid product injected.

However, the area of necrosis may not be fully delineated for up to 2 weeks after injection. These two complications may be difficult to distinguish,

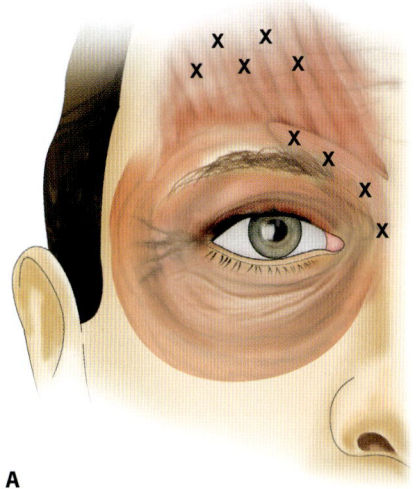

A

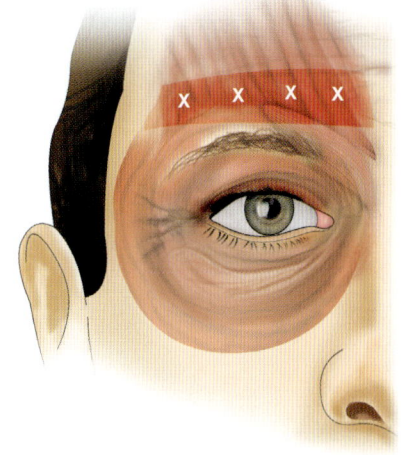

B

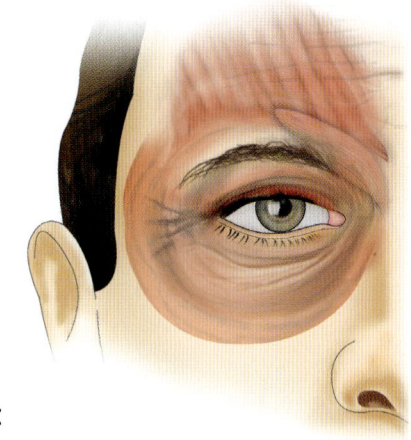

C

Figure 10-11. (A) Treatment of the forehead and glabellar rhytids must preserve sufficient tone of the lower frontalis muscle to avoid undesired descent of the brow. (B) Treatment of the lower frontalis muscle within 2 cm of the orbital rim (shaded area) creates an adynamic muscle mass over the glide plane space. (C) Loss of lower frontalis muscle tone allows additional brow ptosis.

and a prudent surgeon should treat the patient with conservative local wound care, oral antibiotic and antiviral medications, and close follow-up until the area has healed.

Conclusion

As patients seeking cosmetic improvement of the face become younger, they will frequently have less severe brow and forehead issues. In addition, they are less inclined to undergo larger procedures but are more willing to accept temporary and subtle but rapid or immediate improvements in the appearance of the brow and forehead. Some patients may elect to use these nonsurgical approaches as primary treatment, but most view these lesser procedures as methods to delay more invasive surgical procedures. The prudent surgeon will incorporate these nonsurgical techniques into his or her practice and use them to develop a trusting relationship with the patient, until the time when a more invasive procedure is acceptable to the patient.

The conditions required of a surgeon are . . . [h]e should be agreeable; bold in safe things, fearful of dangers; that he avoid bad cures or practices. . . .
Guy de Chauliac (1300–1368)

Suggested Readings

1. Kornstein AN. Soft-tissue reconstruction of the brow with Restylane. Plast Reconstr Surg 2005;116: 2017–2020.
2. Costantino PD, Hiltzik DH, Moche J, Preminger A. Minimally invasive brow suspension for facial paralysis. Arch Facial Plast Surg 2003;5:171–174.
3. Carruthers J, Carruthers A. A prospective, randomized, parallel group study analyzing the effect of BTX-A (Botox) and nonanimal sourced hyaluronic acid

(NASHA, Restylane) in combination compared with NASHA (Restylane) alone in severe glabellar rhytides in adult female subjects: treatment of severe glabellar rhytides with a hyaluronic acid derivative compared with the derivative and BTX-A. Dermatol Surg 2003;29:802–809.

4. Parkes ML, Kamer FM, Bassilios M. Surgical treatment of the ptotic brow. Laryngoscope 1976;86:1435–1436.

INDEX

Information in figures and tables is indicated by *f* and *t*.